case files™

Obstetrics & Gynecology

NOTICE

Medicine is an ever-changing science. As new research and clinical experience broaden our knowledge, changes in treatment and drug therapy are required. The authors and the publisher of this work have checked with sources believed to be reliable in their efforts to provide information that is complete and generally in accord with the standards accepted at the time of publication. However, in view of the possibility of human error or changes in medical sciences, neither the authors nor the publisher nor any other party who has been involved in the preparation or publication of this work warrants that the information contained herein is in every respect accurate or complete, and they disclaim all responsibility for any errors or omissions or for the results obtained from use of the information contained in this work. Readers are encouraged to confirm the information contained herein with other sources. For example and in particular, readers are advised to check the product information sheet included in the package of each drug they plan to administer to be certain that the information contained in this work is accurate and that changes have not been made in the recommended dose or in the contraindications for administration. This recommendation is of particular importance in connection with new or infrequently used drugs.

case files™

Obstetrics & Gynecology

EUGENE C. TOY, MD
The John S. Dunn, Senior Academic Chief
Obstetrics/Gynecology Residency Program
Christus-St. Joseph Hospital
Clerkship Director, Assistant Clinical Professor
The University of Texas-Houston Medical School
Houston, Texas

BENTON BAKER III, MD
Director of Graduate Medical Education
Christus-St. Joseph Hospital
Professor of Obstetrics and Gynecology
The University of Texas-Houston Medical School
Houston, Texas

PATTI JAYNE ROSS, MD
Course Director
Junior Obstetrics/Gynecology Clerkship
Department of Obstetrics, Gynecology,
and Reproductive Sciences
Professor of Obstetrics and Gynecology
The University of Texas-Houston Medical School
Houston, Texas

LARRY C. GILSTRAP III, MD
Professor and Chairman
Department of Obstetrics, Gynecology,
and Reproductive Sciences
Emma Sue Hightower Professor of
Obstetrics & Gynecology
The University of Texas-Houston Medical School
Houston, Texas

**Lange Medical Books /
McGraw-Hill**

MEDICAL PUBLISHING DIVISION

New York Chicago San Francisco
Lisbon London Madrid Mexico City
Milan New Delhi San Juan Seoul
Singapore Sydney Toronto

Case Files™: Obstetrics and Gynecology

Copyright © 2003 by The **McGraw-Hill Companies**, Inc. All rights reserved. Printed in the United States of America. Except as permitted under the United States Copyright Act of 1976, no part of this publication may be reproduced or distributed in any form or by any means, or stored in a data base or retrieval system, without the prior written permission of the publisher.

Case Files is a trademark of the McGraw-Hill Companies, Inc.

4 5 6 7 8 9 0   DOC/DOC   0 9 8 7 6 5

ISBN 0-07-140284-5

This book was set in Times New Roman by ATLIS Graphics and Design.
The editor was Catherine A. Johnson.
Project management was provided by Andover Publishing Services.
The production supervisor was Catherine H. Saggese
The interior designer was Patrice Sheridan.
The cover designer was Mary McKeon.
The index was prepared by Andover Publishing Services.
RR Donnelley was printer and binder.

This book is printed on acid-free paper.

Cataloging-in-Publication data is on file for this title at the Library of Congress.

To my loving and supportive wife, Terri, and my four delightful children, Andy, Michael, Allison, and Christina, who provide me with daily inspiration.

—ECT

With love and gratitude, to Mom, Joy, Ben, Anne, Jessica, Jim, John, and Col. Alvin Sholk.

—BB III

To the residents, faculty, and staff at Christus–St. Joseph Hospital.

—ECT AND BB III

To Dr. James Knight, and Tulane Medical School, for giving me the opportunity to fulfill my dreams. To my parents, Mary and Jimmy Ross, for their love, inspiration, and devotion.

—PJR

To my wife and three daughters, Lori, Lisa, and Erin, and my seven grandchildren.

—LCG III

Finally, to the wonderful medical students from the University of Texas-Houston Medical School who graciously gave constructive feedback and enthusiastically received this curriculum.

—THE AUTHORS

◈ CONTENTS

CONTRIBUTORS

Nichole Fleming Cole, MD
Chief Resident in Obstetrics/Gynecology
Christus–St. Joseph Hospital, Houston, Texas
Approach to Galactorrhea
Approach to Adnexal Masses and Struma Ovarii
Ruptured Corpus Luteum

Valeria T. Fullwood, MD
Chief Resident in Obstetrics/Gynecology
Christus–St. Joseph Hospital, Houston, Texas
Approach to Preterm Labor
Approach to Pyelonephritis in Pregnancy
Approach to Preterm Premature Rupture of Membranes

Konrad P. Harms, MD
Chief Resident in Obstetrics/Gynecology
Christus–St. Joseph Hospital, Houston, Texas
Approach to Preeclampsia
Approach to Abdominal Pain in Pregnancy
Approach to Hirsutism

Christina M. Hines, MD
Resident in Obstetrics/Gynecology
Christus–St. Joseph Hospital, Houston, Texas
Approach to Primary Amenorrhea
Approach to Delayed Puberty

Joseph Bram Johns, MD
Chief Resident in Obstetrics/Gynecology
Christus–St. Joseph Hospital, Houston, Texas
Approach to Ectopic Pregnancy
Approach to Urinary Tract Infections
Approach to Deep Venous Thrombosis in Pregnancy

George T. Kuhn, MD
Faculty, Obstetrics/Gynecology residency program
Vice Chairman, Department of Obstetrics and Gynecology
Christus–St. Joseph Hospital, Houston, Texas
Approach to Pruritus (Cholestasis) in Pregnancy
Approach to the Palpable Breast Mass
Approach to the Abnormal Mammogram

Carl E. Lee II, MD
Resident in Obstetrics/Gynecology
Christus–St. Joseph Hospital, Houston, Texas
Approach to Herpes Simplex Virus in Pregnancy
Approach to Septic Abortion

John C. McBride, MD
Faculty, Obstetrics/Gynecology Residency Program
Christus–St. Joseph Hospital, Houston, Texas
Approach to Salpingitis
Approach to Anemia in Pregnancy
Approach to Postpartum Hemorrhage

Robert K. Morris, Jr., MD
Faculty, Obstetrics/Gynecology Residency Program
Christus–St. Joseph Hospital
Assistant Professor, Department of Obstetrics and Gynecology
The University of Texas–Houston Medical School
Houston, Texas
Approach to Emergency Contraception
Adolescent Health Maintenance
Approach to Breast Infections

Cristo Papasakelariou, MD
Director of Endoscopic and Vaginal Surgery
Obstetrics/Gynecology Residency Program
Christus–St. Joseph Hospital, Houston, Texas
Clinical Professor of Obstetrics and Gynecology
University of Texas Medical Branch Galveston Medical School
Galveston, Texas
Approach to Infertility
Approach to Intrauterine Adhesions
Approach to Tubal Factor Infertility

Kimberly S. Rutter, MD
Resident in Obstetrics/Gynecology
Christus–St. Joseph Hospital, Houston, Texas
Thyroid Storm in Pregnancy
Approach to Abnormal Serum Screening in Pregnancy

Faith M. Whittier, MD
Faculty, Obstetrics/Gynecology Residency Program
Christus–St. Joseph Hospital, Houston, Texas
Approach to Postmenopausal Bleeding
Approach to Uterine Leiomyomata

INTRODUCTION

Mastering the cognitive knowledge within a field such as obstetrics and gynecology is a formidable task. It is even more difficult to draw on that knowledge, to procure and filter through the clinical and laboratory data, to develop a differential diagnosis, and finally to make a rational treatment plan. To gain these skills, the student often learns best at the bedside, guided and instructed by experienced teachers, and inspired toward self-directed, diligent reading. Clearly, there is no replacement for education at the bedside. Unfortunately, clinical situations usually do not encompass the breadth of the specialty. Perhaps the best alternative is a carefully crafted patient case designed to stimulate the clinical approach and decision making. In an attempt to achieve that goal, we have constructed a collection of clinical vignettes to teach diagnostic or therapeutic approaches relevant to obstetrics and gynecology. Most importantly, the explanations for the cases emphasize the mechanisms and underlying principles, rather than merely rote questions and answers.

This book is organized for versatility: It allows the student "in a rush" to go quickly through the scenarios and check the corresponding answers, and it provides more detailed information for the student who wants thought-provoking explanations. The answers are arranged from simple to complex: a summary of the pertinent points, the bare answers, an analysis of the case, an approach to the topic, a comprehension test at the end for reinforcement and emphasis, and a list of resources for further reading. The clinical vignettes are purposely placed in random order to simulate the way that real patients present to the practitioner. A listing of cases is included in Section III to aid the students who desire to test their knowledge of a specific area, or who want to review a topic including basic definitions. Finally, we intentionally did not use a multiple choice question (MCQ) format in our clinical case scenarios, since clues (or distractions) are not available in the real world. Nevertheless, several MCQs are included at the end of each case discussion (comprehension questions) to reinforce concepts or introduce related topics.

HOW TO GET THE MOST OUT OF THIS BOOK

Each case is designed to simulate a patient encounter with open-ended questions. At times, the patient's complaint is different from the most concerning issue, and sometimes extraneous information is given. The answers are organized into four different parts:

PART I:

1. **Summary:** The salient aspects of the case are identified, filtering out the extraneous information. Students should formulate their summary from the case before looking at the answers. A comparison to the summation in the answer will help to improve their ability to focus on the important data, while appropriately discarding the irrelevant information—a fundamental skill in clinical problem solving.

2. A **Straightforward Answer** is given to each open-ended question.

3. The **Analysis of the Case** is comprised of two parts:

    a) **Objectives of the Case:** A listing of the two or three main principles that are crucial for a practitioner to manage the patient. Again, the students are challenged to make educated "guesses" about the objectives of the case upon initial review of the case scenario, which helps to sharpen their clinical and analytical skills.

    b) **Considerations:** A discussion of the relevant points and brief approach to the **specific** patient.

PART II:

Approach to the Disease Process: It consists of two distinct parts:

    a) **Definitions:** Terminology pertinent to the disease process.

    b) **Clinical Approach:** A discussion of the approach to the clinical problem in general, including tables, figures, and algorithms.

PART III:

Comprehension Questions: Each case contains several multiple-choice questions, which reinforce the material, or which introduce new and related concepts. Questions about material not found in the text will have explanations in the answers.

PART IV:

Clinical Pearls: Several clinically important points are reiterated as a summation of the text. This allows for easy review, such as before an examination.

◈ ACKNOWLEDGMENTS

The clerkship curriculum that evolved into the ideas for this book was inspired by two talented and forthright students, Philbert Yau and Chuck Rosipal, who have since graduated from medical school. I am greatly indebted to my editor, Catherine Johnson, whose exuberance, experience, and vision helped to shape the text. I appreciate McGraw-Hill's believing in the concept of teaching through clinical cases, and I would like to especially acknowledge John Williams, the director of editing. I am also thankful to Niels Buessem for his excellent production expertise.

I thank Gerald Suh and Johnny Buckles for their friendship and advice, and Benton Baker III, MD, for his friendship, mentorship, and example.

I greatly appreciate each of the wonderful contributors who have given a practical flavor to the clinical discussions, especially Drs. Cristo Papasakelariou and John C. McBride. At Christus–St. Joseph Hospital, I am grateful to Dorothy Mersinger for her excellent advice and support. At the University of Texas–Houston Medical School, I would like to thank Yaki B. Bryant for her dedication in working with the medical students.

Eugene C. Toy, MD

How to Approach Clinical Problems

PART 1.   APPROACH TO THE PATIENT

The transition from textbook and/or journal article learning to the application of the information in a specific clinical situation is one of the most challenging tasks in medicine. It requires retention of information, organization of the facts, and recall of a myriad of data in precise application to the patient. The purpose of this book is to facilitate this process. The first step is gathering information, also known as establishing the database. This includes taking the history; performing the physical examination; and obtaining selective laboratory examinations or special evaluations, such as urodynamic testing and/or imaging tests. Of these, the historical examination is the most important and useful. Sensitivity and respect should always be exercised during the interview of patients.

CLINICAL PEARL

The history is usually the single most important tool in obtaining a diagnosis. The art of seeking the information in a nonjudgmental, sensitive, and thorough manner cannot be overemphasized.

History

1. Basic information:
    a. Age must be recorded because some conditions are more common at certain ages; for instance, pregnant women younger than 17 years or older than 35 years are at greater risk for preterm labor, preeclampsia, or miscarriage.
    b. Gravidity: Number of pregnancies including current pregnancy (includes miscarriages, ectopic pregnancies, and stillbirths).
    c. Parity: Number of pregnancies that have ended at gestational age(s) greater than 20 weeks.
    d. Abortuses: Number of pregnancies that have ended at gestational age(s) less than 20 weeks (includes ectopic

pregnancies, induced abortions, and spontaneous abortions).

CLINICAL PEARL

Some practitioners use a 4-digit parity system to designate the # **T**erm deliveries, # **P**reterm deliveries, # **A**bortuses, and # **L**ive births (TPAL system). For example, G2 P1001 indicates GRAVIDITY = 2 (two pregnancies including the current one), PARITY 1001 = 1 prior term delivery, no preterm deliveries, no abortuses, and 1 living.

2. Last menstrual period (LMP): The **first** day of the last menstrual period. In obstetric patients, the certainty of the LMP is important in determining the gestational age. The estimated gestational age (EGA) is calculated from the LMP or by ultrasound. A simple rule for calculating the expected due date (EDD) is to subtract 3 months from the LMP and add 7 days to the first day of the LMP (example: an LMP of 1 November would equal an EDD of 8 August).

3. Chief complaint: What is it that brought the patient into the hospital or office? Is it a scheduled appointment, or an unexpected symptom, such as abdominal pain or vaginal bleeding in pregnancy? The duration and character of the complaint, associated symptoms, and exacerbating and relieving factors should be recorded. The chief complaint engenders a differential diagnosis, and the possible etiologies should be explored by further inquiry. For example, if the chief complaint is postmenopausal bleeding, the concern is endometrial cancer. Thus, some of the questions should be related to the risk factors for endometrial cancer, such as hypertension, diabetes, anovulation, early age of menarche, late age of menopause, obesity, infertility, nulliparity, and so forth.

CLINICAL PEARL

The first line of any obstetric presentation should include **age, gravidity, parity, LMP, estimated gestational age, and chief complaint.**

Example: A 32-year-old G3 P1011 woman, whose LMP was April 2 and who has a pregnancy with an estimated gestational age of 32 4/7 weeks' gestation, complains of lower abdominal cramping.

4. Past gynecologic history:
   a. Menstrual history
      i. Age of menarche (should normally be older than 9 years and younger than 16 years).
      ii. Character of menstrual cycles: Interval from the first day of one menses to the first day of the next menses (normal is 28 ± 7 days, or between 21 and 35 days).
      iii. Quantity of menses: Menstrual flow should last less than 7 days (or be less than 80 mL in total volume). If menstrual flow is excessive, then it is called menorrhagia.
      iv. Irregular **AND** heavy menses is called menometrorrhagia.
   b. Contraceptive history: Duration, type, and last use of contraception, and any side effects.
   c. Sexually transmitted diseases: A positive or negative history of herpes simplex virus, syphilis, gonorrhea, *Chlamydia,* human immunodeficiency virus (HIV), pelvic inflammatory disease, or human papilloma virus. Number of sexual partners, whether a recent change in partners, and use of barrier contraception.

5. Obstetric history: Date and gestational age of each pregnancy at termination, and outcome; if induced abortion, then gestational age and method. If delivered, then whether the de-

livery was vaginal or cesarean; if applicable, type of cesarean (low-transverse versus classical). All complications of pregnancies should be listed.

6. Past medical history: Any illnesses, such as hypertension, hepatitis, diabetes mellitus, cancer, heart disease, pulmonary disease, and thyroid disease, should be elicited. Duration, severity, and therapies should be included. Any hospitalizations should be listed with reason for admission, intervention, and location of hospital.

7. Past surgical history: Year and type of surgery should be elucidated and any complications documented. Type of incision (laparoscopy versus laparotomy) should be recorded.

8. Allergies: Reactions to medications should be recorded, including severity and temporal relationship to medication. Immediate hypersensitivity should be distinguished from an adverse reaction.

9. Medications: A list of medications, dosage, route of administration and frequency, and duration of use should be obtained. Prescription, over-the-counter, and herbal remedies are all relevant. Use or abuse of illicit drugs, tobacco, or alcohol should also be recorded.

10. Review of systems: A systematic review should be performed but focused on the more common diseases. For example, in pregnant women, the presence of symptoms referable to preeclampsia should be queried, such as headache, visual disturbances, epigastric pain, or facial swelling. In an elderly woman, symptoms suggestive of cardiac disease should be elicited, such as chest pain, shortness of breath, fatigue, weakness, or palpitations.

CLINICAL PEARL

In every pregnancy greater than 20 weeks' gestation, the patient should be questioned about symptoms of preeclampsia (headaches, visual disturbances, dyspnea, epigastric pain, and face/hand swelling).

Physical Examination

1. General appearance: Cachetic versus well-nourished, anxious versus calm, alert versus obtunded.

2. Vital signs: Temperature, blood pressure, heart rate, and respiratory rate. Height and weight are often placed here.

3. Head and neck examination: Evidence of trauma, tumors, facial edema, goiter, and carotid bruits should be sought. Cervical and supraclavicular nodes should be palpated.

4. Breast examination: Inspection for symmetry, skin or nipple retraction with the patient's hands on her hips (to accentuate the pectoral muscles), and with arms raised. With the patient supine, the breasts should then be palpated systematically to assess for masses. The nipple should be assessed for discharge, and the axillary and supraclavicular regions should be examined for adenopathy.

5. Cardiac examination: The point of maximal impulse (PMI) should be ascertained, and the heart auscultated at the apex of the heart as well as base. Heart sounds, murmurs, and clicks should be characterized. Systolic flow murmurs are fairly common in pregnant women due to the increased cardiac output, but significant diastolic murmurs are unusual.

6. Pulmonary examination: The lung fields should be examined systematically and thoroughly. Wheezes, rales, rhonchi, and bronchial breath sounds should be recorded.

7. Abdominal examination: The abdomen should be inspected for scars, distension, masses or organomegaly (i.e., spleen or liver), and discoloration. For instance, the Grey–Turner sign of discoloration at the flank areas may indicate intra-abdominal or retroperitoneal hemorrhage. Auscultation of bowel sounds should be accomplished to identify normal versus high-pitched, and hyperactive versus hypoactive sounds. The abdomen should be percussed for the presence of shifting dullness (indicating ascites). Careful palpation should begin initially away from the area of pain, involving one hand on top of the other, to assess for masses, tenderness, and peritoneal signs. Tenderness should be recorded on a scale (for example, 1 to 4, where 4 is the most severe pain). Guarding, and whether it is voluntary or involuntary, should be noted.

8. Back and spine examination: The back should be assessed for symmetry, tenderness, or masses. In particular, the flank regions are important to assess for pain on percussion since that may indicate renal disease.

9. Pelvic examination (adequate preparation of the patient is crucial including counseling about what to expect, adequate lubrication, and sensitivity to pain and discomfort):
   a. The external genitalia should be observed for masses or lesions, discoloration, redness, or tenderness. Ulcers in this area may indicate herpes simplex virus, vulvar carcinoma, or syphilis; a vulvar mass at the 5:00 or 7:00 o'clock positions can suggest a Bartholin gland cyst or abscess. Pigmented lesions may require biopsy since malignant melanoma is not uncommon in the vulvar region.
   b. Speculum examination: The vagina should be inspected for lesions, discharge, estrogen effect (well-ruggated versus atrophic), and presence of a cystocele or a rectocele. The appearance of the cervix should be described, and masses, vesicles, or other lesions should be noted.
   c. Bimanual examination: Initially, the index and middle finger of the one gloved hand should be inserted into the pa-

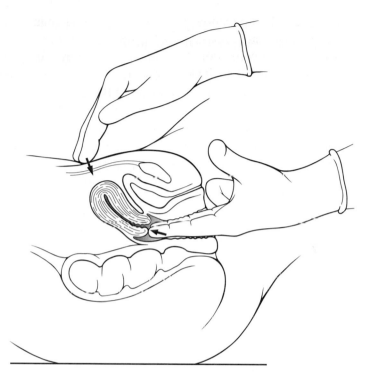

Figure I–1.   Bimanual pelvic examination. The examiner evaluates the patient's uterus by palpating her cervix vaginally while simultaneously assessing her uterine fundus abdominally.

tient's vagina underneath the cervix, while the clinician's other hand is placed on the abdomen at the uterine fundus. With the uterus trapped between the two hands, the examiner should identify whether there is cervical motion tenderness, and evaluate the size, shape, and directional axis of the uterus. The adnexa should then be assessed with the vaginal hand in the lateral vaginal fornices. The normal ovary is approximately the size of a walnut. (Figure I–1).

d. Rectal examination: A rectal examination will reveal masses in the posterior pelvis, and may identify occult blood in the stool. Nodularity and tenderness in the uterosacral ligament can be signs of endometriosis. The posterior uterus and palpable masses in the cul-de-sac can be identified by rectal examination.

10. Extremities and skin: The presence of joint effusions, tenderness, skin edema, and cyanosis should be recorded.

11. Neurologic examination: Patients who present with neurologic complaints usually require a thorough assessment including evaluation of the cranial nerves, strength, sensation, and reflexes.

CLINICAL PEARL

The vaginal examination assesses the anterior pelvis, whereas the rectal examination is directed at the posterior pelvis.

12. Laboratory assessment for obstetric patients:
   a. Prenatal laboratory tests usually include:
      i. CBC, or complete blood count, to assess for anemia and thrombocytopenia.
      ii. Blood type, Rh, and antibody screen is of paramount importance for all pregnant women; for those women who are Rh negative, Rhogam is administered at 28 weeks' gestation and at delivery (if the baby proves Rh positive) to prevent isoimmunization.
      iii. Hepatitis B surface antigen: Indicates that the patient is infectious. At birth, the newborn should be given hepatitis B immune globulin (HBIG) and hepatitis B vaccine in an attempt to prevent neonatal hepatitis.
      iv. Rubella titer: If the patient is not immune to rubella, she should be vaccinated immediately postpartum; because it is a live-attenuated vaccine, this immunization is not given during pregnancy.

      v.   Syphilis nontreponemal test (RPR or VDRL): A positive test necessitates confirmation with a treponemal test, such as MHATP or FTA-ABS. Treatment during pregnancy is crucial to prevent congenital syphilis; penicillin is the agent of choice. Pregnant women who are allergic to penicillin usually undergo desensitization and receive penicillin.

      vi.   Human immunodeficiency virus test: The screening test is usually the ELISA and, when positive, will necessitate the Western blot or other confirmatory test.

      vii.   Urine culture or urinalysis: To assess for asymptomatic bacteriuria, which complicates 6% to 8% of pregnancies.

      viii.   Pap smear: To assess for cervical dysplasia or cervical cancer; involves both ectocervical component and endocervical sampling (Figure I–2). Some clinicians prefer the liquid-based media because it may provide better cellular sampling and allows for HPV subtyping.

      ix.   Endocervical assays for gonorrhea and/or *Chlamydia trachomatis* for high-risk patients.

   b.   Timed prenatal tests:

      i.   Serum screening for neural tube defects or Down syndrome offered; usually performed between 16 to 20 weeks' gestation.

      ii.   Screening for gestational diabetes at 26 to 28 weeks; generally consists of a 50-g oral glucose load and assessment of the serum glucose level after 1 hour.

      iii.   Some practitioners choose to repeat the complete blood count, cervical cultures, or syphilis serology in the third trimester.

      iv.   If the culture strategy for group B streptococcus is adopted, then introital cultures are obtained at 35 to 37 weeks' gestation.

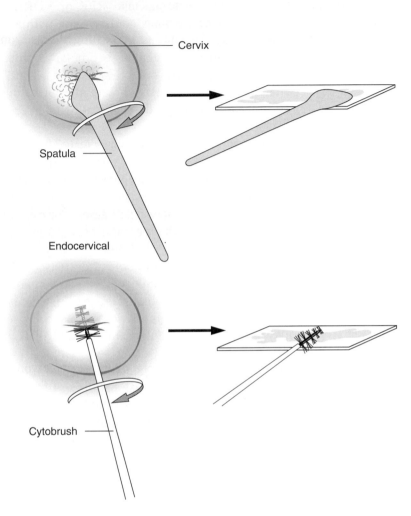

Figure I–2. Pap smear with ectocervical and endocervical component. The spatula is used to sample the exocervix; the endobrush is used to retrieve cells from the endocervix, which are applied to the slide and fixative is applied.

13. Laboratory tests for gynecologic patients:

   A. Dependent on age, presence of coexisting disease, and chief complaint.

   B. Common scenarios:
      i.   Threatened abortion: Quantitative hCG and/or progesterone levels may help to establish the viability of a pregnancy and risk of ectopic pregnancy.
      ii. Menorrhagia due to uterine fibroids: CBC, endometrial biopsy, and Pap smear. The endometrial biopsy is performed to assess for endometrial cancer and the Pap smear for cervical dysplasia or cancer.
      iii. A woman 55 years or older with an adnexal mass: CA-125 and CEA tumor markers for epithelial ovarian tumors.

14. Imaging procedures:
   a. Ultrasound examination:
      i.   Obstetric patients: Ultrasound is the most commonly used imaging procedure in pregnant women. It can be used to establish the viability of the pregnancy, number of fetuses, location of the placenta, or establish the gestational age of the pregnancy. Targeted examinations can help to examine for structural abnormalities of the fetus.
      ii. Gynecologic patients: Adnexal masses evaluated by sonography are assessed for size and echogenic texture; simple (fluid filled) versus complex (fluid and solid components) versus solid. The uterus can be characterized for presence of masses, such as uterine fibroids, and the endometrial stripe can be measured. In postmenopausal women, a thickened endometrial stripe may indicate malignancy. Fluid in the cul-de-sac may indicate ascites. The gynecologic ultrasound examination usually also includes inves-

tigation of the kidneys, because hydronephrosis may suggest a pelvic process (ureteral obstruction).

CLINICAL PEARL

Sonohysterography is a special ultrasound examination of the uterus that involves injecting a small amount of saline into the endometrial cavity to better define the intrauterine cavity. It can help to identify endometrial polyps or submucous myomata.

    b.   Computed tomography (CT) scan:
- i.   Because of the radiation concerns, this procedure is usually not performed on pregnant women unless sonography is not helpful, and it is deemed necessary.
- ii.   The CT scan is useful in women with possible abdominal and/or pelvic masses, and may help to delineate the lymph nodes and retroperitoneal disorders.

    c.   Magnetic resonance imaging (MRI):
- i.   Identifies soft tissue planes very well and may assist in defining müllerian defects, such as vaginal agenesis or uterine didelphys (condition of double uterus and double cervix), and in selected circumstances may also aid in the evaluation of uterine fibroids.
- ii.   May be helpful in establishing the location of a pregnancy, such as in differentiating a normal pregnancy from a cervical pregnancy.

    d.   Intravenous pyelogram (IVP):
- i.   Intravenous dye is used to assess the concentrating ability of the kidneys, the patency of the ureters, and the integrity of the bladder.
- ii.   It is also useful in detecting hydronephrosis, ureteral stone, or ureteral obstruction.

    e.   Hysterosalpingogram (HSG):
        i.   A small amount of radiopaque dye is introduced through a transcervical cannula and radiographs are taken.
        ii.   It is useful for the detection of intrauterine abnormalities (submucous fibroids or intrauterine adhesions) and patency of the fallopian tubes (tubal obstruction or hydrosalpinx).

PART 2.   APPROACH TO CLINICAL PROBLEM SOLVING

There are typically four distinct steps that a clinician undertakes to solve most clinical problems systematically:

1. Making the diagnosis.
2. Assessing the severity and/or stage of the disease.
3. Rendering a treatment based on the stage of the disease.
4. Following the patient's response to the treatment.

Making the Diagnosis

The diagnosis is made by careful evaluation of the database, analysis of the information, assessment of the risk factors, and development of the list of possibilities (the differential diagnosis). The process includes knowing which pieces of information are meaningful and which may be thrown out. Experience and knowledge help to guide the physician to "key in" on the most important possibilities. A good clinician also knows how to ask the same question in several different ways, and use different terminology. For example, patients at times may deny having been treated for "pelvic inflammatory disease," but will answer affirmatively to being hospitalized for "a tubal infection." Reaching a diagnosis may be achieved by systematically reading about each possible cause and disease. The patient's presentation is then matched up against each of these possibilities, and each is either placed high up on the list as a potential etiology, or moved lower down because of disease prevalence, the patient's presentation, or other clues. A patient's risk factors may influence the probability of a diagnosis.

Usually, a long list of possible diagnoses can be pared down to two to three most likely ones, based on selective laboratory or imaging tests. For example, a woman who complains of lower abdominal pain AND has a history of a prior sexually transmitted disease may have salpingitis; another patient who has abdominal pain, amenorrhea, AND a history of prior tubal surgery may have an ectopic pregnancy. Furthermore, yet another woman with a one-day history of periumbilical pain localizing to the right lower quadrant may have acute appendicitis.

CLINICAL PEARL

The first step in clinical problem solving is **making the diagnosis.**

Assessing the Severity of the Disease

After ascertaining the diagnosis, the next step is to characterize the severity of the disease process; in other words, describe "how bad" a disease is. With malignancy, this is done formally by staging the cancer. Most cancers are categorized from stage I (least severe) to stage IV (most severe). Some diseases, such as preeclampsia, may be designated as mild or severe. With other ailments, there is a moderate category. With some infections, such as syphilis, the staging depends on the duration and extent of the infection, and follows along the natural history of the infection (i.e., primary syphilis, secondary, latent period, and tertiary/neurosyphilis).

CLINICAL PEARL

The second step is to **establish the severity or stage of disease.** There is usually prognostic or treatment significance based on the stage.

Treating Based on Stage

Many illnesses are stratified according to severity because prognosis and treatment often vary based on the severity. If neither the prognosis nor the treatment was influenced by the stage of the disease process, there would not be a reason to subcategorize a disease as mild or severe. As an example, a pregnant woman at 32 weeks' gestation with mild preeclampsia is at less risk from the disease than if she developed severe preeclampsia (particularly if the severe preeclampsia were pulmonary edema or eclampsia). Accordingly, with mild preeclampsia, the management may be expectant, letting the pregnancy continue while watching for any danger signs (severe disease). In contrast, if severe preeclampsia complicated this same 32-week pregnancy, the treatment would be magnesium sulfate to prevent seizures (eclampsia) and, most importantly, **delivery.** It is primarily delivery that "cures" the preeclampsia. In this disease, severe preeclampsia means both maternal and fetal risks are increased. As another example, urinary tract infections may be subdivided into lower tract infections (cystitis) that are treated by oral antibiotics on an outpatient basis, versus upper tract infections (pyelonephritis) that generally require hospitalization and intravenous antibiotics.

Bacterial vaginosis (BV), which has been associated with preterm delivery, endometritis, and vaginal cuff cellulitis (following hysterectomy), does not have a severe or mild substaging. The presence of BV may slightly increase the risk of problems, but neither the prognosis nor the treatment is affected by "more" BV or "less" BV. Hence, the student should approach a new disease by learning the mechanism, clinical presentation, staging, and the treatment based on stage.

CLINICAL PEARL

The third step is that, for most conditions, **the treatment is tailored** to the extent or "stage" of the disease.

Following the Response to Treatment

The final step in the approach to disease is to follow the patient's response to the therapy. The "measure" of response should be recorded and monitored. Some responses are clinical, such as improvement (or lack of improvement) in a patient's abdominal pain, temperature, or pulmonary examination. Obviously, the student must work on being more skilled in eliciting the data in an unbiased and standardized manner. Other responses may be followed by imaging tests, such as a CT scan to establish retroperitoneal node size in a patient receiving chemotherapy, or a tumor marker, such as the CA-125 level in a woman receiving chemotherapy for ovarian cancer. For syphilis, it may be the results of the nonspecific treponemal antibody test RPR titer over time. The student must be prepared to know what to do if the measured marker does not respond according to what is expected. Is the next step to retreat, or to reconsider the diagnosis, or to repeat the metastatic work-up, or to follow up with another more specific test?

CLINICAL PEARL

The fourth step is to **monitor treatment response or efficacy,** which may be measured in different ways. It may be symptomatic (patient feels better), or based on physical examination (fever), a laboratory test (CA-125 level), or an imaging test (ultrasound size of ovarian cyst).

PART 3. APPROACH TO READING

The clinical problem-oriented approach to reading is different from the classic "systematic" research of a disease. Patients rarely present with a clear diagnosis; hence, the student must become skilled in applying the textbook information to the clinical setting. Furthermore, a reader retains more information when reading with a purpose. In other words, the student should read with the goal of answering specific questions. There are several fundamental questions that facilitate **clinical thinking.** These are:

1. What is the most likely diagnosis?
2. What should be your next step?
3. What is the most likely mechanism for this process?
4. What are the risk factors for this condition?
5. What are the complications associated with the disease process?
6. What is the best therapy?
7. How would you confirm the diagnosis?

CLINICAL PEARL

Reading with the purpose of answering the seven fundamental clinical questions improves retention of information and facilitates the application of "book knowledge" to "clinical knowledge."

What Is the Most Likely Diagnosis?

The method of establishing the diagnosis has been covered in the previous section. One way of attacking this problem is to develop standard "approaches" to common clinical situations. It is helpful to understand the most common causes of various presentations, such as "the most common cause of postpartum hemorrhage is uterine atony." (Clinical Pearls appear at the end of each case.)

The clinical scenario would be something such as:

> *An 18-year-old G1 P0 woman undergoes an uncomplicated vaginal delivery at term. After the placenta is delivered, she has 1500 cc of vaginal bleeding. What is the most likely diagnosis?*

With no other information to go on, the student would note that this woman has postpartum hemorrhage (blood loss of greater than 500 mL with a vaginal delivery). Using the "most common cause" information, the student would make an educated guess that the patient has **uterine atony.**

However, what if the scenario also included the following phrase?

The uterus is noted to be firm.

CLINICAL PEARLS

The most common cause of postpartum hemorrhage is uterine atony. Thus, the first step in patient assessment and management is uterine massage to check if the uterus is boggy.

If the uterus is firm, and the woman is still bleeding, then the clinician should consider a genital tract laceration.

Now, the student would use the clinical pearl: "The most common cause of postpartum hemorrhage with a firm uterus is a genital tract laceration."

What Should Be Your Next Step?

This question is difficult because the next step has many possibilities; the answer may be to obtain more diagnostic information, stage the illness, or introduce therapy. It is often a more challenging question than "What is the most likely diagnosis?" because there may be insufficient information to make a diagnosis and the next step may be to pursue more diagnostic information. Another possibility is that there is enough information for a probable diagnosis, and the next step is to stage the disease. Finally, the most appropriate answer may be to treat. Hence, from clinical data, a judgment needs to be rendered regarding how far along one is on the road of:

Make a dx → Stage the disease → Treat based on stage → Follow response

Frequently, the student is taught to "regurgitate" the information that someone has written about a particular disease, but is not skilled at giving the next step. This talent is learned optimally at the bedside, in a supportive environment, with freedom to make educated guesses, and with constructive feedback. A sample scenario describes a student's thought process as follows.

1. **Make the diagnosis:** "Based on the information I have, I believe that Ms. Smith has a pelvic inflammatory disease because she is not pregnant and has lower abdominal tenderness, cervical motion tenderness, and adnexal tenderness."
2. **Stage the disease:** "I don't believe that this is severe disease, since she does not have high fever, evidence of sepsis, or peritoneal signs. An ultrasound has already been done showing no abscess (tubo-ovarian abscess would put her in a severe category)."
3. **Treat based on stage:** "Therefore, my next step is to treat her with intramuscular ceftriaxone and oral doxycycline."

4. **Follow response:** "I want to follow the treatment by assessing her pain (I will ask her to rate the pain on a scale of 1 to 10 every day), her temperature, and abdominal examination, and reassess her in 48 hr."

In a similar patient, when the clinical presentation is unclear, perhaps the best "next step" may be diagnostic in nature, such as laparoscopy to visualize the tubes. This information is sometimes tested by the dictum, "the gold standard for the diagnosis of acute salpingitis is laparoscopy to visualize the tubes, and particularly seeing purulent material drain from the tubes."

CLINICAL PEARL

Usually, the vague query, "What is your next step?" is the most difficult question, because the answer may be diagnostic, staging, or therapeutic.

What Is the Likely Mechanism for This Process?

This question goes further than making the diagnosis, but also requires the student to understand the underlying mechanism for the process. For example, a clinical scenario may describe an 18-year-old woman at 24 weeks' gestation who develops dyspnea 2 days after being treated for pyelonephritis. The student must first diagnose the acute respiratory distress syndrome, which often occurs 1 to 2 days after antibiotics are instituted. Then, the student must understand that the endotoxins that arise from gram-negative organisms cause pulmonary injury, leading to capillary leakage of fluid into the pulmonary interstitial space. The mechanism is, therefore, endotoxin-induced "capillary leakage." Answers that a student may also entertain, but would be less likely to be causative, include: pneumonia, pulmonary embolism, or pleural effusion.

The student is advised to learn the mechanisms for each disease process, and not merely memorize a constellation of symptoms. In other words, rather than solely committing to memory the classic presentation of pyelonephritis (fever, flank tenderness, and pyuria), the student should understand that gram-negative rods, such as *Escherichia*

coli, would ascend from the external genitalia to the urethra to the bladder. From the bladder, the bacteria would ascend further to the kidneys
and cause an infection in the renal parenchyma. The involvement of the
kidney now causes fever (versus an infection of only the bladder, which
usually does not induce a fever) and flank tenderness—a systemic response not seen with lower urinary tract infection (i.e., bacteriuria or
cystitis). Furthermore, the body's reaction to the bacteria brings about
leukocytes in the urine (pyuria).

What Are the Risk Factors for This Process?

Understanding the risk factors helps the practitioner to establish a diagnosis and to determine how to interpret tests. For example, understanding the risk factor analysis may help to manage a 55-year-old
woman with postmenopausal bleeding after an endometrial biopsy
shows no pathologic changes. If the woman does not have any risk factors for endometrial cancer, the patient may be observed because the
likelihood for uterine malignancy is not so great. On the other hand, if
the same 55-year-old woman were diabetic, had a long history of
anovulation (irregular menses), was nulliparous, and was hypertensive,
a practitioner should pursue the postmenopausal bleeding further, even
after a normal endometrial biopsy. The physician may want to perform
a hysteroscopy to visualize the endometrial cavity directly, and biopsy
the abnormal appearing areas. Thus, the presence of risk factors helps
to categorize the likelihood of a disease process.

CLINICAL PEARL

When patients are at high risk for a disease based on risk factors, more testing may be indicated.

What Are the Complications of This Process?

Clinicians must be cognizant of the complications of a disease, so that
they will understand how to follow and monitor the patient. Sometimes,
the student will have to make the diagnosis from clinical clues, and then
apply his or her knowledge of the consequences of the pathologic
process. For example, a woman who presents with lower abdominal

pain, vaginal discharge, and dyspareunia is first diagnosed as having pelvic inflammatory disease or salpingitis (infection of the fallopian tubes). Long-term complications of this process would include ectopic pregnancy or infertility from tubal damage. Understanding the types of consequences also helps the clinician to be aware of the dangers to a patient. One life-threatening complication of a tubo-ovarian abscess (which is the end-stage of a tubal infection leading to a collection of pus in the region of the tubes and ovary) is rupture of the abscess. The clinical presentation is shock with hypotension, and the appropriate therapy is immediate surgery. In fact, not recognizing the rupture is commonly associated with patient mortality. The student applies this information when she or he sees a woman with a tubo-ovarian abscess on daily rounds, and monitors for hypotension, confusion, apprehension, and tachycardia. The clinician advises the team to be vigilant for any signs of abscess rupture, and to be prepared to undertake immediate surgery should the need arise.

What Is the Best Therapy?

To answer this question, the clinician needs to reach the correct diagnosis, and assess the severity of the condition, and then he or she must weigh the situation to reach the appropriate intervention. For the student, knowing exact dosages is not as important as understanding the best medication, the route of delivery, mechanism of action, and possible complications. It is important for the student to be able to verbalize the diagnosis and the rationale for the therapy. A common error is for the student to "jump to a treatment," like a random guess, and, therefore, he or she is given "right or wrong" feedback. In fact, the student's guess may be correct, but for the wrong reason; conversely, the answer may be a very reasonable one, with only one small error in thinking. Instead, the student should verbalize the steps so that feedback may be given at every reasoning point.

For example, if the question is "What is the best therapy for a 19-year-old woman with a nontender ulcer of the vulva and painless adenopathy who is pregnant at 12 weeks' gestation?" The incorrect manner of response is for the student to blurt out "azithromycin." Rather, the student should reason it in a way such as the following: "The most common cause of a nontender infectious ulcer of the vulva is syphilis. Painless adenopathy is usually associated. In pregnancy, penicillin is the only effective therapy to prevent congenital syphilis. Therefore, the best treatment for this woman with probable syphilis is intramuscular penicillin (after confirming the diagnosis)."

CLINICAL PEARL

Therapy should be logical based on the severity of disease. Antibiotic therapy should be tailored for specific organism(s).

How Would You Confirm the Diagnosis?

In the previous scenario, the woman with a nontender vulvar ulcer is likely to have syphilis. Confirmation can be achieved by serology (RPR or VDRL test) and specific treponemal test; however, there is a significant possibility that patients with primary syphilis may not have developed an antibody response yet, and have negative serology. Thus, confirmation of the diagnosis would be attained with darkfield microscopy. The student should strive to know the limitations of various diagnostic tests, and the manifestations of disease.

SUMMARY

1. There is no replacement for a meticulous history and physical examination.
2. There are four steps to the clinical approach to the patient: making the diagnosis, assessing severity, treating based on severity, and following response.
3. There are seven questions that help to bridge the gap between the textbook and the clinical arena.

REFERENCES

Cunningham FG, Gant NF, Leveno KJ, Gilstrap LC III, Hauth JC, Wenstrom KD. Prenatal care. In: Williams obstetrics, 21st ed. New York: McGraw-Hill. 2001:221–247.

Moore GJ. Obstetric and gynecologic evaluation. In: Hacker NF and Moore JG, eds. Essentials of obstetrics and gynecology, 3rd ed. Philadelphia: Saunders. 1998:12–26.

Stenchever MA. History, physical examination, and preventive health care. In: Stenchever MA, Droegemueller W, Herbst AL, Mishell DR, eds. Comprehensive gynecology, 4th ed. St. Louis: Mosby-Year Book. 2001:607–631.

Clinical
Cases

A 48-year-old G3 P3 woman complains of a 2-year history of loss of urine four to five times each day, typically occurring 2 to 3 sec after coughing, sneezing, or lifting; additionally, she notes dysuria and the urge to void during these episodes. These events cause her embarrassment and interfere with her daily activities. The patient is otherwise in good health. A urine culture performed 1 month previously was negative. On examination, she is slightly obese. Her blood pressure is 130/80, her heart rate is 80 beats per min, and her temperature 99°F. The breast examination is normal without masses. Her heart has a regular rate and rhythm without murmurs. The abdominal examination reveals no masses or tenderness. A midstream voided urinalysis is unremarkable.

◆ **What is your next step?**

◆ **What is the most likely diagnosis?**

◆ **What is the best initial treatment?**

ANSWERS TO CASE 1: Urinary Incontinence

Summary: A 48-year-old multiparous woman complains of urinary incontinence, which is possibly related to stress activities. There is a prominent urge component, and a delay from the Valsalva maneuver to the loss of urine.

◆ **Next step:** Evaluate the urinary incontinence, including a cystometric examination, to discern the etiology.

◆ **Most likely diagnosis:** Mixed genuine stress and urge incontinence.

◆ **Best initial treatment:** Anticholinergic medication to treat the urge symptoms, and then reassess the symptoms.

Analysis

Objectives

1. Discern between the typical history of genuine stress urinary incontinence (GSUI) versus urge urinary incontinence (UUI).
2. Know that the cystometric examination can be used to distinguish between the two etiologies.
3. Know the treatments for both entities (GSUI and UUI).

Considerations

This patient's history does not offer a straightforward etiology for her urinary incontinence. In particular, genuine SUI cannot be diagnosed, since there is an urge component as well as a several second delay from cough to urine loss. There is no evidence of diabetes or a neuropathy, making overflow incontinence unlikely. The pelvic examination does not reveal a cystocele (bladder bulging into the anterior vagina) or a loss of the normal bladder-urethral angle; both of these findings of pelvic relaxation may be associated with the anatomic problem of

GSUI, the bladder neck being below the abdominal cavity. Even if this patient were to have a cystocele, in reviewing the conflicting history, a prudent practitioner would strongly consider a cystometric examination to differentiate between genuine stress and urge incontinence. An accurate diagnosis is important, since **the therapies for these two conditions are very different, and surgical therapy may actually worsen urge incontinence.**

Note: A classic history and physical examination consistent with GSUI would not require cystometric evaluation, and a surgical procedure, such as a Burch urethropexy, could be performed.

APPROACH TO URINARY INCONTINENCE

Definitions

Urinary incontinence: The involuntary loss of urine that is objectively demonstrable and creates social or hygienic concern.

Genuine stress incontinence: Incontinence through the urethra due to sudden increases in intra-abdominal pressure, in the absence of bladder muscle spasm.

Urge incontinence: Loss of urine due to an uninhibited and sudden bladder detrusor muscle contraction.

Overflow incontinence: Loss of urine associated with an overdistended, hypotonic bladder in the absence of detrusor contractions. This is often associated with diabetes mellitus, spinal cord injuries, or lower motor neuropathies. It may also be caused by urethral edema after pelvic surgery.

Cystometric evaluation: Investigation of pressure and volume changes in the bladder with the filling of known volumes. It is often used to discern between GSUI and UUI.

Normal Physiology

Urinary continence is maintained when the urethral pressure exceeds the intravesicular (bladder) pressure. The bladder and proximal urethra are normally intra-abdominal in position, that is, above the pelvic diaphragm. In this situation, a Valsalva maneuver transmits pressure to both the bladder and proximal urethra so that continence is maintained. In the normal anatomic situation, the urethral pressure exceeds the bladder pressure.

Mechanisms of Incontinence

Genuine stress incontinence: Following trauma and/or other causes of weakness of the pelvic diaphragm (such as childbearing), the proximal urethra may fall below the pelvic diaphragm. When the patient coughs, intra-abdominal pressure is exerted to the bladder, but not to the proximal urethra. **When the bladder pressure equals or exceeds the maximal urethral pressure, then urinary flow occurs.** Because this is a mechanical problem, the patient feels no urge to void, and the loss of urine occurs simultaneously with coughing. There is no delay from cough to incontinence. Urethropexy replaces the proximal urethra back to its intra-abdominal position (Figure 1–1).

Urge incontinence: With uninhibited spasms of the detrusor muscle, the bladder pressure overcomes the urethral pressure. **Dysuria and/or the urge to void are prominent symptoms, reflecting the bladder spasms.** Sometimes, coughing or sneezing can provoke a bladder spasm, so that a several second delay is noted before urine loss.

Overflow incontinence: With an overdistended bladder, coughing will increase the bladder pressure and eventually lead to dribbling or small loss of urine.

Clinical approach: The history, physical examination, urinalysis, and postvoid residual are part of the initial evaluation of urinary incontinence (Table 1–1).

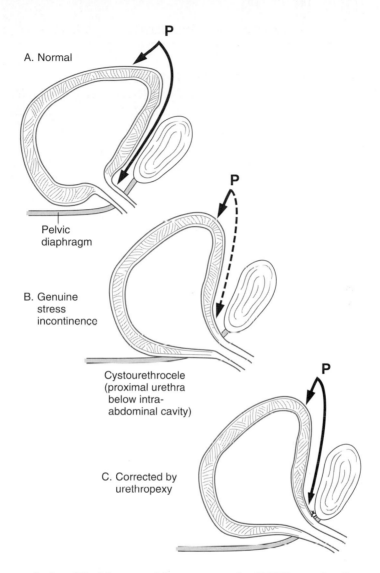

Figure 1–1. Bladder position: normal, GSUI, and after urethropexy. Normally, a Valsalva maneuver causes the increased intra-abdominal pressure (*P*) to be transmitted equally to the bladder and proximal urethra (A). With genuine stress incontinence (GSUI), the proximal urethra has fallen outside the abdominal cavity (B) so that the intra-abdominal pressure no longer is transferred to the proximal urethra, leading to incontinence. After urethropexy (C), pressure is again transmitted to the urethra.

Table 1–1

DIFFERENTIAL DIAGNOSIS OF URINARY INCONTINENCE

	MECHANISM	HISTORY	DIAGNOSTIC TEST	TREATMENT
Genuine stress urinary incontinence	Bladder neck has fallen out of its normal intra-abdominal position	Painless loss of urine concurrent with Valsalva; no urge to void	Physical examination: loss of bladder angle; cystometric examination	Urethropexy (Burch procedure) to return proximal urethra back to intra-abdominal position
Urge incontinence	Detrusor muscle is over-active and contracts unpredictably	Urge component, "I have to go to the bathroom and can't make it there in time"	Cystometric examination showing uninhibited contractions	Anticholinergic medication to relax detrusor muscle (surgery may worsen)
Overflow incontinence	Overdistended bladder due to hypotonic bladder	Loss of urine with Valsalva; dribbling; diabetes or spinal cord injury	Postvoid residual (catheterization) shows large amount of urine	Intermittent self-catheterization
Fistula	Communication between bladder or ureter and vagina	Constant leakage after surgery or prolonged labor	Dye into bladder showing vaginal discoloration	Surgical repair of fistulous tract

Comprehension Questions

Match the following **SINGLE best therapy** (A–G) that will most likely help in the clinical situation described (1.1–1.4):

    A. Burch urethropexy

    B. Oxybutynin (Ditropan, an anticholinergic medication)

C. Placement of ureteral stents
D. Surgical repair of the fistulous tract
E. Propranolol (inderal)
F. Placement of an artificial urethral sphincter
G. Intermittent self-catheterization

[1.1] A 42-year-old woman has long-standing diabetes mellitus and complains of small amounts of urine loss with coughing or lifting.

[1.2] A 39-year-old woman wets her underpants two to three times each day. She feels as though she needs to void, but cannot make it to the restroom in time.

[1.3] A 35-year-old woman has undergone four vaginal deliveries. She notes urinary loss six to seven times a day concurrently with coughing or sneezing. She denies dysuria or an urge to void.

[1.4] A 55-year-old woman notes constant wetness from her vagina following a total vaginal hysterectomy.

Answers

[1.1] **G.** This patient has long-standing diabetes mellitus, which is a risk factor for a neurogenic bladder leading to overflow incontinence. Other causes include spinal cord injury or multiple sclerosis. These patients generally do not feel the urge to void and accumulate large amounts of urine in their bladders. The best therapy for overflow incontinence (neurogenic bladder) is intermittent self-catheterization.

[1.2] **B.** This woman's prominent urge component makes urge incontinence the most likely diagnosis, best treated with anticholinergic medications.

[1.3] **A.** This clinical presentation is consistent with genuine SUI and is best treated by urethropexy. There is some evidence that vaginal deliveries may increase the incidence of GSUI due to trauma to the pelvic diaphragm.

[1.4] **D.** Constant wetness after a pelvic operation suggests a fistula, such as vesicovaginal fistula, which is best treated with surgical repair.

CLINICAL PEARLS

 The primary treatment of genuine stress incontinence is surgical, whereas the best treatment of urge incontinence is medical.

 Cystometric or urodynamic evaluation helps to differentiate genuine from urge incontinence.

 A postvoid catheterization showing a large residual volume suggests overflow incontinence.

 Loss of urine occurs when the intravesicular pressure equals (or exceeds) the sphincter pressure.

REFERENCES

Bhatia NN. Genitourinary dysfunction: pelvic organ prolapse, urinary incontinence, and infections. In: Hacker NF and Moore JG, eds. Essentials of obstetrics and gynecology, 3rd ed. Philadelphia: Saunders. 1998:455–476.

Stenchever MA and Fenner DE. Urogynecology: physiology of micturition, diagnosis of voiding dysfunction and incontinence: surgical and nonsurgical treatment. In: Stenchever MA, Droegemueller W, Herbst AL, Mishell DR, eds. Comprehensive gynecology, 4th ed. St. Louis: Mosby-Year Book. 2001:607–631.

CASE 2

A 66-year-old woman comes in for a routine physical examination. Her menopause occurred at age 51 years, and she is currently taking an estrogen pill along with a progestin pill each day. The past medical history is unremarkable. Her family history includes one maternal cousin with ovarian cancer. On examination, she is found to have a blood pressure of 120/70, heart rate of 70 beats per min, and temperature of 98°F. She weighs 140 lb and is 5′4″ tall. The thyroid is normal to palpation. Examination of her breasts reveals no masses or discharge. The abdominal, cardiac, and lung evaluations are within normal limits. The pelvic examination shows a normal, multiparous cervix, a normal-sized uterus, and no adnexal masses. She had undergone mammography 3 months previously.

◆ **What is your next step?**

◆ **What would be the most common cause of mortality for this patient?**

ANSWERS TO CASE 2: Health Maintenance, Age 66 Years

Summary: A 66-year-old woman presents for health maintenance. A mammogram has been performed 3 months previously.

◆ **Next step:** Each of the following should be performed: Pap smear, stool for occult blood, colonoscopy or barium enema/flexible sigmoidoscopy, pneumococcal vaccine, influenza vaccine, tetanus vaccine (if not within 10 yr), cholesterol screening, fasting blood sugar, bone mineral density screening, and urinalysis.

◆ **Most common cause of mortality:** Cardiovascular disease.

Analysis

Objectives

1. Understand which health maintenance studies should be performed for a 66-year-old woman.
2. Know the most common cause of mortality for a woman in this age group.
3. Understand that preventive maintenance consists of cancer screening, immunizations, and screening for common diseases.

Considerations

The approach to health maintenance includes three parts: 1) cancer screening, 2) immunizations, and 3) addressing common diseases for the particular patient group. For a 66-year-old woman, this includes a Pap smear for cervical cancer screening, annual mammography for breast cancer screening, colon cancer screening (annual stool tetst for occult blood and either intermittent colonoscopy or barium enema/flexible sigmoidoscopy), tetanus booster every 10 yr, the pneumococcal vaccine, and a yearly influenza immunization. Screening for hypercholesterolemia every 5 yr up to age 75 years, and fasting blood sugar levels every 3 yr are also recommended. Because urosepsis is common in geriatric patients, a urinalysis is also usually performed. Osteoporosis screening is indicated for women over the age of 65. Finally, the most common cause of mortality in a woman in this age group is cardiovascular disease.

APPROACH TO HEALTH MAINTENANCE IN OLDER WOMEN

Definitions

Screening test: A device used to identify asymptomatic disease in the hope that early detection will lead to an improved outcome. An optimal screening test has high sensitivity and specificity, is inexpensive, and is easy to perform.

Primary prevention: Identifying and modifying risk factors in people who have never had the disease of concern.

Secondary prevention: Actions taken to reduce morbidity or mortality once a disease has been diagnosed.

Cost effectiveness: A comparison of resources expended (dollars) in an intervention versus the benefit, which may be measured in life-years, or quality-adjusted life years.

Clinical Approach

In each age group, particular screening tests are recommended (Table 2–1).

Rationale

When the patient does not have any apparent disease or complaint, then the goal of medical intervention is disease prevention. One method of targeting diseases is by using the patient's age. For example, the most common cause of death for a 16-year-old person is a motor vehicle accident; hence the teenage patient would be well served by the physician encouraging him or her to wear seat belts and to avoid alcohol intoxication when driving. In contrast, a 56-year-old woman will most likely die of cardiovascular disease, so the physician should focus on exercise, weight loss, and screening for hyperlipidemia.

Table 2–1

SCREENING BASED ON AGE (YEARS)

	13 TO 18	19 TO 39	40 TO 64	65+
Cancer screening	Pap smear if sexually active	Annual Pap smear	Annual Pap smear *Age 50:* stool for occult blood, barium enema with flexible sigmoidoscopy q 5 yr, or colonoscopy every 10 yr, annual mammography*	Annual Pap smear Annual stool for occult blood Colonoscopy or barium enema with flexible sigmoidoscopy every 5 yr Annual mammography*
Immunizations	Tetanus booster once between ages 11–16 yr	Tetanus every 10 yr	Tetanus every 10 yr *Age 50:* annual influenza vaccine	Tetanus every 10 yr Pneumococcal vaccine Annual influenza vaccine
Other diseases	Motor vehicle accidents Depression Firearms	Cardio-vascular diseases	Cholesterol screening every 5 yr @ age 45 Fasting blood sugar every 3 yr @ 45	Cholesterol screening every 5 yr @ age 45 Fasting blood sugar every 3 yr @ 45 Bone mineral density study @ 65
Most common causes of mortality	1. Motor vehicle accidents 2. Homicide 3. Suicide	1. Motor vehicle accidents 2. Cardio-vascular disease 3. AIDS	1. Cardio-vascular disease 2. Cancer	1. Heart disease 2. Cancer 3. Cerebrovas-cular disease

*Some experts recommend mammography beginning at age 40 years whereas others question its efficacy in decreasing mortality.
Adapted from ACOG Committee Opinion 246, 2000. Washington, DC: ACOG, 2000.

Comprehension Questions

For each of the patient scenarios listed below (2.1–2.4), assign one or more answers (A-J) pertaining to health maintenance. *Note:* More than one answer may be used.

    A. Influenza vaccine
    B. Pneumococcal vaccine
    C. Barium enema with flexible sigmoidoscopy
    D. Mammography every year
    E. Pneumococcal vaccine
    F. Chest radiograph
    G. Urinalysis
    H. Pap smear
    I. Fasting blood sugar
    J. Bone mineral density study

[2.1] A 16-year-old girl engaged in one episode of sexual intercourse two years ago, but is currently not sexually active.

[2.2] A 44-year-old woman denies any health problems.

[2.3] A 59-year-old woman has mild osteoarthritis.

[2.4] A woman, aged 69 years, has mild hypertension controlled with an antihypertensive agent.

Answers

[2.1] **H.** A Pap smear should be initiated at age 18 years or when sexually active, whichever occurs first.

[2.2] **H.** A Pap smear for cancer screening is the only indicated test.

[2.3] **A, C, D, H,** and **I.** After the age of 50 years, annual mammography, colon cancer screening, and influenza vaccination are recommended. After age 45, a fasting blood sugar every 3 yr is recommended. Some experts prefer colonoscopy to air-contrast barium enema/flexible sigmoidoscopy.

[2.4] **A, B, C, D, E, G, H, I,** and **J.** All the listed screening tests are indicated after age 65 years except chest x-ray.

CLINICAL PEARLS

 The basic approach to health maintenance is threefold: 1) cancer screening, 2) age-appropriate immunizations, and 3) screening for common diseases.

 The most common cause of mortality in a woman younger than 20 years is motor vehicle accidents.

 The most common cause of mortality of a woman older than 39 years is cardiovascular disease.

 Major conditions in women aged 65 years and older include osteoporosis, heart disease, breast cancer, and depression.

REFERENCES

Peterson HB. Principles of screening. In: Holzman GB, Rinehart RD, Dunn LJ, eds. Precis: primary and preventive care. Washington, DC: ACOG; 1999:15–21.

American College of Obstetricians and Gynecologists. Primary and preventive care: periodic assessments. ACOG Committee Opinion 246. Washington, DC: 1999.

American College of Obstetricians and Gynecologists. Bone density screening for osteoporosis. ACOG Committee Opinion 270. Washington, DC: 2002.

◈ **CASE 3**

After a 4-hour labor, a 31-year-old G4 P3 woman undergoes an un-eventful vaginal delivery of a 7 lb 8 oz infant over an intact perineum. During her labor, she is noted to have mild variable decelerations and accelerations that increase 20 beats per min (bpm) above the baseline heart rate. At delivery, the male baby has Apgar scores of 8 at 1 min, and 9 at 5 min. Slight lengthening of the cord occurs after 28 min along with a small gush of blood per vagina. As the placenta is being deliv-ered, a shaggy, reddish, bulging mass is noted at the introitus around the placenta.

◆ **What is the most likely diagnosis?**

◆ **What is the most likely complication to occur in this patient?**

ANSWERS TO CASE 3: Uterine Inversion

Summary: A 31-year-old G4 P3 woman has a normal vaginal delivery of her baby, and after slight lengthening of the cord, a reddish mass is noted bulging in the introitus.

◆ **Most likely diagnosis:** Uterine inversion.

◆ **Most likely complication:** Postpartum hemorrhage.

Analysis

Objectives

1. Know the signs of spontaneous placental separation.
2. Recognize the clinical presentation of uterine inversion
3. Understand that the most common cause of uterine inversion is undue traction of the cord before placental separation.

Considerations

This patient's history reveals that the first and second stages of labor are normal. The third stage of labor (placental delivery) reaches close to the upper limits of normal. The evidence for placental separation is never definite. **The four signs of placental separation are: 1) gush of blood, 2) lengthening of the cord, 3) globular and firm shape of the uterus, and 4) the uterus rises up to the anterior abdominal wall.** In this case, although there is not good evidence for placental separation, traction on the cord is exerted, which results in an inverted uterus. The reddish bulging mass noted adjacent to the placenta is the endometrial surface; hence, the mass will have a shaggy appearance and be all around the placenta. Other masses and/or organs may at times prolapse, such as vaginal or cervical tissue, but these will have a smooth appearance.

APPROACH TO INVERTED UTERUS

Definitions

Third stage of labor: From delivery of infant to the delivery of the placenta (upper limits of normal is 30 min).

Abnormally retained placenta: Third stage of labor that has exceeded 30 min.

Uterine inversion: A "turning inside out" of the uterus; whereupon the fundus of the uterus moves through the cervix, into the vagina (Figure 3–1).

Signs of placental separation: Cord lengthening, gush of blood, globular uterine shape, and uterus lifting up to the anterior abdominal wall.

Clinical Approach

After a vaginal delivery, 95% of women experience spontaneous placenta separation within 30 min. Because the uterus and placenta are no longer joined, the placenta is usually in the lower segment of the uterus, just inside the cervix, and the uterus is often contracted. The umbilical cord lengthens due to the placenta having dropped into the lower portion of the uterus. The gush of blood represents bleeding from the placental bed, usually coinciding with placental separation. If the placenta has not separated, excessive force on the cord may lead to uterine inversion. Massive hemorrhage usually results; thus, in this situation, the practitioner must be prepared for rapid volume replacement. Although it was classically taught by some that the shock was out of proportion to the actual amount of blood loss, this is not the case. In other words, **shock is due to massive hemorrhage!**

  The best method of averting a uterine inversion is to await spontaneous separation from the placenta from the uterus before placing traction on the umbilical cord. Even after one or two of the signs of placental separation are present, the operator should be cautious not to put undue tension on the cord. At times, part of the placenta may separate, revealing the gush of blood, but the remaining attached placenta

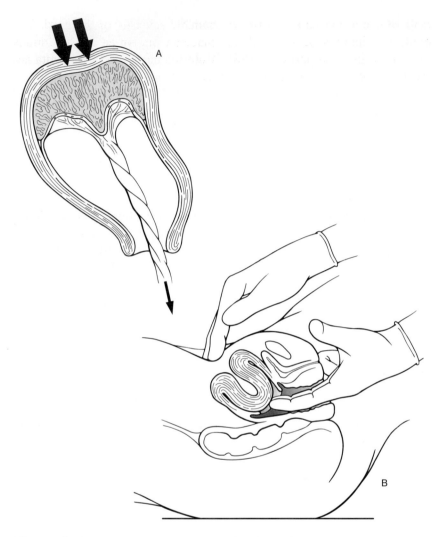

Figure 3–1.   Inverted uterus. Uterine inversion can occur when excessive umbilical cord traction is exerted on a fundally implanted, unseparated placenta (A). Upon recognition, the operator attempts to reposition the inverted uterus using cupped fingers (B).

may induce a uterine inversion or traumatic severing of the cord. The grand-multiparous patient with the placenta implanted in the fundus (top of uterus) is at particular risk for uterine inversion. A placenta accreta, an abnormally adherent placenta, is also a risk factor.

Treatment

With the diagnosis of an inverted uterus, immediate assistance—including that of an anesthesiologist—is essential because a uterine relaxation anesthetic agent, such as halothane (for uterine replacement), and/or emergency surgery may be necessary. If the placenta has already separated, the recently inverted uterus may sometimes be replaced by using the gloved palm and cupped fingers. Two intravenous lines should be started as soon as possible and preferably prior to placental separation, since profuse hemorrhage may follow placental removal. Terbutaline or magnesium sulfate can also be utilized to relax the uterus if necessary prior to uterine replacement. Upon replacing the uterine fundus to the normal location, the relaxation agents are stopped, and then uterotonic agents, such as oxytocin, are given. Placement of the clinician's fist inside the uterus to maintain the normal structure of the uterus is important.

Note: **Even with optimal treatment of uterine inversion, hemorrhage is almost a certainty.**

Comprehension Questions

[3.1] Which of the following placental implantation sites would most likely predispose to an inverted uterus?

A. Fundal
B. Anterior
C. Posterior
D. Lateral
E. Lower segment

[3.2] Which of the following would be the next step after a 30-min
third stage of labor?

  A. Initiate oxytocin
  B. Wait for an additional 30 min
  C. Hysterectomy
  D. Attempt a manual extraction of the placenta
  E. Estrogen intravaginally

[3.3] Which of the following is LEAST likely to be a risk factor for
uterine inversion?

  A. Short umbilical cord
  B. Atonic uterus
  C. Nonseparated placenta
  D. Attenuated umbilical cord
  E. Grand-multiparity

[3.4] A 33-year-old G5 P5 woman who is being induced for
preeclampsia delivers a 9 lb baby. Upon delivery of the placenta,
uterine inversion is noted. The physician attempts to replace the
uterus, but the cervix is tightly contracted, preventing the fundus
of the uterus from being repositioned. Which of the following is
the best therapy for this patient?

  A. Vaginal hysterectomy
  B. Dührssen's incisions of the cervix
  C. Halothane anesthesia
  D. Discontinue the magnesium sulfate
  E. Infuse oxytocin intravenously

Answers

[3.1] **A.** A fundally implanted placenta predisposes to uterine inversion.

[3.2] **D.** After 30 min, the placenta is abnormally retained, and a manual extraction is generally attempted.

[3.3] **D.** An attenuated umbilical cord leads to severing of the cord with traction and in a way protects against uterine inversion, whereas an unusually sturdy cord may predispose to uterine inversion.

[3.4] **C.** A uterine relaxing agent (such as halothane anesthesia) is the best initial therapy for a nonreducible uterus. Dührssen's incisions are used to treat the entrapped fetal head of a breech vaginal delivery.

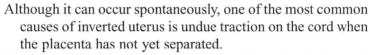

CLINICAL PEARLS

Although it can occur spontaneously, one of the most common causes of inverted uterus is undue traction on the cord when the placenta has not yet separated.

The signs of placental separation are 1) gush of blood, 2) lengthening of the cord, 3) globular-shaped uterus, and 4) the uterus rising to the anterior abdominal wall.

Hemorrhage is a common complication of an inverted uterus.

The upper limit of normal for the third stage of labor (time between delivery of the infant to delivery of the placenta) is 30 min.

REFERENCES

Hayashi RH. Genitourinary dysfunction: pelvic organ prolapse, urinary incontinence, and infections. In: Hacker NF and Moore JG, eds. Essentials of obstetrics and gynecology, 3rd ed. Philadelphia: Saunders. 1998:335–337.

Cunningham FG, Gant NF, Leveno KJ, Gilstrap LC III, Hauth JC, Wenstrom KD. Obstetrical hemorrhage. In: Williams obstetrics, 21st ed. New York: McGraw-Hill. 2001:619–669.

A 49-year-old woman complains of irregular menses over the past 6 months, feelings of inadequacy, vaginal dryness, difficulty sleeping, and episodes of warmth and sweating at night. On examination, her BP is 120/68, heart rate is 90/min, and temperature is 99°F. Her thyroid gland is normal to palpation. The cardiac and lung examinations are unremarkable. The breasts are symmetric, without masses or discharge. Examination of the external genitalia does not reveal any masses.

◆ **What is the most likely diagnosis?**

◆ **What is your next diagnostic step?**

ANSWERS TO CASE 4: Perimenopause

Summary: A 49-year-old woman complains of irregular menses, feelings of inadequacy, sleeplessness, and episodes of warmth and sweating.

◆ **Most likely diagnosis:** Climacteric (perimenopausal state).

◆ **Next diagnostic step:** Serum follicle stimulating hormone (FSH) and luteinizing hormone (LH).

Analysis

Objectives

1. Understand the normal clinical presentation of women in the perimenopausal state.
2. Understand that elevated serum FSH and LH levels help to confirm the diagnosis.
3. Know that estrogen replacement therapy is usually effective in treating the hot flushes.
4. Know the risks of continuous estrogen-progestin therapy.

Considerations

This 49-year-old woman complains of irregular menses, feelings of inadequacy, and intermittent sensations of warmth and sweating. This constellation of symptoms is consistent with the perimenopause, or climacteric. Between the age of 40 and 51 years, the majority of women begin to experience symptoms of hypoestrogenemia, primarily hot flushes. Hot flushes, which are the typical vasomotor change due to decreased estrogen levels, are associated with skin temperature elevation and sweating lasting for 2 to 4 min. The low estrogen concentration also has an effect on the vagina by decreasing the epithelial thickness, leading to atrophy and dryness. Elevated serum FSH and LH levels are helpful in confirming the diagnosis of the perimenopause. Treatment for hot flushes includes estrogen replacement therapy with progestin.

When a woman still has her uterus, the addition of progestin to estrogen replacement is important in preventing endometrial cancer.

Note: The selective estrogen receptor modulator (SERM), raloxifene, does not treat hot flushes.

APPROACH TO THE MENOPAUSE

Definitions

Menopause: The point in time in a woman's life when there is cessation of menses due to follicular atresia occurring after age 40 years (mean age 51 years).
Perimenopause (climacteric): The transitional 2 to 4 yr spanning from immediately before to immediately after the menopause.
Hot flushes: Irregular unpredictable episodes of increased skin temperature and sweating lasting about 3 to 4 min.
Premature ovarian failure: The cessation of ovarian function due to atresia of follicles prior to age 40 years. At ages younger than 30 years, autoimmune diseases or karyotypic abnormalities should be considered.

Physiology

At about 47 years of age, most women experience perimenopausal symptoms due to the ovaries' impending failure. Symptoms include irregular menses due to anovulatory cycles; vasomotor symptoms, such as hot flushes; and decreased estrogen and androgen levels. Because ovarian inhibin levels are decreased, FSH levels rise even before estradiol levels fall. The decreased estradiol concentrations lead to vaginal atrophy, bone loss, and vasomotor symptoms. **While most clinicians agree that estrogen replacement therapy is currently the best treatment for the vasomotor symptoms and to prevent osteoporosis,** recent published data raises concerns about the risks of this therapy. The Women's Health Initiative Study of continuous estrogen-progestin treatment reported a small but significant increased risk of breast cancer, heart disease, pulmonary embolism, and stroke. Women on hormone replacement therapy had fewer fractures and a lower incidence of colon cancer.

It should be noted that there is no evidence of adverse effects from short-term (<6mo) of estrogen therapy for the acute relief of menopausal symptoms. For women who cannot or choose not to take estrogen the antihypertensive agent clonidine may help with the vasomotor symptoms. A selective estrogen receptor modulator (SERM), such as raloxifene, is helpful in preventing bone loss, but does not alter the hot flushes. **Weight-bearing exercise, calcium and vitamin D supplementation, and estrogen replacement are important cornerstones in maintaining bone mass.** Because the FSH responds to the inhibin and not to estrogen, the FSH level cannot be used to *titrate* the estrogen replacement dose. In other words, the FSH concentration is still elevated even though the estrogen replacement may be sufficient.

Other diseases that are important to consider in the perimenopausal woman include hypothyroidism, diabetes mellitus, hypertension, and breast cancer. Women in this stage of life may also experience depression, whether spontaneous in its onset or situational due to grief or midlife adjustments. The practitioner should advocate aerobic exercise at least three times a week, again, with weight-bearing exercise being advantageous for the prevention of osteoporosis. Bone mineral density (BMD) testing, such as by dual-energy x-ray absorptiometry (DEXA), is useful in the early identification of osteoporosis and osteopenia. BMD testing is indicated for all postmenopausal women aged 65 years or older, and postmenopausal women at risk for osteoporosis and presenting with a bone fracture. Alcohol abuse may be seen in up to 10% of postmenopausal women, and requires clinical suspicion to establish the diagnosis.

Comprehension Questions

Match the following **single** best mechanism (A–H) to each of the clinical situations described (4.1–4.6). Each answer may be used once, more than once, or not at all.

    A. Gonadotropin receptor insensitivity
    B. Pituitary dysfunction
    C. Ovarian failure
    D. Ovarian cortical atrophy syndrome
    E. Peritoneal interference with ovulation

F. Hypothalamic dysfunction
G. Estrogen excess
H. Immune down-regulation of ovary

[4.1] A 51-year-old woman with oligomenorrhea and hot flushes.

[4.2] A 22-year-old nonpregnant woman with galactorrhea and hyper-prolactinemia.

[4.3] A 25-year-old woman slightly obese, slightly hirsute, and with a long history of irregular menses.

[4.4] An 18-year-old female with infantile breast development has not started her menses. She has some webbing of the neck region.

[4.5] A 19-year-old nonpregnant woman marathon runner with amenorrhea.

[4.6] A 33-year-old woman who has not started her menses since a vaginal delivery 1 year previously complicated by postpartum hemorrhage. She was unable to breastfeed.

Answers

[4.1] **C.** Ovarian failure due to follicular atresia is the reason for oligo-ovulation in the perimenopausal years.

[4.2] **F.** Both hypothyroidism and hyperprolactinemia may cause hy-pothalamic dysfunction, which inhibits gonadotropin-releasing hormone pulsations, which in turn inhibit pituitary FSH and LH release. The lack of gonadotropins leads to hypoestrogenic amen-orrhea.

[4.3] **G.** In polycystic ovarian syndrome, women are often obese and hirsute, have anovulation and insulin resistance, but an estrogen excess.   Progestin given to these women will induce vaginal bleeding.

[4.4] **C.** Ovarian failure is the most likely etiology in this female with probable Turner's syndrome (45,X). It would be reflected by elevated gonadotropin levels, and streaked ovaries.

[4.5] **F.** Excessive exercise causes hypothalamic dysfunction.

[4.6] **B.** Sheehan's syndrome is anterior pituitary hemorrhagic necrosis associated with postpartum hemorrhage.

CLINICAL PEARLS

◈ Hot flushes and irregular menses after the age of 45 years are most likely due to the climacteric, and the symptoms usually respond to estrogen replacement therapy.

◈ The most common location of an osteoporosis-associated fracture is the thoracic spine as a compression fracture.

◈ Weight-bearing exercise, calcium and vitamin D supplementation, and estrogen replacement therapy are the important cornerstones in the prevention of osteoporosis.

◈ Progestin should be added to estrogen replacement therapy when a woman has her uterus, to prevent endometrial cancer.

◈ Continuous estrogen-progestin therapy may be associated with a small but significant risk of cardiovascular disease and breast cancer.

REFERENCES

Wren BG. Menopause. In: Hacker NF and Moore JG, eds. Essentials of obstetrics and gynecology, 3rd ed. Philadelphia: Saunders. 1998:602–607.

Mishell DR. Menopause. In: Stenchever MA, Droegemueller W, Herbst AL, Mishell DR, eds. Comprehensive gynecology, 4th ed. St. Louis: Mosby-Year Book. 2001:1217–1258.

American College of Obstetricians and Gynecologists. Bone density screening for osteoporosis. ACOG Committee Opinion 270. Washington, DC: 2002.

Writing Group for the Women's Health Initiative Investigators. Risks and benefits of estrogen plus progestin in healthy postmenopausal women. JAMA 2002;288(3):321–333.

A 28-year-old woman is brought into the emergency room with a blood pressure of 60/40. The patient's husband states that she had 2 days of nausea and vomiting, fever to 102°F, and myalgias. On examination, the patient appears lethargic and has mental confusion. Her skin has a sunburn-like rash diffusely. Auscultation of her heart reveals tachycardia. The lung examination demonstrates slight crackles at the lung bases. The abdomen is slightly tender throughout without any discernible masses. The uterus is nontender and the adnexa are normal to palpation. The laboratory evaluation reveals a hemoglobin level of 15 g/dL and a serum creatinine of 2.1 mg/dL.

◆ **What is the most likely diagnosis?**

◆ **What is the next step in therapy?**

ANSWERS TO CASE 5: Toxic Shock Syndrome

Summary: A 28-year-old woman has fever to 102°F, myalgias, vomiting, hypotension, confusion, and a sunburn-like rash. She has evidence of hemoconcentration and renal insufficiency.

◆ **Most likely diagnosis:** Toxic shock syndrome.

◆ **Next step in therapy:** Isotonic intravenous fluids, intravenous nafcillin, monitor urine output and blood pressure, and support blood pressure with dopamine if needed.

Analysis

Objectives

1. Recognize the manifestations of shock.
2. Understand that *Staphylococcus aureus,* acting through an exotoxin, causes toxic shock syndrome (TSS).
3. Understand that aggressive fluid resuscitation and intravenous nafcillin (or vancomycin) are fundamental in the treatment of TSS.

Considerations

The most significant issue for this patient is the hypotension, since her blood pressure is 60/40. Her mean arterial pressure is 47 mm Hg, which is insufficient to maintain cerebral perfusion. **Regardless of the etiology, the blood pressure needs to be supported immediately.** Because the patient has a fever of 102°F with the hypotension, and no history of hemorrhage or pregnancy (ectopic), septic shock is the most likely diagnosis. **The first step in resuscitation should therefore be addressed at supporting the blood pressure, with aggressive use of intravenous isotonic fluids.** A Foley catheter measuring urine output can help to assess urine output and indirectly kidney perfusion, particularly since the patient has an elevated serum creatinine level. The goal is to keep the mean arterial blood pressure at least 65 mm Hg to perfuse her vital organs. Ideally, this patient would have a urine output of at least 25 to 30 mL per hr (depending on the degree of renal insufficiency). Furthermore, this woman most likely has toxic shock syndrome (TSS) since she has myalgias, fever, nausea and vomiting, and **sunburn-like rash.** Desquamation of the skin would be even more typical for TSS.

APPROACH TO TOXIC SHOCK SYNDROME

Definitions

Toxic shock syndrome (TSS): an acute febrile illness usually caused by the exotoxin of *Staphylococcus aureus* that leads to multiorgan dysfunction.

Shock: Condition of circulatory insufficiency where tissue perfusion needs are not met.

Septic shock: Circulatory insufficiency due to infection or the body's response to infection, commonly caused by gram-negative endotoxins.

Mean arterial pressure (MAP) = [(2 × Diastolic blood pressure) + (1 × Systolic blood pressure)]/3

Pathophysiology

Toxic shock syndrome (TSS) was first described by Todd in 1978 in children who died due to *S. aureus* infections. Since the 1980s, 95% of patients with TSS were young healthy, menstruating women, with *S. aureus* isolated in the vast majority of cases. **The use of barrier contraceptives and tampons are predisposing factors.** The TSS exotoxin-1 leads to the syndrome possibly due to tumor necrosis factors and interleukins and other cytokines. The *S. aureus* organisms are in the vagina, and the exotoxins enter the circulation through microulcerations of the vagina. Most women experience a flu-like illness, fever, rash, sore throat, vomiting, and diarrhea. **The skin changes are most characteristic: the intense sunburn-like rash develops during the**

first 48 hr, and after several days becomes maculopapular, similar to a drug-related rash. After 10 days, the rash typically **desquamates** including involvement of the palms and soles.

The management of TSS includes copious intravenous fluids with close monitoring of urine output and blood pressure. At times, invasive hemodynamic monitoring with a central venous catheter or Swan-Ganz line is needed. **Intravenous nafcillin or methicillin is usually the best antibiotic therapy; when the diagnosis is unclear, an aminoglycoside agent is often added for gram-negative coverage.** Dopamine or dobutamine are sometimes required when fluids alone are insufficient to maintain the blood pressure. Rarely, a toxic shock–like picture may be caused by other organisms such as group A beta-hemolytic streptococcus.

Comprehension Questions

[5.1] Each of the following statements about toxic shock syndrome (TSS) is true except:

   A. The symptoms are largely caused by an exotoxin.
   B. Intravenous nafcillin is the initial antibiotic of choice.
   C. Tampon use is a predisposing factor.
   D. *S. aureus* is typically cultured from the blood.
   E. The vagina is a common site of infection.

[5.2] Which of the following describes the usual sequence of skin changes in TSS?

   A. Sunburn rash to desquamation to maculopapular rash
   B. Maculopapular rash to sunburn rash to desquamation
   C. Sunburn rash to maculopapular rash to desquamation
   D. Hypotension to sunburn rash

[5.3] Each of the following is a typical manifestation of TSS except:

   A. Hypotension
   B. Elevated serum creatinine

C. Elevated serum bilirubin level
D. Elevated serum liver function test
E. Thrombophilia

[5.4] Each of the following is a fundamental principle for the treatment of septic shock except:

A. Remove the nidus of infection
B. Plasmaphoresis
C. Fluid resuscitation
D. Support the blood pressure

Answers

[5.1] **D.** The *S. aureus* organism is usually isolated from the vagina and not from the blood, since its effects are mediated by the exotoxins. The most common location of the organisms is the vagina, and often there is vaginal erythema present.

[5.2] **C.** The typical sequence of changes in skin lesions of toxic shock syndrome are sunburn-like rash to maculopapular rash to desquamation.

[5.3] **E.** Usually, TSS causes thrombocytopenia rather than thrombophilia (elevated platelet count). Dysfunction of the kidneys or liver is also common.

[5.4] **B.** Plasmaphoresis is not a major part of the treatment of septic shock.

CLINICAL PEARLS

◈ The initial treatment of septic shock includes aggressive intravenous fluids and antibiotic therapy.

◈ The sunburn-like rash and/or desquamation is typical for *Staphylococcal aureus* infections.

◈ The initial antibiotic therapy for serious *S. aureus* infections is generally intravenous nafcillin or methicillin unless methicillin resistance is suspected, in which case vancomycin is used.

REFERENCES

Lebherz TB. Infectious and benign diseases of the vagina, cervix, and vulva. In: Hacker NF and Moore JG, eds. Essentials of obstetrics and gynecology, 3rd ed. Philadelphia: Saunders. 1998:400.

Droegemueller W. Infections of the lower genital tract. In: Stenchever MA, Droegemueller W, Herbst AL, Mishell DR, eds. Comprehensive gynecology, 4th ed. St. Louis: Mosby-Year Book. 2001:641–705.

Cunningham FG, Gant NF, Leveno KJ, Gilstrap LC III, Hauth JC, Wenstrom KD. Puerperal infection. In: Williams obstetrics, 21st ed. New York: McGraw-Hill. 2001:671–688.

A 26-year-old G1 P0 woman at 39 weeks' gestation is admitted in labor. She is noted to have uterine contractions every 7 to 10 min. Her antepartum history is significant for a nonimmune rubella status. On examination, her BP is 110/70 and heart rate (HR) is 80/minute. The estimated fetal weight is 7 lb. On pelvic examination, she has been noted to have a change in cervical examinations from 4-cm dilation to 7-cm over the last 2 hr. The pelvis is assessed to be adequate on digital examination.

◆ **What is your next step in the management of this patient?**

ANSWERS TO CASE 6: Labor (Normal Active Phase)

Summary: A 26-year-old G1 P0 woman at term with an adequate pelvis on clinical pelvimetry, nonimmune rubella status, is in labor. Her cervix has changed from 4-cm to 7-cm dilation over 2 hr with uterine contractions noted every 7 to 10 min.

◆ **Next step in management:** Continue to observe the labor.

Analysis

Objectives

1. Know the normal labor parameters in the latent and active phase for nulliparous and multiparous patients.
2. Be familiar with the management of common labor abnormalities and know that normal labor does not require intervention.
3. Know that rubella vaccination, as a live-attenuated preparation, should not be administered during pregnancy.

Considerations

This 29-year-old G1 P0 woman is at term (defined as between 37 to 42 completed weeks from the last menstrual period). She is in the active phase of labor (generally ≥ 4 cm of dilation) and her cervix has changed from 4 cm to 7 cm over 2 hr; her contractions are only every 7 to 10 min. Because she is nulliparous, the expectation is that her cervix will dilate at a rate of at least 1.2 cm per hr during the active phase of labor. She has met these norms by a change of 1.5 cm/hr (3 cm over 2 hr). The uterine contraction pattern appears suboptimal, but it is the change in the cervix per time and *not* the uterine contraction pattern that dictates normalcy in labor. **Because she has had a normal labor, the appropriate management is to observe her course without intervention.** The clinical pelvimetry is accomplished by digital palpation of the pelvic bones. This patient's pelvis was judged to be adequate. Unfortunately, this estimation is not very precise, and in clinical practice, the clinician would generally observe the labor of a nulliparous patient. Finally, the nonimmune rubella status should alert the practitioner to immunize for rubella during the postpartum time (since the rubella vaccine is live-attenuated and is contraindicated during pregnancy).

APPROACH TO LABOR EVALUATION

Definitions

Labor: Cervical change accompanied by regular uterine contractions.

Latent phase: The initial part of labor where the cervix mainly effaces (thins) rather than dilates (usually cervical dilation less than 4 cm).

Active phase: The portion of labor where dilation occurs more rapidly, usually when the cervix is greater than 4-cm dilation.

Protraction of active phase: Cervical dilation in the active phase that is less than expected (normal ≥ 1.2 cm/hr for a nulliparous woman, and ≥ 1.5 cm/hr for a woman who has had at least one vaginal delivery).

Arrest of active phase: No progress in the active phase of labor for 2 hr.

Stages of labor: First stage: onset of labor to complete dilation of cervix. Second stage: complete cervical dilation to delivery of infant. Third stage: delivery of infant to delivery of placenta.

Clinical Approach to Labor

The assessment of labor is based on cervical change versus time (Table 6–1). Normal labor should be expectantly managed. **When a labor abnormality is diagnosed, then the 3 Ps should be evaluated (powers, passenger, pelvis).** When inadequate "powers" are thought to be the etiology, then oxytocin may be initiated to augment the uterine contraction strength and/or frequency. When the latent phase exceeds the upper limits of normal, then it is called a **prolonged latent phase.** When the cervix has exceeded 4 to 5 cm, particularly with near-

Table 6–1

NORMAL LABOR PARAMETERS

	NULLIPARA (LOWER LIMITS OF NORMAL)	MULTIPARA (LOWER LIMITS OF NORMAL)
Latent phase (less than 4 cm dilation)	≤ 18–20 hr	≤ 14 hr
Active phase	≥ 1.2 cm/hr	≥ 1.5 cm/hr
Second stage of labor (complete dilation to expulsion of infant)	≤ 2 hr ≤ 3 hr if epidural	≤ 1 hr ≤ 2 hr if epidural
Third stage of labor	≤ 30 min	≤ 30 min

Adapted from Friedman EA. Labor: evaluation and management, 2nd ed. East Norwalk, CT: Appleton-Century-Crofts; 1978.

complete effacement, then the active phase has been reached. When there is cervical dilation but less than the minimum expected change, then this is called **protraction of active phase.** When the cervix does not dilate for 2 hr in the active phase, then it is called **arrest of active phase.**

When there is cephalopelvic disproportion, where the pelvis is too small for the fetus (either due to an abnormal pelvis or an excessively large baby), then cesarean delivery must be considered. When the "powers" are thought to be the factor, then intravenous oxytocin may be initiated via a dilute titration. **Clinically adequate uterine contractions are defined as contractions every 2 to 3 min, firm on palpation, and lasting for at least 40 to 60 sec** (Figure 6–1). Some clinicians choose to use internal uterine catheters to evaluate the adequacy of the powers. One common assessment tool is to examine a 10-min window and add each contraction's rise above baseline (each mm Hg rise is called a Montevideo unit). A calculation that meets or exceeds **200 Montevideo units** is commonly accepted as an adequate uterine contraction pattern (Figure 6–2).

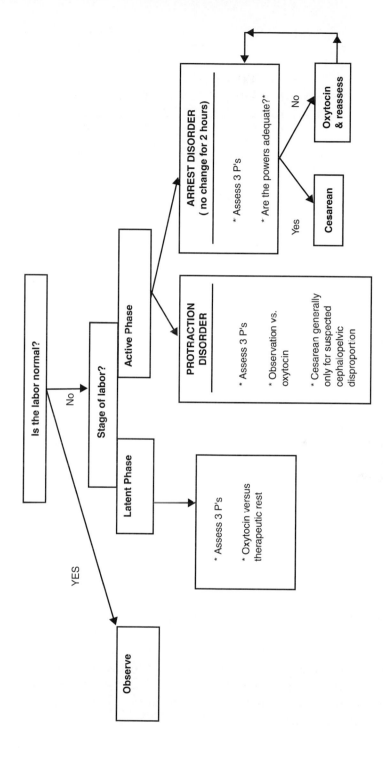

Figure 6–1. Algorithm for the management of labor.

* Adequate contractions generally > 200 Montevideo units or clinically contractions q 2-3 minutes, firm, lasting 40-60 seconds

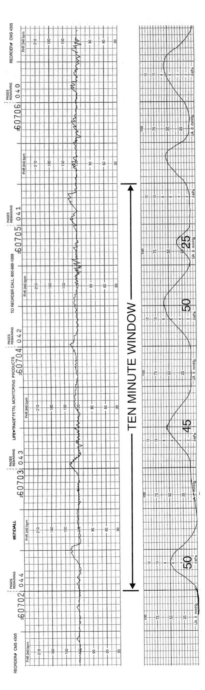

Figure 6–2. Calculating Montevideo units. The Montevideo units are calculated by the sum of the amplitudes (in mm Hg) above baseline of the uterine contractions within a 10-min window.

Comprehension Questions

[6.1] A 31-year old G2 P1 woman at 39 weeks' gestation complains of painful uterine contractions that are occurring every 3 to 4 min. She has only changed her cervix from 1-cm dilation to 2-cm dilation over 3 hr. Which one of the following management plans is most appropriate?

   A. Cesarean delivery
   B. Intravenous oxytocin
   C. Observation
   D. Fetal scalp pH monitoring
   E. Intranasal gonadotropin therapy

[6.2] A 26-year-old G2 P1 woman at 41 weeks' gestation has been pushing for 3 hr without progress. Throughout this time, her vaginal examination has remained completely dilated, completely effaced, and 0 station, with the head persistently in the occiput posterior (OP) position. Each of the following statements accurately describes the situation except:

   A. The occiput posterior position is frequently associated with an anthropoid pelvis.
   B. The labor progress is abnormal if the patient does not have an epidural catheter for analgesia, but is still within normal limits if epidural analgesia is being used.
   C. The patient is best described as having an arrest of descent.
   D. The bony part of the fetal head is likely to be at the plane of the ischial spines.

[6.3] A 31-year-old G2 P1 woman at 40 weeks' gestation has pro-
gressed in labor from 5-cm to 6-cm cervical dilation over 2 hr.
Which of the following best describes the labor?

A. Prolonged latent phase
B. Prolonged active phase
C. Arrest of active phase
D. Protracted active phase
E. Normal labor

[6.4] A 24-year-old G2 P1 woman at 39 weeks' gestation presents with
painful uterine contractions. She also complains of dark, vaginal
blood mixed with some mucus. Which of the following describes
the most likely etiology of her bleeding?

A. Placenta previa
B. Placenta abruption
C. Bloody show
D. Vasa previa
E. Cervical laceration

Answers

[6.1] **C.** Patient is still in the (normal) latent phase, upper limit is 14 hr.
Fetal scalp pH monitoring is a method of obtaining a small
amount of capillary blood from the fetal scalp to assess for fetal
acidemia.

[6.2] **B.** A 3-hr second stage of labor is still abnormal, even with
epidural analgesia. An anthropoid pelvis, which predisposes to
the persistent fetal occiput-posterior position, is characterized by
a pelvis with an anterior-posterior diameter greater than the transverse diameter with prominent ischial spines and a narrow anterior segment.

[6.3] **D.** Protracted active phase means some progress but less than expected (1.5 cm/hr) in the active phase of labor.

[6.4] **C.** Bloody show or loss of the cervical mucus plug is often a sign of impending labor. The sticky mucus admixed with blood can differentiate bloody show from antepartum bleeding.

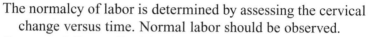

CLINICAL PEARLS

The normalcy of labor is determined by assessing the cervical change versus time. Normal labor should be observed.

Cesarean delivery (for labor abnormalities) in the absence of clear cephalopelvic disproportion is generally reserved for arrest of active phase with adequate uterine contractions.

Adequate uterine contractions is not a precise definition, but is commonly judged as greater than 200 Montevideo units with an internal uterine pressure catheter, or by uterine contractions every 2 to 3 min, firm on palpation, and lasting at least 40 to 60 sec.

In general, latent labor occurs when the cervix is less than 4-cm dilated, and active labor when the cervix is greater than 4-cm dilated.

REFERENCES

Cunningham FG, Gant NF, Leveno KJ, Gilstrap LC III, Hauth JC, Wenstrom KD. Dystocia: abnormal labor and fetopelvic disproportion. In: Williams obstetrics, 21st ed. New York: McGraw-Hill. 2001:425–450.

Ross MF and Hobel CJ. Normal labor, delivery, and the puerperium. In: Hacker NF and Moore JG, eds. Essentials of obstetrics and gynecology, 3rd ed. Philadelphia: Saunders. 1998:150–159.

An 18-year-old G1 P0 woman, who is pregnant at 7 weeks' gestation by last menstrual period, complains of a 2-day history of vaginal spotting and lower abdominal pain. She denies a history of sexually transmitted diseases. On examination, her BP is 130/60 and HR 70 beats per min, and temperature is 99°F. Her neck is supple and the heart examination is normal. The lungs are clear bilaterally. The abdomen is nontender and no masses are palpated. On pelvic examination, the uterus is 4-week size and nontender. There are no adnexal masses on pelvic examination. The quantitative beta-hCG level is 700 mIU/mL (Third International Standard) and a transvaginal ultrasound reveals an empty uterus and no adnexal masses.

◆ **What is your next step in the management of this patient?**

ANSWERS TO CASE 7: Threatened Abortion

Summary: An 18-year-old woman at 7 weeks' gestation by LMP complains of a 2-day history of vaginal spotting and lower abdomen pain. The physical examination reveals a 4-week sized uterus and unremarkable adnexa. The beta-hCG level is 700 mIU/mL and no intrauterine gestational sac is noted on endovaginal sonography.

◆ **Next step in management:** Follow up beta-hCG in 48 hr.

Analysis

Objectives

1. Understand the concept of the hCG discriminatory zone or threshold, and its utility with transvaginal sonography.
2. Understand the principle of obtaining a follow-up hCG level when a patient is asymptomatic and has an hCG level that is below the discriminatory zone.
3. Know that a normal ultrasound examination does not rule out the presence of an ectopic pregnancy.

Considerations

This 18-year-old woman complains of lower abdominal pain and vaginal spotting, which in a woman of childbearing potential **should be considered an ectopic pregnancy until otherwise proven.** She does not have a history of sexually transmitted diseases, which if present would be a risk factor for an ectopic pregnancy. The physical examination is unremarkable and ultrasound does not show any adnexal masses. Significantly, the hCG level is below the threshold whereby transvaginal sonography should reveal an intrauterine pregnancy (hCG threshold of 1500 to 2000 mIU/mL). Thus, the goal is to establish whether this pregnancy is a normal intrauterine gestation or an abnormal pregnancy. This may be accomplished by following serial hCG levels. After 48 hr, if the follow-up hCG level rises by at least 66%, then the patient most likely has a normal intrauterine pregnancy. If the follow-up hCG does not rise by 66% (particularly if it rises by only 20%), then she most likely has an abnormal pregnancy. The subnormal rise in hCG does not indicate whether the abnormal pregnancy is in the uterus or the tube. Notably, the gestational age based on last menstrual period is not very reliable. **Thus, the hCG levels and transvaginal ultrasound are generally the best tools for evaluating a possible ectopic pregnancy.**

APPROACH TO THREATENED ABORTION

Definitions

Threatened abortion: Pregnancy with vaginal spotting during the first half of pregnancy. This does not delineate the viability of the pregnancy.

Ectopic pregnancy: Pregnancy outside of the normal uterine implantation site. Most of the time, this means a pregnancy in the fallopian tube.

Human chorionic gonadotropin: "The pregnancy hormone," which is a glycoprotein that is secreted by the chorionic villi of a pregnancy. It is the hormone on which pregnancy tests are based. The normal pregnancy will have a logarithmic rise in early pregnancy. Usually the beta-subunit is assayed to prevent cross-reactivity with LH.

HCG threshold: Level of serum hCG such that an intrauterine pregnancy should be seen on ultrasound. For endovaginal sonography, this level is 1500 to 2000 mIU/mL. When an intrauterine pregnancy is not seen on sonography *and* the hCG level exceeds the threshold, then it is highly probable that an ectopic pregnancy is present.

Clinical Approach

The possibility of ectopic pregnancy must be considered when assessing a pregnant woman with vaginal spotting and/or lower abdominal pain. It is of paramount importance to determine if the woman is hypotensive, volume depleted, or has severe abdominal or adnexal pain. These patients will most likely need laparoscopy or laparotomy since

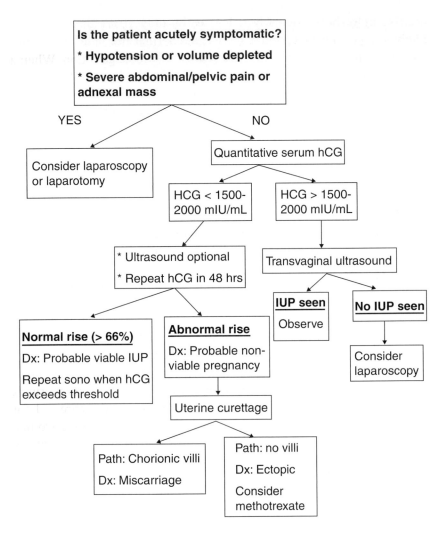

Figure 7–1.   Algorithm for the management of suspected ectopic pregnancy.

ectopic pregnancy is probable. For asymptomatic women, the quantitative human chorionic gonadotropin (hCG) level is useful. When the hCG level is below the threshold for sonographic visualization of an intrauterine gestational sac, then a repeat hCG level is generally performed in 48 hr to establish the viability of the pregnancy. Another option would be a single progesterone level: levels greater than 25 ng/mL almost always indicate a normal intrauterine gestation, whereas values less than 5 ng/mL usually correlate with a nonviable gestation. When a nonviable pregnancy is diagnosed either by an abnormal hCG rise or a single progesterone assay (< 5ng/mL), it is still unclear whether the patient has a spontaneous abortion or an ectopic pregnancy. Many clinicians will perform a uterine curettage at this time to assess whether the patient has a miscarriage (histologic confirmation of chorionic villi) or an ectopic pregnancy (no villi from the curettage). Women with asymptomatic, small (< 3.5 cm) ectopic pregnancies are ideal candidates for intramuscular methotrexate.

When the hCG level is greater than the ultrasound threshold, then a transvaginal sonogram will dictate the next step. A patient in whom an intrauterine gestational sac is seen may be sent home with a diagnosis of threatened abortion and should have close follow-up. There is still a significant risk of miscarriage. **When the hCG level is above the threshold, and there is no sonographic evidence of intrauterine pregnancy, the risk of ectopic pregnancy is high** (about 85%), and thus laparoscopy is often undertaken to diagnose and treat the ectopic pregnancy. Because an intrauterine gestation is possible in this circumstance (about 15% of the time), methotrexate is usually not given; however, a high hCG level in the face of a sonographically empty uterus is almost always caused by an extrauterine gestation. (See Figure 7–1 for one example of a management scheme). Finally, Rh-negative women with threatened abortion, spontaneous abortion, or ectopic pregnancy should receive Rhogam to prevent isoimmunization.

Comprehension Questions

[7.1] Each of the following is a risk factor for the development of an ectopic pregnancy except:

A. Prior chlamydial cervical infection
B. History of a tubal ligation and currently pregnant
C. Prior ectopic pregnancy
D. Infertility
E. Combination oral contraceptive pill use

[7.2] A 32-year-old woman is diagnosed with an ectopic pregnancy based on hCG levels that have plateaued in the range of 1400 mIU/mL and no chorionic villi found on uterine curettage. She is given 50 mg/m^2 of methotrexate intramuscularly. Five days later, she complains of increased lower abdominal pain. Her blood pressure and heart rate are normal. Her abdomen shows some tenderness in the lower quadrants without guarding or rebound. Which of the following is the best course of action?

A. Immediate laparotomy
B. Repeat dose of methotrexate
C. Observation
D. Folic acid rescue
E. Epidural analgesia

[7.3] An 18-year-old woman who is brought to the emergency room complains of vaginal spotting and lower abdominal pain. Her abdominal and pelvic examinations are normal. The hCG level is 700 mIU/mL and transvaginal sonogram shows no intrauterine gestational sac and no adnexal masses. Which of the following statements is most accurate regarding this patient's situation?

A. She has an unruptured ectopic pregnancy.
B. She has a viable intrauterine pregnancy that is too early to assess on ultrasound.
C. She has a nonviable intrauterine pregnancy.
D. There is insufficient information to draw a conclusion about the viability of this pregnancy.
E. An MRI scan would be useful in further assessing the possibility of an ectopic pregnancy.

[7.4] A 22-year-old woman who is pregnant at 5 weeks' gestation complains of severe lower abdominal pain. On examination, she is noted to have a blood pressure of 86/44 and heart rate of 120 bpm. Her abdomen is tender. The pelvic examination is difficult to perform due to guarding. The hCG level is 500 mIU/mL and the transvaginal sonogram reveals no intrauterine gestational sac and no adnexal masses. There is some free fluid in the cul-de-sac. Which of the following is the best management for this patient?

A. Repeat hCG level in 48 hr to assess for a rise of 66%
B. Check the serum progesterone level
C. Immediate surgery
D. Intramuscular methotrexate
E. Repeat sonography in 48 hr

Answers

[7.1] **E.** The use of combination oral contraceptives tends to prevent all pregnancies, both ectopic and intrauterine, and is not a risk factor. A history of a tubal ligation by itself does not increase the risk of ectopic pregnancy. However, if a woman has had a tubal ligation and then becomes pregnant, then there is a significant risk of tubal pregnancy. Prior ectopic pregnancy greatly increases the risk of future ectopic pregnancy.

[7.2] **C.** Many women treated with methotrexate will have mild abdominal pain, and may be observed in the absence of severe peritoneal signs, hypotension, or overt signs of rupture.

[7.3] **D.** There is insufficient information in this scenario to establish viability of the pregnancy. A repeat hCG in 48 hr may be able to assess the state of the pregnancy.

[7.4] **C.** Surgery is indicated since this patient is hypotensive and tachycardic, and likely has a ruptured ectopic pregnancy.

CLINICAL PEARLS

 When the hCG level is above the threshold and no intrauterine pregnancy is seen on transvaginal ultrasound, the patient most likely has an ectopic pregnancy.

 Early in the course of a normal intrauterine pregnancy, the beta-hCG should rise by at least 66% over 48 hr.

 The presence of a true intrauterine gestational sac on ultrasound makes the risk of ectopic pregnancy very unlikely.

Surgery is usually the best therapy in a patient with an early pregnancy who is hypotensive or has severe adnexal pain.

REFERENCES

Palmieri A, Moore JG, DeCherney AH. Ectopic pregnancy. In: Hacker NF and Moore JG, eds. Essentials of obstetrics and gynecology, 3rd ed. Philadelphia: Saunders. 1998:487–498.

Mishell DR. Ectopic pregnancy. In: Stenchever MA, Droegemueller W, Herbst AL, Mishell DR, eds. Comprehensive gynecology, 4th ed. St. Louis: Mosby-Year Book. 2001:443–478.

CASE 8

A 35-year-old G5 P4 woman at 39 weeks' gestation is undergoing a vaginal delivery. She had a history of a previous myomectomy and one prior low transverse cesarean delivery. The delivery of the baby is uneventful. The placenta does not deliver after 30 min, and a manual extraction of the placenta is undertaken. The placenta seems to be firmly adherent to the uterus.

◆ **What is the most likely diagnosis?**

◆ **What is your next step in management for this patient?**

ANSWERS TO CASE 8: Placenta Accreta

Summary: A 35-year-old G5 P4 woman at term with a prior history of a myomectomy and cesarean delivery is undergoing a vaginal delivery. The retained placenta is firmly adherent to the uterus when there is an attempt at manual extraction.

◆ **Most likely diagnosis:** Placenta accreta.

◆ **Next step in management for this patient:** Hysterectomy.

Analysis

Objectives

1. Know the risk factors for and the clinical diagnosis of placenta accreta.
2. Understand that hysterectomy is usually the best treatment for placenta accreta.

Considerations

This patient has had two previous uterine incisions, which increases the risk of placenta accreta. **The placenta is noted to be very adherent to the uterus, which is the clinical definition of placenta accreta, although the histologic diagnosis requires a defect of the decidua basalis layer.** The usual management of true placental accreta is **hysterectomy** since attempts to remove a firmly attached placenta often lead to hemorrhage and/or maternal death. Conservative management of placenta accreta, such as removal of as much placenta as possible and packing the uterus, often leads to excess mortality as compared to immediate hysterectomy.

APPROACH TO PLACENTA ACCRETA

Definitions

Placenta accreta: Abnormal adherence of the placenta to the uterine wall due to an abnormality of the decidua basalis layer of the uterus. The placental villi are attached to the myometrium.
Placenta increta: The abnormally implanted placenta penetrates into the myometrium.
Placenta percreta: The abnormally implanted placenta penetrates entirely through the myometrium to the serosa.

Clinical Approach

Risk factors for placental adherence include low-lying placentation or placenta previa, prior cesarean delivery or uterine curettage, or prior myomectomy. Antepartum bleeding may occur. With complete placenta accreta, there may be no bleeding and only a retained placenta. Undue traction on the cord may lead to uterine inversion. With a retained placenta, clinicians will usually attempt a manual extraction of the placenta, in an effort to find a cleavage plane between the placenta and the uterus. With placenta accreta, no cleavage plane is found. **Hysterectomy is usually the best choice in this circumstance.** Because the placenta is so firmly adherent, attempts to conserve the uterus, such as curettage of the placenta or removing the placenta "piecemeal," are often unsuccessful, and may lead to hemorrhage and exsanguination.

Placenta accreta should be suspected in circumstances of placenta previa, particularly with a history of a prior cesarean delivery (Table 8–1). The greater the number of prior cesareans in the face of current placenta previa, the higher the risk of accreta. For example, a woman with **three or more prior cesarean deliveries and a low-lying anterior placenta suggestive of partial previa or a known placenta previa has up to a 40% to 50% chance of having placenta accreta!** Some practitioners advise performing ultrasound examinations to assess the placental location in those women who have had a prior cesarean delivery. When the placenta is anterior or low-lying in position,

Table 8–1

RISK FACTORS FOR PLACENTA ACCRETA

Placenta previa
Implantation over the lower uterine segment
Prior cesarean scar or other uterine scar
Uterine curettage
Down syndrome

there is a greater risk of accreta. One caution is that a low-lying placenta or placenta previa diagnosed in the second trimester may resolve
in the third trimester, as the lower uterine segment grows more rapidly,
a phenomenon known as "transmigration of the placenta."

Comprehension Questions

Match the single most likely placental abnormality described (A–E) to
the clinical situation (8.1–8.3).

    A. Placenta accreta
    B. Placenta increta
    C. Placenta percreta
    D. Placenta polyp
    E. Placental hemangioma

[8.1] A 33-year-old G5 P4 woman at 38 weeks' gestation has had three
       prior cesarean deliveries and is currently suspected of having a
       placenta previa.

[8.2] A 25-year-old woman at 34 weeks' gestation is noted to have a
       placenta previa. Upon cesarean section, bluish tissue densely ad-
       herent between the uterus and maternal bladder is noted.

[8.3] When the placenta of a certain patient is sent for histologic analy-
       sis, the pathologist states that there is a defective decidua basalis

layer where the placenta villi abut against the myometrium of the uterus.

[8.4] A 32-year-old woman undergoes myomectomy for symptomatic uterine fibroids, all of which are subserosal. The endometrial cavity was not entered during the procedure. Which of the following statements is most likely to be correct regarding the risk of placental accreta?

A. Her risk of accreta is most likely to be increased due to the myomectomy.
B. Her risk of accreta is most likely to be decreased due to the myomectomy.
C. Her risk of accreta is most likely not affected by the myomectomy.
D. If the myomectomy incisions are anterior, then she has an increased risk of a placental polyp.

Answers

[8.1] **A.** Although the risks of placental accreta, increta, or percreta are all increased, placenta accreta is more common than either increta or percreta.

[8.2] **C.** The blue tissue densely adherent between the uterus and bladder is very characteristic of a percreta, where the placenta penetrates entirely through the myometrium to the serosa and adheres to the bladder.

[8.3] **A.** Placenta abutting against myometrium is placenta accreta; villi into myometrium would be increta; villi penetrating through myometrium to serosa would be percreta.

[8.4] **C.** In general, myomectomy incisions on the serosal (outside) surface of the uterus do not predispose to accreta, since the endometrium is not disturbed.

CLINICAL PEARLS

The usual management of placenta accreta (abnormal adherence of the placenta to the uterus) is hysterectomy.

Placenta previa is associated with a defect in the decidua basalis.

The risk of placenta accreta increases in a woman with a prior uterine incision and placenta previa. The greater the number of cesareans, the higher the risk of accreta.

Low-lying or marginal placenta previa diagnosed in the second trimester will often resolve later in pregnancy, so repeat sonography is prudent.

REFERENCES

Cunningham FG, Gant NF, Leveno KJ, Gilstrap LC III, Hauth JC, Wenstrom KD. Obstetrical hemorrhage. In: Williams obstetrics, 21st ed. New York: McGraw-Hill. 2001;619–670.

Hayashi RH. Postpartum hemorrhage and puerperal sepsis. In: Hacker NF and Moore JG, eds. Essentials of obstetrics and gynecology, 3rd ed. Philadelphia: Saunders. 1998:334.

Placenta Accreta. ACOG Committee Opinion 266. January 2002.

A 22-year-old nulliparous woman complains of a 2-week history of vaginal discharge and vaginal spotting after intercourse. She denies a history of sexually transmitted diseases and currently does not use any contraceptive agents. Her past medical history is unremarkable. Her last menstrual period began 1 week ago and was normal. On examination, her BP is 100/60, HR 80/min, and temperature is 99°F. The heart and lung examinations are normal. Her abdomen is nontender and without masses. Her pelvic examination shows purulent vaginal discharge, which on Gram's stain shows intracellular gram-negative diplococci. Her pregnancy test is negative.

◆ **What is the most likely diagnosis?**

◆ **What is the next step in therapy?**

◆ **What are the complications of this problem?**

ANSWERS TO CASE 9: Gonococcal Cervicitis

Summary: A 22-year-old nonpregnant nulliparous woman complains of a vaginal discharge and postcoital spotting. A purulent vaginal discharge on Gram's stain shows intracellular gram-negative diplococci.

◆ **Most likely diagnosis:** Gonococcal cervicitis.

◆ **Next step in therapy:** Intramuscular ceftriaxone for gonorrhea, and oral azithromycin (or doxycycline) for chlamydial infection.

◆ **Complications of this problem:** Salpingitis, which may lead to infertility or increased risk of ectopic pregnancy. Disseminated gonorrhea is also possible.

Analysis

Objectives

1. Know that gram-negative intracellular diplococci are highly suggestive of *Neisseria gonorrhoeae.*
2. Know the clinical presentation and treatment of gonococcal cervicitis.
3. Understand the complications of gonococcal cervicitis.

Considerations

This 22-year-old nulliparous woman complains of a vaginal discharge and postcoital spotting. The first disease that should be ruled out with abnormal vaginal bleeding is a pregnancy-related disorder, such as ectopic pregnancy or threatened abortion. In this case, the patient's pregnancy test is negative. The purulent vaginal discharge is found to be diagnostic of gonorrhea by Gram's stain. Because of gonorrhea's propensity to invade the endocervix, this woman almost certainly has at least cervicitis. Thus, the endocervix should be sampled for culture or

DNA probe. The next step is to assess the extent of the disease. This patient had no evidence of salpingitis (tubal infection) since she did not have adnexal tenderness. She did not complain of abdominal tenderness or heavy menses (uterine involvement), which would be more indicative of upper genital tract disease. Likewise, she has no joint complaints to indicate gonococcal arthritis, or painful skin lesions to suggest disseminated gonorrhea.

One common treatment for gonococcal cervicitis is ceftriaxone 125 to 250 mg intramuscularly. **Because *Chlamydia* often coexists with gonorrhea, therapy with azithromycin 1 g orally or doxycycline 100 mg twice daily for 7 to 10 days is also indicated.** The gonococcal organisms appear to be confined to the endocervix in this case, but complications can include ascension to the tubes causing infertility (tubal disease) or a development of ectopic pregnancy in the future.

APPROACH TO CERVICITIS

Definitions

Mucopurulent cervicitis: Yellow exudative discharge arising from the endocervix with 10 or more polymorphonucleocytes per high-power field on microscopy.
Lower genital tract: The vulva, vagina, and cervix.
Upper genital tract: The uterine corpus, fallopian tubes, and ovaries.

Clinical Approach

An infection of the cervix is analogous to an infection of the urethra in the male. Thus, sexually transmitted pathogens, **such as *Chlamydia trachomatis, Neisseria gonorrhoeae,* or herpes simplex virus,** may infect the cervix. Gonococcal and chlamydial organisms have a propensity for the columnar cells of the endocervix. Often, erythema of the endocervix is noted, leading to friability; these patients may complain of **postcoital spotting.** Mucopurulent cervical discharge is a common complaint, again analogous to the exudative urethral discharge of the

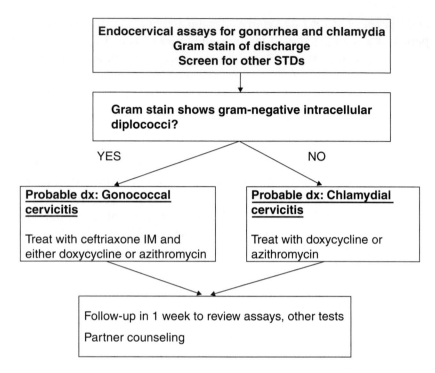

Figure 9–1.   Algorithm for the evaluation of mucopurulent cervical discharge.

male. **The most common organism implicated in mucopurulent cervical discharge is** *Chlamydia trachomatis,* **although gonorrhea may also be a pathogen.**

When a patient presents with this type of cervical discharge, Gram's stain may be done; if evidence of gonorrhea is present, that is, **intracellular gram-negative diplococci, then treatment should be directed toward gonococcal disease** (ceftriaxone 125 to 250 mg IM). Because of the **frequency of coexisting chlamydial infection,** azithromycin 1 g orally or doxycycline 100 mg orally BID for 7 to 10 days is also often given. If the Gram's stain of the cervical discharge is negative, then antimicrobial therapy directed at *Chlamydia* is warranted. Nevertheless, cultures or tests for both organisms should be performed. If the symptoms resolve, no follow-up cultures need to be done (see Figure 9–1 for one suggested management scheme). Finally, the patient and partner should be counseled and offered testing for other sexually transmitted organisms such as HIV, syphilis, and hepatitis B and C.

Gonococcal cervicitis may lead to more serious complications. The organism may ascend and infect the fallopian tubes, causing salpingitis. The **term pelvic inflammatory disease is usually synonymous with acute salpingitis.** The tubal infection in turn predisposes the patient to infertility and ectopic pregnancies due to tubal occlusion and/or adhesions. The gonococcal organism may lead to **an infectious arthritis, usually involving the large joints, and classically is migratory.** In fact, in the United States, gonorrhea is the most common cause of septic arthritis in young women. Disseminated gonorrhea can occur also; affected individuals will usually have eruptions of painful pustules with an erythematous base on the skin. The diagnosis is made by Gram's stain and culture of the pustules.

Comprehension Questions

[9.1]   An 18-year-old woman has a yellowish vaginal discharge. On examination, the cervix is erythematous and the discharge reveals numerous leukocytes. Which is the most likely etiology?

A. *Neisseria* gonorrhea
B. *Chlamydia trachomatis*
C. Ureaplasma species
D. Bacterial vaginosis

[9.2]   A 22-year-old woman, who uses a barrier method for contraception, complains of lower abdominal tenderness and dyspareunia. On laparoscopy, hyperemic fallopian tubes are noted. Which of the following is least likely to be an isolated pathogen in this process?

A. *Neisseria* gonorrhea
B. *Chlamydia trachomatis*
C. *Peptostreptococcus*
D. *Actinomyces* species

[9.3] A 34-year-old woman is diagnosed as having a vaginitis based on a "fishy odor" to her vaginal discharge and vaginal pruritus. The cervix is normal in appearance. Which of the following most likely corresponds to the etiology?

A. *Neisseria* gonorrhea
B. *Chlamydia trachomatis*
C. Both
D. Neither

[9.4] A 21-year-old college student has a sexually transmitted pharyngitis. Which of the following most likely corresponds to the etiology?

A. *Neisseria* gonorrhea
B. *Chlamydia trachomatis*
C. Both
D. Neither

[9.5] A 28-year-old woman has multiple painful pustules erupting throughout the skin of her body. Which of the following most likely corresponds to the etiology?

A. *Neisseria* gonorrhea
B. *Chlamydia trachomatis*
C. Both
D. Neither

[9.6] Which of the following maternal cervical infections causes blindness in the newborn?

A. *Neisseria* gonorrhea
B. *Chlamydia trachomatis*
C. Both
D. Neither

Answers

[9.1] **B.** Chlamydial cervicitis is the most common cause of mucopurulent cervical discharge.

[9.2] **D.** This patient has salpingitis; common organisms include *Gonorrhoeae, Chlamydia,* gram-negative rods, and anaerobes. *Actinomyces* is an organism associated with IUD use, but is not commonly encountered.

[9.3] **D.** Neither gonorrhea nor chlamydial infection typically cause vaginitis. This patient likely has bacterial vaginosis, based on the fishy odor.

[9.4] **A.** Gonococcal pharyngitis is diagnosed by swabbing the throat. *Chlamydia* are not a common cause of pharyngitis.

[9.5] **A.** Disseminated gonococcal disease will lead to multiple pustules on the skin. Chlamydial infection is not a common cause of a disseminated process.

[9.6] **C.** Both chlamydial infection and gonorrhea may cause conjunctivitis and blindness.

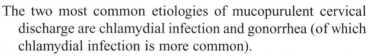

CLINICAL PEARLS

◈ The two most common etiologies of mucopurulent cervical discharge are chlamydial infection and gonorrhea (of which chlamydial infection is more common).

◈ Gram-negative intracellular diplococci are highly suggestive of *Neisseria gonorrhoeae.*

◈ *Chlamydia* often coexists with gonococcal cervicitis.

◈ Ceftriaxone treats gonorrhea, whereas doxycycline or azithromycin treat chlamydial infections.

REFERENCES

Droegemueller W. Infections of the lower genital tract. In: Stenchever MA, Droegemueller W, Herbst AL, Mishell DR, eds. Comprehensive gynecology, 4th ed.
St. Louis: Mosby-Year Book. 2001:641–706.

Lebherz TB. Infectious and benign diseases of the vagina, cervix, and vulva. In:
Hacker NF and Moore JG, eds. Essentials of obstetrics and gynecology, 3rd ed.
Philadelphia: Saunders. 1998:401.

A 35-year-old woman at 8 weeks' gestation complains of crampy lower abdominal pain and vaginal bleeding. She states that the pain was intense last night, and that something that looked like liver passed per vagina. After that, the pain subsided tremendously as did the vaginal bleeding. On examination, her BP is 130/80, HR 90/min, and temperature is 98°F. Her abdominal examination is unremarkable. The pelvic examination reveals normal external female genitalia. The cervix is closed and nontender, and no adnexal masses are appreciated.

◆ **What is the most likely diagnosis?**

◆ **What is the your next step in management?**

ANSWERS TO CASE 10: Completed Spontaneous Abortion

Summary: A 35-year-old woman at 8 weeks' gestational age had intense crampy lower abdominal pain and vaginal bleeding last night; after passing what looked like "liver," her pain and bleeding subsided tremendously. On examination, her cervix is closed.

◆ **Most likely diagnosis:** Completed abortion.

◆ **Next step in management:** Follow hCG levels to zero.

Analysis

Objectives

1. Know the typical characteristics of the different types of spontaneous abortions.
2. Understand the clinical presentations of and the treatments for the different types of abortions.

Considerations

This woman is pregnant at 8 weeks' gestation, which is in the first trimester. She noted intense cramping pain the night before and passed something that looked like liver to her. This may be tissue, although the gross appearance of presumed tissue can be misleading. The patient's pain and bleeding have subsided since the passage of the "liver." This fits with the complete expulsion of the pregnancy tissue. **The clinical picture of passage of tissue, resolution of cramping and bleeding, and a closed cervical os are consistent with a completed abortion.** To confirm that all of the pregnancy (trophoblastic) tissue has been expelled from the uterus, the clinician should follow serum quantitative hCG levels. It is expected that the hCG levels should halve every 48 to 72 hr. If the hCG levels plateau instead of falling, then the patient has residual pregnancy tissue (which may be either an incomplete abortion or an ectopic pregnancy). Notably, this patient is of advanced maternal age, and spontaneous abortions are more common in older patients. The most common cause identified with spontaneous abortion is a chromosomal abnormality of the embryo.

APPROACH TO SPONTANEOUS ABORTION

Definitions

Threatened abortion: A pregnancy less than 20 weeks' gestation associated with vaginal bleeding, generally without cervical dilation.

Inevitable abortion: A pregnancy less than 20 weeks' gestation associated with cramping, bleeding, and cervical dilation; there is no passage of tissue.

Incomplete abortion: A pregnancy less than 20 weeks' gestation associated with cramping, vaginal bleeding, an open cervical os, and some passage of tissue per vagina but also some retained tissue in utero. The **cervix remains open** due to the continued uterine contractions; the uterus continues to contract in an effort to expel the retained tissue.

Completed abortion: A pregnancy less than 20 weeks' gestation in which all the products of conception have passed; the **cervix is generally closed.** Because all the tissue has passed, the uterus no longer contracts, and the cervix closes.

Missed abortion: A pregnancy less than 20 weeks' gestation with embryonic or fetal demise but no symptoms such as bleeding or cramping.

Clinical Approach

The history, physical examination, and/or sonography usually point to the category of spontaneous abortion (Table 10–1). Women with threatened abortion should be instructed to bring in any passed tissue for histologic analysis.

Table 10-1

CLASSIFICATION OF SPONTANEOUS ABORTIONS

TERMINOLOGY	HISTORY	PASSAGE OF TISSUE?	CERVICAL OS	VIABILITY OF PREGNANCY?	TREATMENT
Threatened abortion	Vaginal bleeding	No	Closed	Uncertain; up to 50% will miscarry	Transvaginal ultrasound and hCG levels
Inevitable abortion	Cramping, bleeding	No	Open	Abortion is inevitable	D&C vs. expectant management
Incomplete abortion	Cramping, bleeding (still continuing)	Some but not all tissue passed	Open	Nonviable	D&C
Complete abortion	Cramping, bleeding previously now subsided	All tissue passed	Closed	Nonviable	Follow hCG levels to negative
Missed abortion	No symptoms	No	Closed	Nonviable (diagnosed on ultrasound)	D&C vs. expectant management

Note: An inevitable abortion must be differentiated from an incompetent cervix. With an inevitable abortion, the uterine contractions (cramping) lead to the cervical dilation. **With an incompetent cervix, the cervix opens spontaneously without uterine contractions and, therefore, affected women present with *painless* cervical dilation.** This disorder is treated with a **surgical ligature** at the level of the internal cervical os (cerclage). Hence, one of the main features used to distinguish between an incompetent cervix and an inevitable abortion is the presence or absence of uterine contractions.

The treatment of an incomplete abortion, characterized by the passage of tissue and an open cervical os, is dilatation and curettage of the uterus. The primary complications of persistently retained tissue are bleeding and infection. A completed abortion is suspected by the history of having passed tissue and experiencing cramping abdominal pain, now resolved. The cervix is closed. Serum hCG levels are still followed to confirm that no further chorionic villi are contained in the uterus.

Comprehension Questions

Match the single most likely diagnosis (A–F) with the clinical scenario (10.1–10.4).

   A. Threatened abortion
   B. Inevitable abortion
   C. Incomplete abortion
   D. Complete abortion
   E. Missed abortion
   F. None of the above

[10.1]   A 19-year-old G1 P0 woman at 14 weeks' gestation, who had a prior cervical conization procedure, states that she has had felt no abdominal cramping. She has a cervical dilation of 3 cm and effacement of 90%.

[10.2] A 33-year-old woman complains of vaginal bleeding and passage of a whitish substance along with something "meat-like." She continues to have cramping, and her cervix is 2 cm dilated.

[10.3] A 20-year-old G2 P1 woman at 12 weeks' gestation has had no problems with this pregnancy. No fetal heart tones are heard on Doppler, and an ultrasound reveals an embryo of 10-week size and no fetal cardiac activity.

[10.4] A 28-year-old G3 P2 woman at 22 weeks' gestation is noted to have vaginal spotting, and fetal heart tones are in the 140 to 145 bpm range.

Answers

[10.1] **F.** Incompetent cervix is the most likely diagnosis since she had painless dilation. Cervical conization is a risk factor.

[10.2] **C.** An open cervical os, a history of passing tissue, and continued cramping are consistent with an incomplete abortion.

[10.3] **E.** The patient had no symptoms, which is consistent with a missed abortion.

[10.4] **F.** This patient does not have an abortive process since she is 22 weeks' gestation; she has *antepartum bleeding.* Abortions are described as less than 20 weeks' gestation.

CLINICAL PEARLS

When a pregnant woman has an open cervical os with uterine cramping and history of passage of tissue, she usually has an incomplete abortion, best treated by uterine curettage.

The typical history of a completed abortion is resolution of cramping and vaginal bleeding following passage of tissue, and the finding of a small firm uterus and a closed cervical os.

The most common cause of a first trimester miscarriage is a fetal karyotypic abnormality.

Incompetent cervix, which is suspected with painless cervical dilation, is best treated with a cervical cerclage (stitch).

REFERENCES

Bennett MJ. Abortion. In: Hacker NF and Moore JG, eds. Essentials of obstetrics and gynecology, 3rd ed. Philadelphia: Saunders. 1998:477–486.

Mishell DR. Spontaneous and recurrent abortion. In: Stenchever MA, Droege-mueller W, Herbst AL, Mishell DR, eds. Comprehensive gynecology, 4th ed. St. Louis: Mosby-Year Book. 2001:413–442.

A 25-year-old G2 P1 woman is delivering at 42 weeks' gestation. She is moderately obese, but the fetus appears clinically to be of about 3700 g weight. After a 4-hr first stage of labor, and a 2-hr second stage of labor, the fetal head delivers but is noted to be retracted back toward the patient's introitus. The fetal shoulders do not deliver, even with maternal pushing.

◆ **What is your next step in management?**

◆ **What is a likely complication that can occur because of this situation?**

ANSWERS TO CASE 11: Shoulder Dystocia

Summary: A 25-year-old obese G2 P1 woman is delivering at 42 weeks' gestation; the fetus appears clinically to be 3700 g (average weight). After a 4-hr first stage of labor, and a 2-hr second stage of labor, the head delivers but the shoulders do not easily deliver.

◆ **Next step in management:** McRobert's maneuver (hyperflexion of the maternal hips onto the maternal abdomen and/or suprapubic pressure).

◆ **Likely complication:** A likely maternal complication is postpartum hemorrhage; a common neonatal complication is a brachial plexus injury such as an Erb's palsy.

Analysis

Objectives

1. Understand the risk factors for shoulder dystocia.
2. Understand that shoulder dystocia is an obstetric emergency, and be familiar with the initial maneuvers used to manage this condition.
3. Know the neonatal complications that can occur with shoulder dystocia.

Considerations

The patient is multiparous and obese, both of which are risk factors for shoulder dystocia. There is no indication of **gestational diabetes,** which would also be a significant risk factor. The patient is post-term at 42 weeks, which increases the likelihood of fetal macrosomia. The patient's prolonged second stage of labor (upper limits for a multiparous patient is 1 hr without and 2 hr with epidural analgesia) may be a nonspecific indicator of impending shoulder dystocia. Nevertheless, the diagnosis is straightforward in that the fetal shoulders are described as not easily delivering. The fetal head is retracted back toward the maternal introitus, the "turtle sign." Because most shoulder dystocia events are unpredictable, as in this case, the clinician must be proficient in the management of this entity, particularly because of the potential for fetal injury.

APPROACH TO SHOULDER DYSTOCIA

Definitions

Shoulder dystocia: Inability of the fetal shoulders to deliver spontaneously, usually due to the impaction of the anterior shoulder behind the maternal symphysis pubis.

McRobert's maneuver: The maternal thighs are sharply flexed against the maternal abdomen to straighten the sacrum relative to the lumbar spine and rotate the symphysis pubis anteriorly toward the maternal head (Figure 11–1).

Suprapubic pressure: The operator's hand is used to push on the suprapubic region in a downward or lateral direction in an effort to push the fetal shoulder into an oblique plane and from behind the symphysis pubis.

Erb's palsy: A brachial plexus injury involving the C5–6 nerve roots, which may result from the downward traction of the anterior shoulder; the baby usually has weakness of the deltoid and infraspinatus muscles as well as the flexor muscles of the forearm. The arm often hangs limply by the side and is internally rotated.

Management of Shoulder Dystocia

Because of the unpredictability and urgency of shoulder dystocia, the clinician must rehearse its management and be ready when the situation is encountered. **Shoulder dystocia should be suspected with fetal macrosomia, maternal obesity, prolonged second stage of labor, and gestational diabetes.** However, it must be noted that almost one-half of all cases occur in babies weighing less than 4000 g, and shoulder dystocia is frequently unsuspected. Significant fetal hypoxia may occur

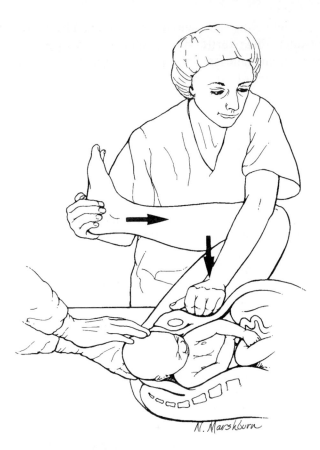

Figure 11–1. Maneuvers for shoulder dystocia. The McRobert's maneuver involves flexing the maternal thighs against the abdomen. Suprapubic pressure attempts to push the fetal shoulders into an oblique plane.

(Reproduced, with permission, from Cunningham FG et al. Williams obstetrics, 21st ed. New York: McGraw-Hill; 2001: 462.)

Table 11–1
COMMON MANEUVERS FOR THE TREATMENT
OF SHOULDER DYSTOCIA

McRobert's maneuver
Suprapubic pressure
Woodscrew maneuver
Delivery of the posterior arm
Zavanelli maneuver

with undue delay from the delivery of the head to the body. Moreover, **excessive traction on the fetal head may lead to a brachial plexus injury to the baby.** It should be recognized that brachial plexus injury can occur with vaginal delivery not associated with shoulder dystocia, or even with cesarean delivery. Shoulder dystocia is not resolved with more traction, but by maneuvers to relieve the impaction of the anterior shoulder (Table 11–1). The diagnosis is made when external rotation of the fetal head is difficult, and the fetal head may retract back toward the maternal introitus, the **"turtle sign."** The first actions are nonmanipulative of the fetus, such as the McRobert's maneuver and suprapubic pressure. **Fundal pressure should be avoided** when shoulder dystocia is diagnosed because of the increased associated neonatal injury. Other maneuvers include the Wood's corkscrew (progressively rotating the posterior shoulder in 180° in a corkscrew fashion), delivery of the posterior arm, and the Zavanelli maneuver (cephalic replacement with immediate cesarean section).

One area of controversy is the practice of cesarean delivery in certain circumstances in an attempt to avoid shoulder dystocia; indications include macrosomia diagnosed on ultrasound, particularly with maternal gestational diabetes. Because of the imprecision of estimated fetal weights and prediction of shoulder dystocia, there is not uniform agreement regarding this practice. Operative vaginal delivery, such as vacuum or forceps-assisted deliveries in the face of possible fetal macrosomia, may possibly increase the risk of shoulder dystocia.

Comprehension Questions

[11.1] Each of the following is a risk factor for shoulder dystocia except:

    A. Maternal gestational diabetes
    B. Fetal hydrocephaly
    C. Maternal obesity
    D. Fetal macrosomia

[11.2] Each of the following is a maneuver that is useful when encountering shoulder dystocia except:

    A. Cephalic replacement
    B. Suprapubic pressure
    C. Fundal pressure
    D. Intentional fracture of the fetal clavicle
    E. Delivery of the posterior arm

Match the following mechanisms (A–E) to the stated maneuver (11.3–11.5):

    A. Anterior rotation of the symphysis pubis
    B. Decreases the fetal bony diameter from shoulder to axilla
    C. Fracture of the humerus
    D. Displaces the fetal shoulder axis from anterior–posterior to oblique
    E. Separates the maternal symphysis pubis

[11.3] The clinician performs a delivery of the posterior fetal arm.

[11.4] The McRobert's maneuver is utilized.

[11.5] The nurse is instructed to apply the suprapubic pressure maneuver.

Answers

[11.1] **B.** With hydrocephalus, the fetal head is greater than the body; whereas with gestational diabetes, the fetal shoulders and abdomen are disproportionately bigger than the head.

[11.2] **C.** Fundal pressure is contraindicated in shoulder dystocia, since it may be associated with increased maternal or neonatal complications.

[11.3] **B.** With delivery of the posterior arm, the shoulder girdle diameter is reduced from shoulder-to-shoulder to shoulder-to-axilla, which usually allows the fetus to deliver.

[11.4] **A.** The McRobert's maneuver causes anterior rotation of the symphysis pubis and flattening of the lumbar spine.

[11.5] **D.** The rationale of suprapubic pressure is to move the fetal shoulders from the anterior–posterior plane into an oblique plane allowing the shoulders to slip out from under the symphysis pubis.

CLINICAL PEARLS

❖ Shoulder dystocia cannot be predicted nor prevented in the majority of cases.

❖ The biggest risk factor for shoulder dystocia is fetal macrosomia, particularly in a woman who has gestational diabetes.

❖ The estimation of fetal weight is most often inaccurate, as is the diagnosis of macrosomia.

❖ The most common injury to the neonate in a shoulder dystocia is brachial plexus injury, such as Erb's palsy.

❖ The first actions for shoulder dystocia are generally the McRobert's maneuver or suprapubic pressure.

❖ Fundal pressure should not be used once shoulder dystocia is encountered.

REFERENCES

Hayashi RH, Bashore RA. Gap junctions, uterine contractility, and dystocia. In: Hacker NF and Moore JG, eds. Essentials of obstetrics and gynecology, 3rd ed. Philadelphia: Saunders. 1998:308–310.

Cunningham FG, Gant NF, Leveno KJ, Gilstrap LC III, Hauth JC, Wenstrom KD. Dystocia: abnormal presentation, position, and development of the fetus. In: Williams obstetrics, 21st ed. New York: McGraw-Hill. 2001:469–482.

A 45-year-old woman underwent a total abdominal hysterectomy for symptomatic endometriosis 2 days previously. She complains of right flank tenderness. On examination, her temperature is 102°F, HR is 100/min, and BP is 130/90. Her heart and lung examinations are normal. The abdomen is slightly tender diffusely with normal bowel sounds. The incision appears within normal limits. Exquisite right costovertebral angle tenderness is noted.

◆ **What would be your next diagnostic step?**

◆ **What is the most likely diagnosis?**

ANSWERS TO CASE 12: Ureteral Injury after Hysterectomy

Summary: A 45-year-old woman who underwent a total abdominal hysterectomy for symptomatic endometriosis two days previously has right flank tenderness, fever of 102°F, and exquisite costovertebral angle tenderness. The incision appears normal.

◆ **Next step:** Intravenous pyelogram (IVP).

◆ **Most likely diagnosis:** Right ureteral obstruction or injury.

Analysis

Objectives

1. Understand that the urinary tract is sometimes injured in pelvic surgery.
2. Know the common presentations of ureteral and bladder injuries after gynecologic surgery.
3. Know some of the conditions that predispose patients to urinary tract injury.

Considerations

This patient has a clinical picture identical to pyelonephritis; however, because she has recently undergone a hysterectomy, injury to or obstruction of the ureter is of paramount concern. **Endometriosis** tends to obliterate tissue planes, making ureteral injury more likely. The intravenous pyelogram (IVP) is the best initial test to evaluate this disorder. If the same clinical picture were present without the recent surgery, then the most likely diagnosis would be pyelonephritis and the next step would be intravenous antibiotics and urine culture. Finally, the wound is normal, which argues against a wound infection causing the postoperative fever.

APPROACH TO URETERAL INJURIES

Definitions

Cardinal ligament: The attachments of the uterine cervix to the pelvic side walls through which the uterine arteries traverse.

Intravenous pyelogram (IVP):   Radiologic study in which intravenous dye is injected and radiographs are taken of the kidneys, ureters, and bladder.

Hydronephrosis: Dilation of the renal collecting system, which gives evidence of urinary obstruction.

Cystoscopy: Procedure whereby a scope is placed into the bladder via the urethra. Various procedures, such as placement of stents into the ureters, can be performed.

Percutaneous nephrostomy: Placement of a stent into the renal pelvis through the skin under radiologic guidance to relieve a urinary obstruction.

Clinical Approach

Up to 1% of abdominal hysterectomies can be complicated by ureteral injury. **Cancer, extensive adhesions, endometriosis, tubo-ovarian abscess, residual ovaries, and interligamentous leiomyomata are risk factors.** Any gynecologic procedure, including laparoscopy or vaginal hysterectomy, may result in ureteral injury; however, the majority of the injuries are associated with abdominal hysterectomy. **The most common location for ureteral injury is at the cardinal ligament, where the ureter is only 2- to 3-cm lateral to the cervix.** The ureter is just under the uterine artery, "water under the bridge" (Figure 12–1). Other locations of ureteral injuries include the pelvic brim, which occur during the ligation of the ovarian vessels (infundibular pelvic ligament), and at the point at which the ureter enters the bladder (anterior to the vagina, when the vaginal cuff is ligated at the end of the hysterectomy). Ureteral injuries include suture ligation, transsection, crushing with clamps, ischemia-induced damage from stripping the blood supply, and laparoscopic injury.

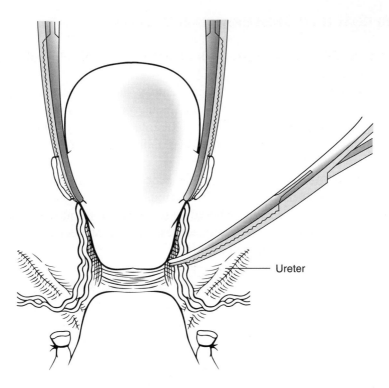

Ureter

Figure 12–1.   Location of ureters during hysterectomy. The ureters are within 2- to 3-cm lateral to the internal cervical os and can be injured on clamping the uterine arteries.

If the IVP shows possible obstruction with hydronephrosis and/or hydroureter (Figure 12–2), the next steps include antibiotic administration *and* cystoscopy to attempt retrograde stent passage. This procedure is performed in the hope that the ureter is kinked but not occluded. Relief of the obstruction is paramount in preventing renal damage. The decision for immediate ureteral repair versus initial percutaneous nephrostomy with later ureteral repair should be individualized.

Comprehension Questions

Match the following processes (A–E) to the most likely clinical situations (12.1–12.4).

A. Vesicovaginal fistula
B. Ureteral ligation
C. Ureteral ischemia leading to injury
D. Ureteral thermal injury
E. Bladder perforation injury

[12.1] A 55-year-old woman undergoes a total abdominal hysterectomy and develops fever and flank tenderness.

[12.2] A 33-year-old woman undergoes pelvic lymphadenectomy for cervical cancer. During the procedure, the right ureter is meticulously and cleanly dissected free and a Penrose drain is placed around it to ensure its safety. She is asymptomatic until postoperative day 9, when she develops profuse nausea and vomiting, and is noted to have ascites on ultrasound.

[12.3] A 55-year-old woman, who underwent a vaginal hysterectomy for third-degree vaginal prolapse 1 month ago, complains of constant leakage of fluid per vagina of 7 days duration.

[12.4] A 44-year-old woman undergoes a right salpingo-ophorectomy laparoscopically. Bipolar cautery is used to ligate the infundibular pelvic ligament. The next day, she complains of fever and flank tenderness.

Answers

[12.1] **B.** Abdominal hysterectomy most likely involves ligating the ureter at the level of the cardinal ligament.

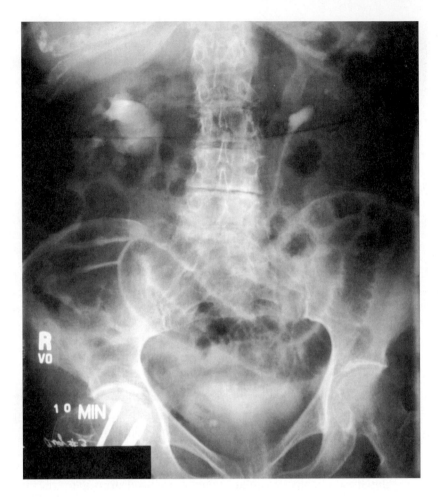

Figure 12–2. Intravenous pyelogram. A. Right hydronephrosis is reflected by dilation of the renal collecting system and hydroureter, whereas the left collecting system is normal.

(Courtesy of Dr. John E. Bertini.)

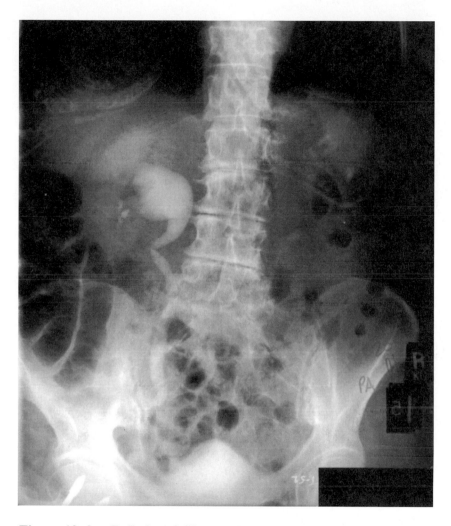

Figure 12–2. B. Delayed film on the same patient shows the right hydroureter more prominently.

(Courtesy of Dr. John E. Bertini.)

[12.2] **C.** Overdissection of the ureter may lead to devascularization injury because the ureter receives its blood supply from various arteries along its course, and flows along its adventitial sheath. Urine in the abdominal cavity is irritating to the intestines and induces nausea and emesis.

[12.3] **A.** Constant urinary leakage after pelvic surgery is a typical history for vesicovaginal fistula (see Case 1).

[12.4] **D.** Thermal injury can spread from the cauterized tissue to surrounding structures.

CLINICAL PEARLS

 Ureteral injury should be suspected when a patient has flank tenderness and fever after a hysterectomy or oophorectomy.

 Meticulous ureteral dissection can lead to devascularization injury to the ureter.

 A fistula should be considered when there is constant leakage of drainage from the vagina.

An intravenous pyelogram (IVP) is the imaging test of choice to assess a postoperative patient with a suspected ureteral injury.

REFERENCES

Gambone JC, Brooks PG, Moore JG. Gynecologic operative techniques. In: Hacker NF and Moore JG, eds. Essentials of obstetrics and gynecology, 3rd ed. Philadelphia: Saunders. 1998:561–564.

Thompson JD. Operative injuries to the ureter: prevention, recognition, and management. In: Thompson JD, Rock JA, eds. TeLinde's operative gynecology, 8th ed. Philadelphia: Lippincott. 1997:1135–1173.

CASE 13

A 66-year-old nulliparous woman who underwent menopause at age 55 years complains of a 2-week history of vaginal bleeding. Prior to menopause, she had irregular menses. She denies the use of estrogen replacement therapy. Her medical history is significant for diabetes mellitus controlled with an oral hypoglycemic agent. On examination, she weighs 190 lb, height 5′3″, BP is 150/90, and temp is 99°F. The heart and lung examinations are normal. The abdomen is obese, and no masses are palpated. The external genitalia appear normal, the uterus is normal size without adnexal masses.

◆ **What is the next step?**

◆ **What is your concern?**

ANSWERS TO CASE 13: Postmenopausal Bleeding

Summary: A 66-year-old diabetic, nulliparous woman complains of postmenopausal vaginal bleeding. Prior to menopause, which occurred at age 55, she had irregular menses. She denies the use of estrogen replacement therapy. Her examination is significant for obesity and hypertension.

◆ **Next step:** Perform an endometrial biopsy.

◆ **Your concern:** Endometrial cancer.

Analysis

Objectives

1. Understand that postmenopausal bleeding requires endometrial sampling to assess for endometrial cancer.
2. Know the risk factors for endometrial cancer.
3. Know that endometrial cancer is staged surgically.

Considerations

This patient has postmenopausal vaginal bleeding. The biggest concern should be endometrial cancer. **She also has numerous risk factors for endometrial cancer including obesity, diabetes, hypertension, prior anovulation (irregular menses), late menopause, and nulliparity.** The endometrial sampling or aspiration can be performed in the office by placing a thin, flexible catheter through the cervix. It is the initial test of choice to assess for endometrial cancer. This patient is not taking unopposed estrogen replacement therapy, which would be another risk factor. If endometrial cancer were diagnosed, the patient would need surgical staging. If the endometrial sampling is negative for cancer, another cause for postmenopausal bleeding, such as atrophic endometrium, is possible. A blind sampling of the endometrium, such as with the endometrial biopsy device, has a 90% to 95% sensitivity for detecting cancer. If this patient, who has so many risk factors for endometrial cancer, were to have a negative endometrial sampling, many practitioners would go to **a direct visualization of the endometrial cavity, such as hysteroscopy.** If the clinician were to elect to observe this patient after the endometrial biopsy, any further bleeding episodes would necessitate further investigation.

APPROACH TO POSTMENOPAUSAL BLEEDING

Definitions

Endometrial sampling (biopsy): A thin catheter is introduced through the cervix into the uterine cavity under some suction to aspirate endometrial cells.

Endometrial polyps: A growth of endometrial glands and stroma, which projects into the uterine cavity, usually on a stalk; it can cause postmenopausal bleeding.

Atrophic endometrium: The most common cause of postmenopausal bleeding is friable tissue of the endometrium or vagina due to low estrogen levels.

Endometrial stripe: Transvaginal sonographic assessment of the endometrial thickness; a thickness greater than 5-mm is abnormal in a postmenopausal woman.

Clinical Approach

Postmenopausal bleeding always needs to be investigated because it can indicate malignant disorders and premalignant conditions, such as endometrial hyperplasia. Notably, complex hyperplasia with atypia is associated with endometrial carcinoma in 30% to 50% of cases.

Approximately 20% of postmenopausal women not on hormonal therapy but complaining of vaginal bleeding will have an endometrial carcinoma. The most common etiology of postmenopausal bleeding is atrophic endometritis or vaginitis; also, vaginal spotting can occur in a patient taking hormonal therapy. However, since endometrial malignancy can coexist with atrophic changes or in women taking hormone

Table 13–1

RISK FACTORS FOR ENDOMETRIAL CANCER

Early menarche
Late menopause
Obesity
Chronic anovulation
Estrogen secreting ovarian tumors
Ingestion of unopposed estrogen
Hypertension
Diabetes mellitus
Personal or family history of breast or ovarian cancer

replacement therapy, **endometrial carcinoma must be ruled out in any patient with postmenopausal bleeding.** Possible methods for assessment of the endometrium include endometrial sampling, hysteroscopy, or vaginal sonography.

Risk factors for endometrial cancer are listed in Table 13–1. They primarily include conditions of estrogen exposure without progesterone. Although endometrial cancer typically affects older women, a woman in her 30s with a history of chronic anovulation, such as polycystic ovarian syndrome, may be affected. **When the endometrial sampling is unrevealing, the patient with persistent postmenopausal bleeding, or with numerous risk factors for endometrial cancer, should undergo further evaluation, such as by hysteroscopy.** Direct visualization of the intrauterine cavity can identify small lesions that may be missed by the office endometrial sampling device. Additionally, endometrial polyps can be identified by hysteroscopy.

Table 13–2

STAGING PROCEDURE FOR ENDOMETRIAL CANCER

Total abdominal hysterectomy, bilateral salpingo-ophorectomy
Omentectomy
Lymph node sampling
Peritoneal washings

Although endometrial cancer is not the most common cause of post-menopausal bleeding, it is usually the one of most concern. Once diagnosed, endometrial cancer is staged surgically (Table 13–2).

Comprehension Questions

[13.1] Each of the following is a risk factor for endometrial cancer except:

    A. Nulliparity
    B. Obesity
    C. Diabetes mellitus
    D. Oral contraceptive use
    E. Hypertension

[13.2] A 60-year-old postmenopausal woman has a Pap smear performed, which reveals normal endometrial cells. Which of the following is the best next step?

    A. Repeat Pap smear in 3 months
    B. Colposcopy
    C. Hormone replacement therapy
    D. Endometrial sampling

[13.3] A 57-year-old postmenopausal woman with hypertension, diabetes, and a history of polycystic ovarian syndrome complains of vaginal bleeding for 2 weeks. The endometrial sampling shows a few fragments of atrophic endometrium. Estrogen replacement therapy is begun. The patient continues to have several episodes of vaginal bleeding 3 months later. Which of the following is the best next step?

    A. Continued observation and reassurance
    B. Unopposed estrogen replacement therapy
    C. Hysteroscopic examination
    D. Endometrial ablation
    E. Serum CA-125 testing

[13.4] Which of the following is the most important therapeutic measure in the treatment of stage I (confined to the uterus) endometrial cancer?

A. Radiation therapy
B. Chemotherapy
C. Immunostimulation therapy
D. Progestin therapy
E. Surgical therapy

Answers

[13.1] **D.** Progestin use will decrease the risk of endometrial cancer.

[13.2] **D. Normal** endometrial cells on the Pap smear of a post-menopausal woman may indicate endometrial cancer. Therefore, an endometrial sampling is indicated.

[13.3] **C.** Persistent postmenopausal bleeding, especially in a woman with risk factors for endometrial cancer, must be pursued. Hysteroscopy is one of the best methods to assess the uterine cavity.

[13.4] **E.** Surgical treatment is a fundamental aspect of the treatment. Radiotherapy is used as an adjunctive treatment, for possible spread.

CLINICAL PEARLS

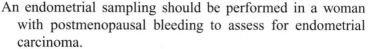

- An endometrial sampling should be performed in a woman with postmenopausal bleeding to assess for endometrial carcinoma.
- Unopposed estrogen is generally the biggest risk factor for the development of endometrial cancer.
- Endometrial cancer is staged surgically and surgery is a fundamental part of its treatment.
- Persistent postmenopausal bleeding warrants further investigation (such as hysteroscopy) even after a normal endometrial sampling.

REFERENCES

Carcinoma of the endometrium. ACOG Technical Bulletin 162. December, 1991.

Heaps JM, Leuchter RS. Uterine corpus cancer. In: Hacker NF and Moore JG, eds. Essentials of obstetrics and gynecology, 3rd ed. Philadelphia: Saunders. 1998:561–564.

Herbst AL. Neoplastic diseases of the uterus. In: Stenchever MA, Droegemueller W, Herbst AL, Mishell DR, eds. Comprehensive gynecology, 4th ed. St. Louis: Mosby-Year Book. 2001:919–954.

A 30-year-old G5 P4 woman at 32 weeks' gestation complains of significant bright red vaginal bleeding. She denies uterine contractions, leakage of fluid, or trauma. The patient states that 4 weeks previously, after she had engaged in sexual intercourse, she experienced some vaginal spotting. On examination, her blood pressure is 110/60 and HR is 80/min. Temperature is 99°F. The heart and lung examinations are normal. The abdomen is soft and uterus nontender. Fetal heart tones are in the range of 140 to 150 bpm.

♦ **What is your next step?**

♦ **What is most likely diagnosis?**

♦ **What will be the long-term management of this patient?**

ANSWERS TO CASE 14: Placenta Previa

Summary: A 30-year-old G5 P4 woman at 32 weeks' gestation complains of painless vaginal bleeding. Four weeks previously, she experienced some postcoital vaginal spotting. The abdomen is soft and uterus nontender. Fetal heart tones are in the range of 140 to 150 bpm.

◆ **Next step:** Ultrasound examination.

◆ **Most likely diagnosis:** Placenta previa.

◆ **Long-term management of this patient:** Expectant management as long as the bleeding is not excessive. Cesarean delivery at 36 to 37 weeks' gestation.

Analysis

Objectives

1. Know the differential diagnosis of antepartum bleeding.
2. Understand that painless vaginal bleeding is consistent with placenta previa.
3. Understand that the ultrasound examination is a good method for assessing placental location.

Considerations

The patient experiences antepartum vaginal bleeding (bleeding after 20 weeks' gestation). Because of the **painless nature of the bleeding** and lack of risk factors for placental abruption, this case is more likely to be placenta previa, defined as the placenta overlying the internal os of the cervix. Placenta abruption (premature separation of the placenta) usually is associated with painful uterine contractions or excess uterine tone. **The history of postcoital spotting earlier during the pregnancy is consistent with previa,** since vaginal intercourse may induce bleeding. The ultrasound examination is performed before a vaginal examination because vaginal manipulation (even a speculum examination) may induce bleeding. Because the patient is hemodynamically stable, and the fetal heart tones are normal, expectant management is the best therapy at 32 weeks' gestation (due to the prematurity risks). If the same patient were at 35 to 36 weeks' gestation, then delivery by cesarean section would be prudent.

APPROACH TO ANTEPARTUM VAGINAL BLEEDING

Definitions

Antepartum vaginal bleeding: Vaginal bleeding occurring after 20 weeks' gestation.
Complete placenta previa: The placenta completely covers the internal os of the uterine cervix (Figure 14–1).
Partial placenta previa: The placenta partially covers the internal cervical os.
Marginal placenta previa: The placenta abuts against the internal os of the cervix.
Low-lying placenta: The edge of the placenta is within 2-3 centimeters of the internal cervical os.
Placental abruption: Premature separation of a normally implanted placenta.

Clinical Approach

Antepartum hemorrhage is defined as significant vaginal bleeding after 20 weeks' gestation. The two most common causes of significant antepartum bleeding are placenta abruption and placenta previa (Table 14–1). **The classic presentation of previa bleeding is *painless* vaginal bleeding after the midsecond trimester, whereas placental abruption frequently presents with painful contractions.** When the patient complains of antepartum hemorrhage, the physician should first rule out placenta previa by ultrasound even **before** a speculum or digital examination, since these maneuvers may induce bleeding.

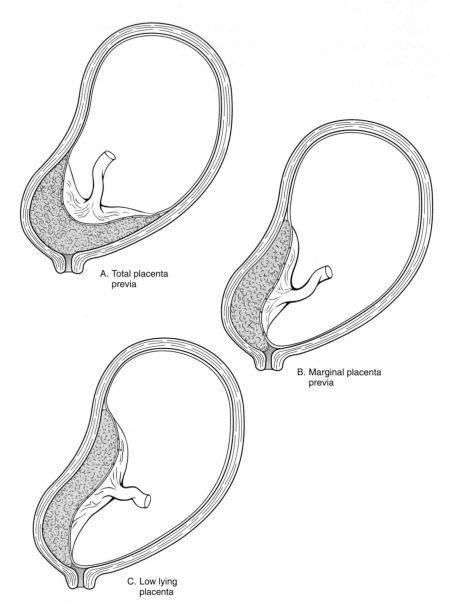

A. Total placenta previa

B. Marginal placenta previa

C. Low lying placenta

Figure 14–1.   Types of placenta previa. Complete placenta previa (A), marginal previa (B), and low-lying placentation (C) are depicted.

Table 14–1
RISK FACTORS FOR PLACENTA PREVIA

Grand-multiparity
Prior cesarean delivery
Prior uterine curettage
Previous placenta previa
Multiple gestation

Ultrasound is an accurate method of assessing placental location. At times, transabdominal sonography may not be able to visualize the placenta, and transvaginal ultrasound is necessary.

The natural history of placenta previa is such that the first episode of bleeding does not usually cause sufficient concern as to necessitate delivery. Hence, a woman with a preterm gestation and placenta previa is usually observed on bed rest with the hope that time may be gained for fetal maturation. Often, the second or third episode of bleeding forces delivery. The bleeding from previa rarely leads to coagulopathy, as opposed to that of placenta abruption. At or near term (36 to 37 weeks), many practitioners will perform an amniocentesis to establish fetal lung maturity; if the fetal lungs appear mature, then delivery will be scheduled. The route of delivery as a general rule is by cesarean section. Because the lower uterine segment is poorly contractile, postpartum bleeding may ensue. Also, invasion of the placenta into the uterus (accreta) is more common with placenta previa.

Comprehension Questions

[14.1] Each of the following is a risk factor of placenta previa except:

    A. Prior cesarean section
    B. Hypertension
    C. Multiple gestation
    D. Prior uterine curettage

[14.2] Each of the following is a typical feature of placenta previa except:

   A. Painless bleeding
   B. Commonly associated with coagulopathy
   C. First episode of bleeding is usually self-limited
   D. Associated with postcoital spotting

[14.3] A 33-year-old woman at 37 weeks' gestation, confirmed by first trimester sonography, presents with moderately severe vaginal bleeding. She is noted on sonography to have a placenta previa. Which of the following is the best management for this patient?

   A. Induction of labor
   B. Tocolysis of labor
   C. Cesarean delivery
   D. Expectant management
   E. Intrauterine transfusion

[14.4] A 22-year-old G1 P0 woman at 34 weeks' gestation presents with moderate vaginal bleeding and no uterine contractions. Which of the following sequence of examinations is most appropriate?

   A. Speculum examination, ultrasound examination, digital examination
   B. Ultrasound examination, digital examination, speculum examination
   C. Digital examination, ultrasound examination, speculum examination
   D. Ultrasound examination, speculum examination, digital examination

[14.5] An 18-year-old woman is noted to have a marginal placenta previa on an ultrasound examination at 22 weeks' gestation. Which of the following is the most appropriate management?

A. Schedule cesarean delivery at 39 weeks.
B. Schedule an amniocentesis at 36 weeks and deliver by cesarean if the fetal lungs are mature.
C. Schedule an MRI examination at 35 weeks to assess for possible percreta involving the bladder.
D. Reassess placental position at 32 weeks
E. Recommend termination of pregnancy

Answers

[14.1] **B.** Hypertension is not a risk factor for placenta previa.

[14.2] **B.** Unlike placenta abruption, placenta previa is not commonly associated with coagulopathy.

[14.3] **C.** The best plan for placenta previa at term is cesarean delivery.

[14.4] **D.** Ultrasound should be performed first to rule out previa, speculum examination second to assess the cervix and look for lacerations, and, then finally, a digital examination should be done.

[14.5] **D.** Very often, a marginal or low lying placenta previa at the early second trimester will resolve by transmigration of the placenta (see Case 8).

CLINICAL PEARLS

❖ Painless antepartum vaginal bleeding suggests the diagnosis of placenta previa.

❖ Ultrasound is the diagnostic test of choice in assessing placenta previa and should be performed before digital or speculum examination.

❖ Cesarean section is the best route of delivery for placenta previa.

❖ Placenta previa in the face of prior cesarean deliveries increases the risk of placenta accreta.

REFERENCES

Goodman JR. Antepartum hemorrhage. In: Hacker NF and Moore JG, eds. Essentials of obstetrics and gynecology, 3rd ed. Philadelphia: Saunders. 1998:187–192.

Cunningham FG, Gant NF, Leveno KJ, Gilstrap LC III, Hauth JC, Wenstrom KD. Obstetrical hemorrhage. In: Williams obstetrics, 21st ed. New York: McGraw-Hill. 2001:619–670.

CASE 15

A 22-year-old G2 P1 woman at 35 weeks' gestation, who admits to cocaine abuse, complains of abdominal pain. She states that she has been experiencing moderate vaginal bleeding, no leakage of fluid per vagina, and has no history of trauma. On examination, her blood pressure is 150/90 and HR is 110 bpm. The fundus reveals tenderness and a moderate amount of dark vaginal blood is noted in the vaginal vault. The ultrasound examination shows no placental abnormalities. The cervix is 1-cm dilated. The fetal heart tones are in the 160 to 170 bpm range.

◆ **What is the most likely diagnosis?**

◆ **What are complications that can occur due to this situation?**

◆ **What is the best management for this condition?**

ANSWERS TO CASE 15: Placental Abruption

Summary: A 22-year-old G2 P1 cocaine user at 35 weeks' gestation complains of abdominal pain and moderate vaginal bleeding. On examination, her blood pressure is 150/90 and HR is 110 bpm. The fundus reveals tenderness. The ultrasound is normal. The fetal heart tones are in the 160 to 170 bpm range.

◆ **Most likely diagnosis:** Placental abruption.

◆ **Complications that can occur:** Hemorrhage, fetal to maternal bleeding, coagulopathy, and preterm delivery.

◆ **Best management for this condition:** Delivery (at 35 weeks, the risks of abruption significantly outweigh the risks of prematurity).

Analysis

See also answers to Case 14.

Objectives

1. Understand that placental abruption and placenta previa are major causes of antepartum hemorrhage.
2. Know the clinical presentation of abruptio placentae.
3. Understand that coagulopathy is a complication of placental abruption.

Considerations

The patient complains of **painful** antepartum bleeding, which is consistent with placental abruption. Also, she has several risk factors for abruptio placentae, such as hypertension and cocaine use (Table 15–1). Because **the natural history of placental abruption is extension of**

Table 15–1

RISK FACTORS FOR ABRUPTIO PLACENTAE

Hypertension (chronic and preeclampsia)
Cocaine use
Short umbilical cord
Trauma
Uteroplacental insufficiency
Submucous leiomyomata
Sudden uterine decompression (hydramnios)
Cigarette smoking
Preterm premature rupture of membranes

the separation, leading to complete shearing of the placenta from the uterus, the best treatment at a gestational age near term (greater than 34 weeks) is delivery. As opposed to the diagnosis of placenta previa, **ultrasound examination is a poor method of assessment for abruption.** This is because the freshly developed blood clot behind the placenta has the same sonographic texture as the placenta itself.

APPROACH TO SUSPECTED PLACENTAL ABRUPTION

Definitions

Concealed abruption: When the bleeding occurs completely behind the placenta and no external bleeding is noted.
Fetomaternal hemorrhage: Fetal blood that enters into the maternal circulation.
Couvelaire uterus: Bleeding into the myometrium of the uterus giving a discolored appearance to the uterine surface.

Clinical Approach

As compared to placenta previa, abruptio placentae is more dangerous and unpredictable. Furthermore, the diagnosis is much more difficult to establish. Ultrasound examination is not helpful in the majority of cases; a normal ultrasound examination does not rule out placental abruption. **There is no one test that is diagnostic of placental abruption, but rather the clinical picture must be taken as a whole.** Thus, a patient at risk for abruptio placentae (a hypertensive patient or one who has recently been involved in a motor vehicle accident) who complains of vaginal bleeding after 20 weeks' gestation must be suspected of having a placental abruption. Furthermore, the bleeding is often associated with uterine pain or hypertonus. The blood may seep into the uterine muscle and cause a reddish discoloration also known as the "Couvelaire uterus." Uterine atony and postpartum hemorrhage after delivery may occur. Upon delivery, a blood clot adherent to the placenta is often seen. **Another complication of abruption is coagulopathy, and when the abruption is of sufficient severity to cause fetal death, coagulopathy is found in one-third or more of cases.** The coagulopathy is secondary to hypofibrinogenemia, and clinically evident bleeding is usually not encountered unless the fibrinogen level is below 100 to 150 mg/dL.

The diagnosis of placental abruption is difficult because the clinical presentation is variable. Although painful vaginal bleeding is the hallmark, preterm labor, stillbirth, and/or fetal heart rate abnormalities also may be seen. Ultrasound diagnosis is not sensitive. A concealed abruption can occur when blood is trapped behind the placenta, so that external hemorrhage is not seen. Serial hemoglobin levels, following the fundal height and assessment of the fetal heart rate pattern, are often helpful. **Fetal-to-maternal hemorrhage is more common with placental abruption,** and some practitioners recommend testing for fetal erythrocytes from the maternal blood. One such test of acid elution methodology is called the **Kleihauer–Betke test,** which takes advantage of the different solubilities of maternal versus fetal hemoglobin.

The management of placental abruption is dependent on the fetal gestational age, fetal status, and the hemodynamic status of the mother. **Delivery is the usual management!** In a woman with a premature fetus and a diagnosis of "chronic abruption," expectant management may be exercised if the patient is stable with no active bleeding or signs of fetal compromise. Although there is no contraindication to vaginal delivery, cesarean section is often the chosen route of delivery for fetal indications. In cases of abruptions that are associated with fetal death and coagulopathy, the vaginal route is most often the safest for the mother. In the latter scenario, blood products and intravenous fluids are given to maintain the hematocrit above 25% to 30% and a urine output of at least 30 mL/hr. These women generally have very rapid labors. Many of these women will manifest hypertension or preeclampsia following volume replacement and it may be necessary to start magnesium sulfate for seizure (eclampsia prophylaxis).

Comprehension Questions

[15.1] In which of the following conditions would consumptive coagulopathy most likely be seen?

A. Placental abruption
B. Placenta previa
C. Gestational diabetes
D. Multifetal gestation
E. Gestational trophoblastic disease

[15.2] In which of the following conditions is ultrasound an accurate and sensitive method of diagnosis?

A. Placental abruption
B. Placenta previa
C. Both
D. Neither

[15.3] Each of the following is a risk factor for abruptio placentae except:

A. Hypertension
B. Premature rupture of membranes
C. Trauma
D. Marijuana use
E. Uterine leiomyomata

[15.4] Which one of the following statements regarding placental abruption is most correct?

A. External bleeding is necessary to make the diagnosis.
B. The clinical presentation is fairly predictable.
C. Couvelaire uterus arises from blood seeping into the myometrium.
D. Vaginal delivery is contraindicated.
E. It is associated with chronic hypertension but not preeclampsia.

Answers

[15.1] **A.** Placental abruption is a common cause of coagulopathy.

[15.2] **B.** Sonography is accurate in identifying previa, but not sensitive in diagnosing placental abruption.

[15.3] **D.** Marijuana, as opposed to cocaine, is not associated with abruption. Uterine leiomyomata, especially submucous ones, predispose patients to placental abruption.

[15.4] **C.** Hidden bleeding is possible (concealed abruption), the clinical picture is highly variable necessitating a high index of suspicion, vaginal delivery is not contraindicated, and it is associated with both chronic hypertension and preeclampsia.

CLINICAL PEARLS

 Painful antepartum bleeding should make one suspicious of placental abruption.

 The major risk factors for abruptio placentae are hypertension, trauma, and cocaine use.

 A concealed abruption may hide significant bleeding without external hemorrhage.

 The most common cause of antepartum bleeding with coagulopathy is abruptio placentae.

 Placental abruption may lead to fetal-to-maternal hemorrhage.

REFERENCES

Goodman JR. Antepartum hemorrhage. In: Hacker NF and Moore JG, eds. Essentials of obstetrics and gynecology, 3rd ed. Philadelphia: Saunders. 1998:187–195.

Cunningham FG, Gant NF, Leveno KJ, Gilstrap LC III, Hauth JC, Wenstrom KD. Obstetrical hemorrhage. In: Williams obstetrics, 21st ed. New York: McGraw-Hill. 2001:619–670.

A 50-year-old G5 P5 woman complains of postcoital spotting over the past 6 months. Most recently, she complains of a malodorous vaginal discharge. She states that she has had syphilis in the past. Her deliveries were all vaginal and uncomplicated. She has smoked 1 pack per day for 20 years. On examination, her BP is 100/80, temp is 99°F, and HR 80 is bpm. Her heart and lung examinations are within normal limits. The abdomen reveals no masses, ascites, or tenderness. Her back examination is unremarkable and there is no costovertebral angle tenderness. The pelvic examination reveals normal external female genitalia. The speculum examination reveals a 3-cm exophytic lesion on the anterior lip of the cervix. No other masses are palpated.

◆ **What is your next step?**

◆ **What is the most likely diagnosis?**

ANSWERS TO CASE 16: Cervical Cancer

Summary: A 50-year-old G5 P5 woman complains of a 6-month history of postcoital spotting and malodorous vaginal discharge. She has had a prior infection with syphilis, and is a smoker. The speculum examination reveals a 3-cm exophytic lesion on the anterior lip of the cervix.

◆ **Next step:** Biopsy of the cervical lesion.

◆ **Most likely diagnosis:** Cervical cancer.

Analysis

Objectives

1. Understand that a cervical biopsy and not a Pap smear (which is actually a screening test) is the best diagnostic procedure when a cervical lesion is seen.
2. Know that postcoital spotting is a symptom of cervical cancer.
3. Know the risk factors for cervical cancer.

Considerations

This 50-year-old woman presents with postcoital spotting. **Abnormal vaginal bleeding is the most common presenting symptom of invasive cervical cancer, and in sexually active women, postcoital spotting is common.** This patient's age is close to the mean age of presentation of cervical cancer, 51 years. She also complains of a malodorous vaginal discharge that is due to the large, necrotic tumor. Notably, the woman does not have flank tenderness, which would be a result of metastatic obstruction of the ureter, leading to hydronephrosis. **A cervical biopsy and not Pap smear is the best diagnostic test to evaluate a cervical mass.** A Pap smear is a screening test and appropriate for a woman with a normal appearing cervix.

Risk factors for cervical cancer in this woman include multiparity, cigarette smoking, and history of a sexually transmitted disease

Table 16–1
RISK FACTORS FOR CERVICAL CANCER

Early age of coitus
Sexually transmitted diseases
Early childbearing
Low socioeconomic status
Human papilloma virus
HIV infection
Cigarette smoking
Multiple sexual partners

(syphilis). Other risk factors not mentioned would be early age of coitus, multiple sexual partners, and HIV infection (Table 16–1).

APPROACH TO CERVICAL CANCER

Definitions

Cervical intraepithelial neoplasia: Preinvasive lesions of the cervix with abnormal cellular maturation, nuclear enlargement, and atypia.
Human papilloma virus: Circular, double-stranded DNA virus that can become incorporated into cervical squamous epithelium, predisposing the cells for dysplasia and/or cancer.
Radical hysterectomy: Removal of the uterus, cervix, and supportive ligaments, such as the cardinal ligament, uterosacral ligament, and proximal vagina.
Radiation brachytherapy: Radioactive implants placed near the tumor bed.
Radiation teletherapy: External beam radiation where the target is at some distance from the radiation source.

Clinical Approach

When a woman presents with **postcoital spotting** or has an abnormal Pap smear, cervical dysplasia or cancer should be suspected. **An**

abnormal Pap smear is usually evaluated by colposcopy with biop-sies, in which the cervix is soaked with 3% or 5% acetic acid solution. The colposcope is a binocular magnifying device that allows visual examination of the cervix. **The majority of cervical dysplasia and cancers arise near the squamocolumnar junction of the cervix.** Many times, cervical intraepithelial lesions will turn white with the addition of acetic acid, the so-called "acetowhite change." Along with the change in color, dysplastic lesions will often have vascular changes, reflecting the more rapidly growing process; in fact, the vascular pattern usually characterizes the severity of the disease. An example of mild vascular pattern is punctations (vessels seen end-on) versus atypical vessels (such as corkscrew and hairpin vessels). A biopsy of the worst-appearing area should be taken during colposcopy for histologic diagnosis. Hence, **the next step to evaluate an abnormal Pap smear is colposcopic examinations with directed biopsies.**

When a woman presents with a cervical mass, biopsy of the mass, not a Pap smear, is appropriate. Because the Pap smear is a screening test, used for asymptomatic women, it is not the best test when a mass is visible. The Papanicolaou test has a false negative rate and may give false reassurance.

When cervical cancer is diagnosed, then the next step is to stage the severity. **Cervical cancer is staged clinically (Table 16–2).** Early cervical cancer (contained within the cervix) may be treated equally well with surgery (radical hysterectomy) or radiation therapy. However, **advanced cervical cancer is best treated with radiotherapy,** consisting of brachytherapy (implants) with teletherapy (whole pelvis radiation) along with chemotherapy to sensitize the tissue to the radiotherapy.

Table 16–2
STAGING PROCEDURE FOR CERVICAL CANCER

Examination under anesthesia
Intravenous pyelogram
Chest radiograph
Barium enema or proctoscopy
Cystoscopy

Cervical cancer often spreads through the cardinal ligaments toward the pelvic sidewalls. It can obstruct one or both ureters leading to hydronephrosis. In fact, **bilateral ureteral obstruction leading to uremia is the most common cause of death due to this disease.**

Comprehension Questions

[16.1] Which of the following HPV subtypes is most likely to be associated with cervical cancer?

    A. 6 and 11
    B. 16 and 18
    C. 55 and 57
    D. 89 and 92

[16.2] Each of the following statements regarding cervical cancer is true except:

    A. The best therapy for advanced cervical cancer is radiotherapy.
    B. Both brachytherapy and teletherapy are important in the treatment of advanced cervical cancer.
    C. The main advantage of radiation therapy over radical hysterectomy in early stage cervical cancer is preservation of sexual function.
    D. The majority of cervical cancers are of squamous cell type.

[16.3] Each of the following is a risk factor for cervical cancer except:

    A. Early age of coitus
    B. Multiparity
    C. Cigarette smoking
    D. Late menopause

[16.4] A 33-year-old woman has a Pap smear showing moderately severe cervical dysplasia (high-grade squamous intraepithelial neoplasia). Which of the following is the best next step?

A. Repeat Pap smear in 3 months
B. Conization of the cervix
C. Colposcopic directed biopsies
D. Radical hysterectomy
E. CT scan of the abdomen and pelvis

Answers

[16.1] **B.** HPV subtypes 6 and 11 are associated with condylomata ac-
cuminata (venereal warts): whereas subtypes 16 and 18 are associated with cervical dysplasia and cancer.

[16.2] **C.** Major advantages of radical hysterectomy over radiotherapy
are preservation of sexual function (due to vaginal agglutina-
tion) and preservation of ovarian function. Radiotherapy may be
performed on women who are poor operative candidates, and is
the best therapy in advanced disease, such as spread to the
pelvic sidewalls or hydronephrosis.

[16.3] **D.** Late menopause is a risk factor for endometrial cancer, not
cervical cancer.

[16.4] **C.** Colposcopic examination with directed biopsies is the next
step to evaluate abnormal cytology on Pap smear.

CLINICAL PEARLS

The main risk factors for cervical cancer are sexually related, especially exposure to human papilloma virus.

Human papilloma virus 16 and 18 are the most commonly isolated subtypes in cervical dysplasia and cancer.

Flank tenderness or leg swelling indicate advanced cervical cancer, which is best treated by radiotherapy with a chemotherapeutic radiosensitizer.

A visible lesion of the cervix should be evaluated by biopsy and not Pap smear.

An abnormal Pap smear is usually evaluated with colposcopic-directed biopsies.

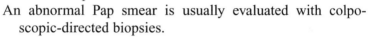
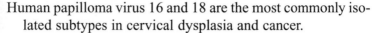

REFERENCES

Savage EW and Leuchter RS. Cervical dysplasia and cancer. In: Hacker NF and Moore JG, eds. Essentials of obstetrics and gynecology, 3rd ed. Philadelphia: Saunders. 1998:645–659.

Herbst AL. Malignant diseases of the cervix. In: Stenchever MA, Droegemueller W, Herbst AL, Mishell DR, eds. Comprehensive gynecology, 4th ed. St. Louis: Mosby-Year Book. 2001:889–918.

Hacker NF. Cervical cancer. In: Berek JS, Hacker NF, eds. Practical gynecologic oncology, 3rd ed. Philadelphia: Lippincott Williams & Wilkins. 2000:345–406.

Diagnosis and treatment of cervical carcinomas. ACOG Practice Bulletin 35, May 2002.

A 24-year-old G2 P2 woman delivered vaginally 8 months previously. Her delivery was complicated by postpartum hemorrhage requiring curettage of the uterus and a blood transfusion of two units of erythrocytes. She complains of amenorrhea since her delivery. She was not able to breast-feed her baby. She denies taking medications or having headaches or visual abnormalities. Her pregnancy test is negative.

◆ **What is the most likely diagnosis?**

◆ **What are other complications that are likely with this condition?**

ANSWERS TO CASE 17: Amenorrhea (Sheehan's Syndrome)

Summary: A 24-year-old G2 P2 woman has had amenorrhea since a vaginal delivery complicated by postpartum hemorrhage and uterine curettage. She was not able to breast-feed after delivery and is not currently pregnant.

◆ **Most likely diagnosis:** Sheehan's syndrome (anterior pituitary necrosis).

◆ **Other complications that are likely with this condition:** Anterior pituitary insufficiency, such as hypothyroidism or adrenocortical insufficiency.

Analysis

Objectives

1. Be able to differentiate Sheehan's syndrome from intrauterine adhesions (Asherman's syndrome).
2. Understand the mechanism of Sheehan's syndrome.
3. Know the other tropic hormones that may be affected by anterior pituitary necrosis.

Considerations

This patient developed amenorrhea from the time of her vaginal delivery that was complicated by postpartum hemorrhage. The initial evaluation should be a pregnancy test (which is negative). The patient also underwent a uterine curettage in the treatment of the postpartum bleeding. In this setting, there are two explanations: 1) Sheehan's syndrome and 2) intrauterine adhesions (Asherman's syndrome). Sheehan's syndrome is caused by hypotension in the postpartum period, leading to hemorrhagic necrosis of the anterior pituitary gland. Asherman's syndrome is caused by the uterine curettage, which damages the decidua basalis layer, rendering the endometrium unresponsive. **The key to dif-**

ferentiating between Sheehan's syndrome and intrauterine adhesions is to assess for whether or not the anterior pituitary is functioning. This patient was not able to breast-feed after the delivery, which suggests that the anterior pituitary was not functioning (lack of prolactin). Had the patient been able to breast-feed, then the most likely diagnosis would have been intrauterine synechiae. Other evidence of anterior pituitary function may include low thyroid hormone, gonadotropin (FSH and LH), or cortisol levels.

APPROACH TO POSTPARTUM AMENORRHEA

Definitions

Amenorrhea: No menses for 6 months.

Sheehan's syndrome: Anterior pituitary hemorrhagic necrosis caused by hypertrophy of the prolactin-secreting cells in conjunction with a hypotensive episode, usually in the setting of postpartum hemorrhage. The bleeding in the anterior pituitary induces pressure necrosis.

Intrauterine adhesions (Asherman's syndrome): Scar tissue that forms in the endometrium, leading to amenorrhea due to unresponsiveness of the endometrial tissue.

Postpartum hemorrhage: Classically defined as bleeding greater than 500 mL for a vaginal delivery and greater than 1000 mL for a cesarean delivery. From a more pathophysiologic standpoint, it is that amount of bleeding that results in, or threatens to result in, hemodynamic instability if left unabated.

Clinical Approach

Amenorrhea can ensue after a term delivery for 2 to 3 months; breast-feeding may inhibit the hypothalamic function, and lead to a greater duration of amenorrhea. **However, in a nonlactating woman, when no menses resumes by 12 weeks after delivery, then pathology must be suspected.** Overall, the most common cause of amenorrhea in the reproductive years is pregnancy. Hence, a pregnancy test is the appropriate

initial test. If the patient does not have a history of postpartum hemorrhage, pursuit of hypothalamic causes, such as hypothyroidism or hyperprolactinemia, are often fruitful. If the patient is somewhat obese, or
has a history of irregular cycles, then polycystic ovarian syndrome
(PCOS) would be entertained. Findings consistent with PCOS include
a positive progestin withdrawal bleed (vaginal bleeding after the ingestion of a progestin, such as medroxyprogesterone acetate or Provera).
**Polycystic ovarian syndrome is characterized by estrogen excess
without progesterone, obesity, hirsutism, and glucose intolerance.
Elevated luteinizing hormone to follicle stimulating hormone ratios
are often seen (for example, LH:FSH of 2:1).** When women are **hypoestrogenic,** then two broad categories of causes are common: hypo-
thalamic/pituitary diseases or ovarian failure. The FSH level can distinguish between these two causes, with an **elevated FSH indicative of
ovarian failure.**

Table 17–1
DIFFERENCES BETWEEN SHEEHAN'S SYNDROME AND ASHERMAN'S SYNDROME

HORMONE FUNCTION	SHEEHAN'S SYNDROME	INTRAUTERINE ADHESIONS
Thyroid hormone (T4)	Low	Normal
TSH	Low	Normal
FSH	Low	Normal
Estradiol levels	Low	Normal
LH surge (biphasic basal body temperature chart)	Absent	Normal biphasic
Cortisol levels	Low	Normal
Prolactin levels (able to breast-feed)	Low (unable to lactate)	Normal
Bleed in response to estrogen and progestin (oral contraceptive)	Yes	No

The patient in this case had amenorrhea after a vaginal delivery, making Sheehan's syndrome or intrauterine adhesions the two most likely causes. Distinguishing between the two entities involves assessing whether the patient has normal or abnormal anterior pituitary function (Table 17–1). Treatment of Sheehan's syndrome consists of replacement of hormones, such as thyroxine, cortisol, and mineralcorticoid, and estrogen and progestin therapy. Intrauterine adhesions are treated by hysteroscopic resection of the scar tissue.

Comprehension Questions

[17.1] Each of the following is a feature of intrauterine synechiae (Asherman's syndrome) except:

A. Usually occurs after uterine curettage
B. Associated with ability to breast-feed after delivery
C. Associated with a monophasic basal body temperature chart
D. Associated with normal cortisol levels

[17.2] Each of the following is consistent with Sheehan's syndrome except:

A. Usually occurs at or soon after a delivery
B. Is caused by an ischemic necrosis of the posterior pituitary gland
C. Is associated with decreased prolactin levels
D. Is often associated with hypothyroidism

[17.3] Which of the following is the best description of the mechanism of intrauterine synechiae (Asherman's syndrome)?

A. Trophoblastic hyperplasia
B. Pituitary engorgement
C. Myometrial scarring
D. Endometrial hypertrophy
E. Disruption of large segments of the endometrium

[17.4] Which of the following is consistent with Sheehan's syndrome?

A. Diabetes insipidus
B. Lack of LH surge
C. Endometrial hyperplasia
D. Endometriosis

Answers

[17.1] **C.** Intrauterine adhesions are associated with a biphasic basal temperature chart that reflects normal pituitary function and normal ovulation, indicating the presence of progesterone, which elevates the temperature.

[17.2] **B.** Sheehan's syndrome involves the **anterior** pituitary.

[17.3] **E.** Large patches of endometrium are defective due to intrauterine adhesions.

[17.4] **B.** No LH surge is seen with Sheehan's syndrome. Diabetes insipidus is a problem of the posterior pituitary (lack of antidiuretic hormone).

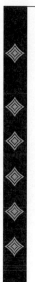

CLINICAL PEARLS

◆ The two most common causes of secondary amenorrhea after postpartum hemorrhage are Sheehan's syndrome and intrauterine adhesions.

◆ A pregnancy test should be the first test in evaluating a woman with secondary amenorrhea.

◆ Normal function of the anterior pituitary points toward intrauterine adhesions.

◆ Hypothyroidism or a monophasic basal body temperature chart suggests Sheehan's syndrome.

◆ The treatment of Sheehan's syndrome is replacement of the hormones governed by the anterior pituitary gland.

◆ The most common cause of ovulatory dysfunction in a reproductive-aged woman is polycystic ovarian syndrome (PCOS). PCOS is characterized by obesity, anovulation, hirsutism, glucose intolerance, and estrogen excess.

REFERENCES

Mishell DR. Primary and secondary amenorrhea. In: Stenchever MA, Droegemueller W, Herbst AL, Mishell DR, eds. Comprehensive gynecology, 4th ed. St. Louis: Mosby-Year Book. 2001:1099–1124.

Schlaff WD and Kletzky OA. Amenorrhea, hyperprolactinemia, and chronic anovulation. In: Hacker NF and Moore JG, eds. Essentials of obstetrics and gynecology, 3rd ed. Philadelphia: Saunders. 1998:583–593.

◈ **CASE 18**

A 22-year-old G3 P2 at 40 weeks' gestation complains of strong uterine contractions. She denies leakage of fluid per vagina. She denies medical illnesses. Her antenatal history is unremarkable. On examination, the BP is 120/80, HR is 85 bpm, and temp is 98°F. The fetal heart rate is in the 140 to 150 bpm range. The cervix is dilated at 5 cm and the vertex is at -3 station. Upon artificial rupture of membranes, fetal bradycardia to the 70 to 80 bpm range is noted for 3 minutes without recovery.

◆ **What is your next step?**

ANSWER TO CASE 18: Fetal Bradycardia (Cord Prolapse)

Summary: A 22-year-old G3 P2 at term is in labor with a cervical dilation of 5-cm dilation; the vertex is at -3 station. Upon artificial rupture of membranes, persistent fetal bradycardia to the 70 to 80 bpm range is noted for 3 minutes.

♦ **Next step:** Vaginal examination to assess for umbilical cord prolapse.

Analysis

Objectives

1. Understand that the first step in the evaluation of fetal bradycardia in the face of rupture of membranes should be to rule out umbilical cord prolapse.
2. Understand that the treatment for cord prolapse is emergent cesarean delivery.
3. Know that an unengaged presenting part, or a transverse fetal lie with rupture of membranes, predisposes to cord prolapse.

Considerations

This patient has had two prior deliveries. She is currently in labor and her cervix is 5-cm dilated. The fetal vertex is at –3 station, indicating that the fetal head is unengaged. With artificial rupture of membranes, fetal bradycardia is noted. This situation is very typical for a cord prolapse, where the umbilical cord protrudes through the cervical os. Usually, the fetal head will fill the pelvis and prevent the cord from prolapsing. However, **with an unengaged fetal presentation, such as in this case, umbilical cord accidents are more likely**. Thus, as a general rule, artificial rupture of membranes should be avoided with an unengaged fetal part. Situations such as with a transverse fetal lie or a footling breech presentation are also predisposing conditions. It is not uncommon for a multiparous patient to have an unengaged fetal head during early labor. The lesson in this case is not to rupture membranes with an unengaged fetal presentation. **With fetal bradycardia, the next step would be a digital examination of the vagina to assess for the umbilical cord, which would feel like a rope-like structure through the cervical os. If the umbilical cord is palpated and the diagnosis of cord prolapse confirmed, the patient should be taken for immediate cesarean delivery.** The physician should keep his or her hand in the vagina to elevate the presenting part, thus keeping pressure off the cord.

APPROACH TO FETAL BRADYCARDIA

Definitions

Engagement: Largest transverse (biparietal) diameter of the fetal head has negotiated the bony pelvic inlet.

Umbilical cord prolapse: Umbilical cord enters through the cervical os presenting in front of the presenting part.

Artificial rupture of membranes: Maneuver used to cause a rent in the fetal chorioamniotic membranes.

Clinical Approach

The onset of fetal bradycardia should be confirmed either by internal fetal scalp electrode or ultrasound, and distinguished from the maternal pulse rate. The initial steps should be directed at improving maternal oxygenation and delivery of cardiac output to the uterus. These maneuvers include 1) placement of the patient on her side to move the uterus from the great vessels, thus improving blood return to the heart; 2) intravenous fluid bolus if the patient is possibly volume depleted; 3) administration of 100% oxygen by face mask; and 4) stopping oxytocin if it is being given (Table 18–1).

Simultaneously with these maneuvers, the practitioner should try to identify the cause of the bradycardia, such as **hyperstimulation with oxytocin.** With this process, the uterus will be tetanic, or the uterine contractions will be frequent (every 1 min); often a beta agonist, such

Table 18–1
STEPS TO TAKE WITH FETAL BRADYCARDIA

Confirm fetal heart rate (versus maternal heart rate)
Vaginal examination to assess for cord prolapse
Positional changes
Oxygen
Intravenous fluid bolus
Discontinue oxytocin

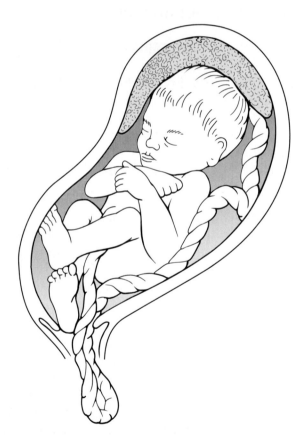

Figure 18–1. Umbilical cord prolapse. A footling breech presentation predisposes to umbilical cord prolapse.

as terbutaline, given intravenously will be helpful. Hypotension due to an epidural catheter is another common cause. Intravenous hydration is the first remedy, and if unsuccessful, then support of the blood pressure with ephedrine, a pressor agent, is often useful. A vaginal examination when the membranes are ruptured is "a must" to identify overt umbilical cord prolapse. A rope-like cord will be palpated, often with pulsations (Figure 18–1). **The best treatment is elevation of the presenting part digitally, and emergent cesarean delivery.** In women with prior cesarean delivery, uterine rupture may manifest as fetal bradycardia.

Comprehension Questions

[18.1] An 18-year-old woman who had undergone a previous low-transverse cesarean delivery is admitted for active labor. During labor, an intrauterine pressure catheter displays normal uterine contractions every 3 min with intensity up to 60 mm Hg. Fetal bradycardia ensues. Which of the following statements is most accurate?

A. The normal intrauterine pressure catheter display makes uterine rupture unlikely.
B. The most common sign of uterine rupture is a fetal heart rate abnormality.
C. If the patient has a uterine rupture, the practitioner should wait to see whether the heart tones return to decide on route of delivery.
D. The intrauterine pressure catheter has been found to be helpful in preventing uterine rupture.

[18.2] Umbilical cord prolapse is least common with which one of the following?

A. Transverse lie
B. Footling breech presentation
C. Frank breech presentation
D. Complete breech presentation
E. Oblique lie

[18.3] Each of the following maneuvers improves oxygenation to the placenta except:

    A. Supine position
    B. Correct hypotension
    C. Correct hypoxia
    D. Stop oxytocin

[18.4] A 33-year-old G2 P1 woman at 39 weeks' gestation in active labor is noted to have a 1-min episode of bradycardia on the external fetal heart rate tracing in the range of 100 bpm, which has not resolved. Her cervix is closed. Which of the following is the best initial step in management of this patient?

    A. Fetal scalp pH assessment
    B. Emergency cesarean delivery
    C. Intravenous atropine
    D. Intravenous terbutaline
    E. Assess maternal pulse

Answers

[18.1] **B.** The most common finding in a uterine rupture is a fetal heart rate abnormality, such as fetal bradycardia, deep variable decelerations, or late decelerations; the intrauterine pressure catheter has not been found to be helpful and sometimes confuses the picture and may delay the diagnosis of uterine rupture. Immediate cesarean section is indicated for suspected uterine rupture.

[18.2] **C.** With the frank breech (hips flexed and knees extended), the buttocks fill the pelvis and decrease the risk of cord prolapse.

[18.3] **A.** The supine position causes uterine compression on the vena cava, which decreases the venous return of blood to the heart, leading to supine hypotension; one important maneuver when encountering fetal heart rate abnormalities is a positional change, such as the lateral decubitus position.

[18.4] **E.** The first step in assessment of the apparent fetal bradycardia is differentiating the heart rate from the maternal pulse.

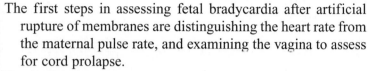

CLINICAL PEARLS

◈ The first steps in assessing fetal bradycardia after artificial rupture of membranes are distinguishing the heart rate from the maternal pulse rate, and examining the vagina to assess for cord prolapse.

◈ The best therapy for umbilical cord prolapse is elevation of the presenting part and emergency cesarean delivery.

◈ The risk of cord prolapse with a vertex presentation or frank breech presentation is very low; the risk with a footling breech or transverse lie is substantially higher.

◈ The most common finding with uterine rupture is a fetal heart rate abnormality.

◈ The best treatment for suspected uterine rupture is immediate cesarean delivery.

REFERENCES

Cunningham FG, Gant NF, Leveno KJ, Gilstrap LC III, Hauth JC, Wenstrom KD. Intrapartum assessment. In: Williams obstetrics, 21st ed. New York: McGraw-Hill. 2001:331–360.

Staisch KJ. Fetal distress assessment during labor. In: Hacker NF and Moore JG, eds. Essentials of obstetrics and gynecology, 3rd ed. Philadelphia: Saunders. 1998:290–297.

◈ **CASE 19**
_____

A 30-year-old parous woman notes a watery breast discharge of 6 months' duration. Her menses have been somewhat irregular. She denies a family history of breast cancer. The patient had been treated previously with radioactive iodine for Grave's disease. Currently, she is not taking any medications. On examination, she appears alert and in good health. The BP is 120/80 and HR is 80 bpm. The breasts are symmetric and without masses. No skin retraction is noted. A white discharge can be expressed from both breasts. No adenopathy is appreciated. The pregnancy test is negative.

◆ **What is the most likely diagnosis?**

◆ **What is your next step?**

ANSWERS TO CASE 19: Galactorrhea Due to Hypothyroidism

Summary: A 30-year-old parous woman with irregular menses notes a watery breast discharge of 6 months' duration. She had been treated previously with radioactive iodine for Grave's disease. The pregnancy test is negative.

◆ **Most likely diagnosis:** Galactorrhea due to hypothyroidism.

◆ **Next step:** Check serum prolactin and TSH levels.

Analysis

Objectives

1. Know the clinical presentation of galactorrhea.
2. Know some of the major causes of hyperprolactinemia.
3. Understand that hyperprolactinemia can induce hypothalamic dysfunction leading to oligo-ovulation and irregular menses.

Considerations

This patient complains of oligomenorrhea and a white, watery breast discharge, which is likely to be milk (galactorrhea). The first investigation should be a pregnancy test. Causes of galactorrhea include a pituitary adenoma, pregnancy, breast stimulation, chest wall trauma, or hypothyroidism. She does not have headaches or visual disturbances. This woman had been treated previously with radioactive iodine for Grave's disease and is not taking thyroid replacement. Thus, she likely has hypothyroidism. With primary hypothyroidism, both the thyroid-releasing hormone (TRH) and thyroid-stimulating hormone (TSH) are elevated. TRH acts as a prolactin-releasing hormone. Hence, elevated TSH and prolactin levels will be noted in this patient. The hyperprolactinemia inhibits hypothalamic GnRH pulsations, leading to oligomenorrhea.

APPROACH TO GALACTORRHEA

Definitions

Galactorrhea: Nonpuerperal watery or milky breast secretion that contains neither pus nor blood. The secretion can be manifested spontaneously or obtained only by breast examination.

Pituitary secreting adenoma: A tumor in the pituitary gland that produces prolactin; symptoms include galactorrhea, headache, and peripheral vision defect (bitemporal hemianopsia).

Clinical Approach

Galactorrhea is a milky breast secretion that occurs in a nonlactating patient. It is usually bilateral. To determine if the breast discharge is truly galactorrhea, a smear under microscope will reveal multiple fat droplets. Patients with galactorrhea often have associated oligomenorrhea or amenorrhea. See Table 19–1 for the different etiologies for hyperprolactinemia.

Galactorrhea and hyperprolactinemia require a careful diagnostic approach. A thorough history and physical should be done. All med-

Table 19–1
CAUSES OF HYPERPROLACTINEMIA

Drugs (tranquilizers, tricyclic antidepressants, antihypertensives, narcotics, OCPs)
Hypothyroidism
Hypothalamic causes (craniopharyngioma, sarcoidosis, histiocytosis, leukemia)
Pituitary causes [microadenoma (< 1 cm), macroadenoma (> 1 cm)]
Hyperplasia of the lactotrophs
Empty sella syndrome
Acromegaly
Renal disease (acute or chronic)
Chest surgery or trauma (breast implants, herpes zoster at the T2 dermatome of the chest)

ications that can stimulate prolactin production should be discontinued. **A magnetic resonance scan is the most sensitive test** to detect pituitary adenomas, providing 1-mm resolution; it can detect virtually all microadenomas. The TRH test is useful for patients with mildly elevated hyperprolactinemia (in the range of 20 to 60ng/mL). Those with a markedly high prolactin level, or those with neurologic symptoms, should have MRI of the pituitary. **Hyperprolactinemia is a common cause of menstrual disturbances.** Hence, a woman with galactorrhea, regular menses, and normal serum prolactin is at low risk for having a prolactinoma. These patients can be followed with annual serum prolactin tests. However, even in the face of normal prolactin assays, women with **oligomenorrhea and galactorrhea** should undergo an anteroposterior and lateral coned-down view of the sella turcica. If necessary, a skull MRI will confirm the diagnosis of empty sella. Patients with secondary amenorrhea and low levels of serum estrogen (<40 pg/mL) have a significantly greater risk of having a pituitary adenoma as well as early onset of **osteoporosis.**

Women with galactorrhea but normal menses and normal serum prolactin levels may be observed. Also, patients with microadenomas who do not wish to conceive and without estrogen deficiency may be expectantly managed. Other patients with pituitary adenomas may be offered medical management versus surgery.

Primary hypothyroidism can lead to hyperprolactinemia and should be treated with thyroxine. Patients with hyperprolactinemia and low estrogen levels were once treated with bromocriptine. However, compliance with this medication was low due to the side effects (orthostatic hypotension, fainting, dizziness, and nausea and vomiting) and high cost. Another alternative is exogenous estrogen. Bromocriptine is particularly useful for patients desiring fertility. Patients with hyperprolactinemia with or without microadenoma with adequate estrogen levels (> 40 pg/mL) and who do not desire pregnancy should be treated with periodic progestin withdrawal.

Surgery involves transsphenoidal microsurgical exploration of the sella turcica with removal of the pituitary adenoma while preserving the functional capacity of the remaining gland. Complications of the surgery include transient diabetes insipidus (occurs in about one-third), hemorrhage, meningitis, cerebrospinal fluid leak, and panhypopituitarism. Cure rate is directly related to the pretreatment prolactin levels (prolactin level of < 100 ng/mL has an excellent prognosis, whereas >200 ng/mL has a poor prognosis). It may be preferable to reduce the size of the macroadenoma with bromocriptine before surgical removal of these tumors. Surgery, which is associated with some adverse effects, is usually reserved as secondary management in patients who have a macroadenoma with complete or partial failure of medical treatment or poor compliance.

Comprehension Questions

[19.1] Each of the following is a cause of hyperprolactinemia except:

    A. Pituitary adenoma
    B. Chest wall trauma
    C. Pregnancy
    D. Hyperthyroidism

[19.2] Each of the following clinical presentations is consistent with a pituitary adenoma except:

    A. Headaches
    B. Galactorrhea
    C. Central visual defect
    D. Amenorrhea

[19.3] Each of the following is a hormone contained in the anterior pituitary gland except:

    A. Follicle-stimulating hormone (FSH)
    B. Prolactin
    C. Thyroid-stimulating hormone (TSH)
    D. Oxytocin

[19.4] A 33-year-old woman with a microadenoma of the pituitary gland becomes pregnant. When she reaches 28 weeks' gestation, she complains of headaches and visual disturbances. Which of the following is the best therapy?

A. Craniotomy and pituitary resection
B. Tamoxifen therapy
C. Oral bromocriptine therapy
D. Expectant management
E. Lumbar puncture

Answers

[19.1] **D.** Hypothyroidism leads to hyperprolactinemia, not hyperthyroidism.

[19.2] **C.** Pituitary adenomas impinge on the optic chiasm, causing deficits of the peripheral vision (bitemporal hemianopsia) and not the central visual field.

[19.3] **D.** Oxytocin and antidiuretic hormone are posterior pituitary hormones.

[19.4] **C.** Bromocriptine therapy is indicated during pregnancy if symptoms (such as headache or visual field abnormalities) arise.

CLINICAL PEARLS

 Galactorrhea in the face of normal menses and a normal prolactin level may be observed.
 The first evaluation in a woman with oligomenorrhea and galactorrhea should be a pregnancy test.
 Osteoporosis is a danger with hypoestrogenemia due to hyperprolactinemia.
 Hypothyroidism can lead to hyperprolactinemia and galactorrhea.
 MRI is the most sensitive imaging test to assess pituitary adenomas.

REFERENCES

Mishell DR. Hyperprolactinemia, galactorrhea, and pituitary adenomas. In: Stenchever MA, Droegemueller W, Herbst AL, Mishell DR, eds. Comprehensive gynecology,. 4th ed. St. Louis: Mosby-Year Book. 2001:1125–1142.

Shlaff WD and Kletzty OA. Amenorrhea, hyperprolactinemia, and chronic anovulation. In: Hacker NF and Moore JG, eds. Essentials of obstetrics and gynecology, 3rd ed. Philadelphia: Saunders. 1998:585–589.

A 24-year-old G1 P0 at 28 weeks' gestation complains of a 2-week duration of generalized pruritus. She denies rashes, exposures to insects, or allergies. Her medications include prenatal vitamins and iron supplementation. On examination, her BP is 100/60, HR is 80 bpm, and weight is 140 lb. She is anicteric. The skin is without rashes. The fetal heart tones are in the 140-bpm range.

♦ **What is the most likely diagnosis?**

ANSWERS TO CASE 20: Pruritus (Cholestasis) of Pregnancy

Summary: A 24-year-old G1 P0 at 28 weeks' gestation complains of a 2-week duration of generalized pruritus. She is anicteric and nor-motensive. The skin is without rashes. The fetal heart tones are in the 140-bpm range.

◆ **Most likely diagnosis:** Cholestasis of pregnancy.

Analysis

Objectives

1. Know the differential diagnosis of pruritus in pregnancy.
2. Understand the clinical presentation of cholestasis of pregnancy.
3. Know that the first line of treatment of cholestasis of pregnancy is an oral antihistamine.

Considerations

This 24-year-old woman, who is at 28 weeks' gestational age, com-plains of generalized pruritus. The systemic location of the itching and lack of rash makes a contact dermatitis unlikely. Another cause of pru-ritus unique to pregnancy is pruritic urticarial papules and plaques of pregnancy (PUPPP), which are erythematous papules and hives begin-ning in the abdominal area and often spreading to the buttocks. This is unlikely, as the patient does not have a rash. This patient's clinical pic-ture does not resemble herpes gestationalis, a condition causing in-tense itching but associated with erythematous blisters on the ab-domen and extremities. Thus, the most likely etiology in this case is intrahepatic cholestasis, a process in which bile salts are incompletely cleared by the liver, accumulate in the body, and are deposited in the dermis, causing pruritus. This disorder usually begins in the third trimester. There are no associated skin rashes, other than excoriations from patient scratching.

APPROACH TO PRURITUS IN PREGNANCY

Definitions

Cholestasis in pregnancy: Intrahepatic cholestasis of unknown etiology in pregnancy whereby the patient usually complains of pruritus with or without jaundice and no skin rash.

Pruritic urticarial papules and plaques of pregnancy (PUPPP): A common skin condition of unknown etiology unique to pregnancy characterized by intense pruritus and erythematous papules on the abdomen and extremities.

Herpes gestationalis: Rare skin condition only seen in pregnancy; it is characterized by intense itching and vesicles on the abdomen and extremities.

Clinical Approach

Pruritus in pregnancy may be caused by many disorders, of which one of the most common is intrahepatic cholestasis of pregnancy, a condition that usually begins in the third trimester. It begins as mild pruritus **without lesions,** usually at night, and gradually increases in severity. The itching is usually more severe on the extremities than on the trunk. It may recur in subsequent pregnancies and with the ingestion of oral contraceptives, suggesting a hormone-related pathogenesis. The disease is common in some ethnic populations such as Swedes, suggesting a genetic basis for the disease process. Increased levels of circulating bile acids confirm the diagnosis. Elevated liver function tests are uncommon and there are no hepatic sequelae in the mother. Cholestasis of pregnancy must be distinguished from viral hepatitis and other causes of pruritus or liver disease. **Cholestasis of pregnancy, especially when accompanied by jaundice, is associated with an increased incidence of prematurity, fetal distress, and fetal loss.** There is also an increased incidence of gallstones associated with the pruritus of pregnancy. The first line of treatment has traditionally been **antihistamines** and cornstarch baths. Other treatments include the bile salt binder, cholestyramine.

Herpes gestationalis, which has no relationship to herpes simplex virus, is a pruritic bullous disease of the skin. It usually begins in the second trimester of pregnancy and the reported incidence is less than 1 in 1000 pregnancies. The etiology is thought to be autoimmune related. The presence of IgG autoantibody directed at the basement membrane has been demonstrated and may result in activation of the classic complement pathway by autoantibodies directed against the basement membrane zone. The clinical features are characterized by intense pruritus followed by extensive patches of cutaneous erythema and subsequent formation of small vesicles and tense bullae. The limbs are affected more often than the trunk. Definitive diagnosis is made by immunofluorescent examination of biopsy specimens. There have been reports of an increased incidence of fetal growth retardation and stillbirth. Transient neonatal herpes gestationalis has also been reported at birth. Treatment has primarily been the use of oral corticosteroids.

The lesions of PUPPP usually begin on the abdomen and spread to the thighs and sometimes the buttocks and arms. The lesions, as their name describes, consist of erythematous urticarial plaques and small papules surrounded by a narrow, pale halo. The incidence of PUPPP is less than 1% of pregnant women. Immunofluorescent studies are negative for both IgG and complement. Histologic findings consist of normal epidermis accompanied by a superficial perivascular infiltrate of lymphocytes and histiocytes associated with edema of the papillary dermis. There are no studies to suggest an adverse effect on fetal and maternal outcome. Therapy includes topical steroids and antihistamines.

Comprehension Questions

[20.1] Each of the following is consistent with intrahepatic cholestasis of pregnancy except:

A. Hepatic transaminase levels in the 2000 U/L range
B. May be associated with jaundice
C. May be associated with an increased perinatal morbidity
D. Almost always resolves after delivery

[20.2] Which of the following best describes the pregnancy outcome with pruritic urticarial papules and plaques of pregnancy (PUPPP)?

A. Somewhat increased perinatal morbidity and mortality
B. Increased preterm delivery rate
C. Increased preeclampsia
D. No effect on pregnancy

[20.3] A 33-year-old woman G1 P0 at 39 weeks' gestation is in labor. She has been diagnosed with herpes gestationalis with the characteristic pruritus and vesicular lesions on the abdomen. Which of the following precautions is best advised for this patient?

A. Cesarean delivery is indicated.
B. Neonatal lesions may be noted and will resolve.
C. Vaginal delivery is permissible if the lesions are not in the introitus region and provided that oral acyclovir is given to the baby.
D. Tocolysis and oral steroid use is advisable until the lesions are healed.

Answers

[20.1] **A.** The hepatic enzymes are normally less than 35 U/L; women with intrahepatic cholestasis may have slightly elevated levels but almost never in the thousands.

[20.2] **D.** PUPPP is not thought to be associated with adverse pregnancy outcomes

[20.3] **B.** Neonatal lesions are sometimes seen with herpes gestationalis, and will resolve. Herpes gestationalis is not the same as herpes simplex virus. The latter would necessitate cesarean delivery to avoid infection to the baby.

CLINICAL PEARLS

◆ The most common cause of generalized pruritus in pregnancy in the absence of skin lesions is cholestasis of pregnancy.

◆ Cholestatic jaundice in pregnancy may be associated with increased adverse pregnancy outcomes.

◆ The lesions of PUPPP usually begin on the abdomen and spread to the thighs and sometimes the buttocks and arms.

REFERENCES

Nuwayhid B, Nguyen T, Khalife S. Medical complications of pregnancy. In: Hacker NF and Moore JG, eds. Essentials of obstetrics and gynecology, 3rd ed. Philadelphia: Saunders. 1998:261–262.

Cunningham FG, Gant NF, Leveno KJ, Gilstrap LC III, Hauth JC, Wenstrom KD. Gastrointestinal disorders In: Williams obstetrics, 21st ed. New York: McGraw-Hill. 2001:1283–1285 and 1431–1434.

CASE 21

A 23-year-old G0 P0 woman complains of lower abdominal tenderness and subjective fever. She states that her last menstrual period started 5 days previously and was heavier than usual. She also complains of dyspareunia of recent onset. She denies vaginal discharge or prior sexually transmitted diseases. On examination, her temp is 100.8°F, BP 90/70, and HR is 90 bpm. Her heart and lung examinations are normal. The abdomen has slight lower abdominal tenderness. No costovertebral angle tenderness is noted. On pelvic examination, the external genitalia are normal. The cervix is somewhat hyperemic, and the uterus as well as adnexa are exquisitely tender. The pregnancy test is negative.

◆ **What is the most likely diagnosis?**

◆ **What are long-term complications that can occur with this condition?**

ANSWERS TO CASE 21: Salpingitis, Acute

Summary: A 23-year-old G0 P0 nonpregnant woman complains of lower abdominal tenderness, subjective fever, heavier menses than usual, and dyspareunia. Her temperature is 100.8°F. The cervix is hyperemic, and the uterus and adnexa are exquisitely tender.

◆ **Most likely diagnosis:** Pelvic inflammatory disease (PID).

◆ **Long-term complications that can occur with this condition:** Infertility or ectopic pregnancy.

Analysis

Objectives

1. Understand the clinical diagnostic criteria of salpingitis.
2. Understand that the long-term complications of salpingitis are infertility, ectopic pregnancy, and chronic pelvic pain.
3. Know that one of the outpatient treatment regimens of salpingitis is intramuscular ceftriaxone and oral doxycycline.

Considerations

This nulliparous woman has lower abdominal pain, adnexal tenderness, and cervical motional tenderness. The presence of cervical motion tenderness is indirect, based on the dyspareunia and hyperemic cervix. The patient also has fever. These are the clinical criteria for pelvic inflammatory disease or salpingitis (infection of the fallopian tubes). Salpingitis is most commonly caused by pathogenic bacteria of the endocervix, which ascend to the tubes. The fallopian tubes can become damaged by the infection, leading to tubal occlusion and infertility or ectopic pregnancy.

APPROACH TO SALPINGITIS

Definitions

Pelvic inflammatory disease: Synonymous with salpingitis, or infection of the fallopian tubes.

Cervical motion tenderness: Extreme tenderness when the uterine cervix is manipulated digitally, which suggests salpingitis.

Ascending infection: Mechanism of upper genital tract infection whereby the offending microorganisms arise from the lower genital tract.

Tubo-ovarian abscess: Collection of purulent material around the distal tube and ovary, which unlike the typical abscess is often treatable by antibiotic therapy rather than requiring surgical drainage.

Clinical Approach

Pelvic inflammatory disease, or salpingitis, usually **involves *Chlamydia,* gonorrhea, and other vaginal organisms, such as anaerobic bacteria.** The mechanism is usually by ascending infection. A common presentation would be a young, nulliparous female complaining of lower abdominal or pelvic pain and vaginal discharge. At times, the patient may also have fever, and nausea and vomiting if the upper abdomen is involved. The cervix is inflamed and, therefore, the patient often complains of **dyspareunia.**

The diagnosis of acute salpingitis is made clinically **by abdominal tenderness, cervical motion tenderness, and adnexal tenderness (Table 21–1).** Confirmatory tests may include a positive gonorrhea or *Chlamydia* culture, or an ultrasound suggesting a tubo-ovarian abscess. Other diseases that must be considered are acute appendicitis, especially if the patient has right-sided abdominal pain and **ovarian torsion, which usually presents as colicky pain** and is associated with an ovarian cyst on ultrasound. Renal disorders, such as pyelonephritis or nephrolithiasis, must also be considered. Right upper quadrant pain may be seen with salpingitis when perihepatic adhesions are present,

Table 21–1

SIGNS AND SYMPTOMS OF ACUTE SALPINGITIS

Abdominal tenderness
Cervical motion tenderness
Adnexal tenderness
Vaginal discharge
Fever
Pelvic mass on examination or ultrasound

the so-called Fitz-Hugh-Curtis syndrome. When the diagnosis is in doubt, the **best method for confirmation is laparoscopy.** The surgeon would look for purulent discharge exuding from the fimbria of the tubes.

The treatment of acute salpingitis depends on whether the patient is a candidate for inpatient versus outpatient therapy. Criteria for outpatient management include low-grade fever, tolerance of oral medication, and the absence of peritoneal signs. The woman must also be compliant. One regimen consists **of intramuscular ceftriaxone, as a single injection, and oral doxycycline** twice a day for 10 to 14 days. It is paramount to reevaluate the patient in 48 hr for improvement. If the patient fails outpatient therapy, or is pregnant, or at the extremes of age, or cannot tolerate oral medication, she would be a candidate for inpatient therapy. One such therapeutic combination is **intravenous cefotetan and doxycycline.** Again, if the patient does not improve within 48 to 72 hr, the clinician should consider laparoscopy to assess the disease.

One important sequelae of salpingitis is tubo-ovarian abscess (TOA). This disorder generally has anaerobic predominance and necessitates the corresponding antibiotic coverage (clindamycin or metronidazole). The physical examination may suggest an adnexal mass, or the ultrasound may reveal a complex ovarian mass. A devastating complication of TOA is **rupture, which is a surgical emergency,** and one that leads to mortality if unattended.

Long-term complications of salpingitis include chronic pelvic pain, involuntary infertility, and ectopic pregnancy. The risk of infertility due to tubal damage is directly related to the number of episodes of PID. The intrauterine contraceptive device (IUD) places the patient at greater risk for PID; whereas oral contraceptive agents (progestin thickens the cervical mucus) decrease the risk of PID.

Comprehension Questions

[21.1] Each of the following are organisms that are commonly cultured from the tubes infected with salpingitis except:

A. *Neisseria gonorrhoeae*
B. *Chlamydia trachomatis*
C. *Peptostreptococcus* species
D. *Treponema pallidum*

[21.2] Which of the following is the most accurate method of diagnosing acute salpingitis?

A. Clinical criteria
B. Sonography
C. CT scan
D. Laparoscopy

[21.3] Each of the following is a risk factor for developing PID except:

A. Nulliparity
B. Multiple sexual partners
C. Oral contraceptive agents
D. Douching

[21.4] A 33-year-old woman with an intrauterine contraceptive device develops symptoms of acute salpingitis. On laparoscopy, sulfur granules appear at the fimbria of the tubes. Which of the following is the most likely organism?

A. *Chlamydia trachomatis*
B. *Norcardia* species
C. *Neisseria gonorrhoeae*
D. *Treponema pallidum*
E. *Actinomyces* species

Answers

[21.1] **D.** Syphilis is not a common cause of salpingitis.

[21.2] **D.** Laparoscopy is considered the "gold standard" in diagnosing salpingitis.

[21.3] **C.** Oral contraceptive agents decrease the risk of PID by virtue of the progestin thickening the cervical mucus and thinning the endometrium.

[21.4] **E.** Sulfur granules are classic for *Actinomyces,* which occurs more often in the presence of an IUD. *Actinomyces israelii* is a gram-positive anaerobe, which is generally sensitive to penicillin.

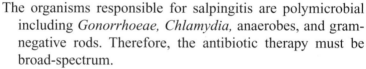
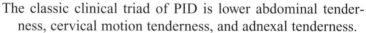

CLINICAL PEARLS

❖ The organisms responsible for salpingitis are polymicrobial including *Gonorrhoeae, Chlamydia,* anaerobes, and gram-negative rods. Therefore, the antibiotic therapy must be broad-spectrum.

❖ The classic clinical triad of PID is lower abdominal tenderness, cervical motion tenderness, and adnexal tenderness.

❖ Laparoscopy is the "gold standard" in the diagnosis of acute salpingitis, by the operator visualizing purulent drainage from the fallopian tubes.

❖ Long-term sequelae of acute salpingitis include chronic pelvic pain, ectopic pregnancy, and involuntary infertility.

REFERENCES

Droegemueller W. Infections of the upper genital tract. In: Stenchever MA, Droegemueller W, Herbst AL, Mishell DR, eds. Comprehensive gynecology, 4th ed. St. Louis: Mosby-Year Book. 2001:641–706.

McGregor JA. Pelvic inflammatory disease. In: Hacker NF and Moore JG, eds. Essentials of obstetrics and gynecology, 3rd ed. Philadelphia: Saunders. 1998:446–454.

A 19-year-old G1 P0 woman at 20 weeks' gestation complains of the acute onset of pleuritic chest pain and severe dyspnea. She denies a history of reactive airway disease or cough. On examination, her temp is 98°F, HR 120 bpm, BP 130/70, and respiratory rate (RR) 40/min. The lung examination reveals clear lungs bilaterally. The heart examination shows tachycardia. The fetal heart tones are in the 140–150-bpm range.

◆ **What test would most likely lead to the diagnosis?**

◆ **What is your concern?**

ANSWERS TO CASE 22: Pulmonary Embolus in Pregnancy

Summary: A 19-year-old G1 P0 woman at 20 weeks' gestation complains of the acute onset of pleuritic chest pain and severe dyspnea. On examination, her HR is 120 bpm and RR 40/min. The lung examination reveals clear lungs bilaterally.

◆ **Test most likely to lead to the diagnosis:** Ventilation-perfusion scan.

◆ **Your concern:** Pulmonary embolism.

Analysis

Considerations

This 19-year-old woman at 20 weeks' gestation complains of the acute onset of severe dyspnea and pleuritic chest pain. The physical examination confirms the respiratory distress due to the tachycardia and tachypnea. The lungs are clear on auscultation, which rules out reactive airway disease or significant pneumonia. The patient also does not complain of cough or fever, further making pneumonia unlikely. Clear lungs also speak against pulmonary edema. Thus, the most likely diagnosis and concern is pulmonary embolism. Although many diagnostic tests should be considered in the initial evaluation of a patient with respiratory distress (such as arterial blood gas, chest radiograph, electrocardiograph), in this case the ventilation-perfusion scan would most likely lead to the diagnosis. If the V-Q scan confirms pulmonary embolism, then the patient should receive anticoagulation to help stabilize the deep venous thrombosis and decrease the likelihood of further embolization. **Pregnancy causes venous stasis due to the mechanical effect of the uterus on the vena cava; additionally, the high estrogen level induces a hypercoagulable state** due to the increase in clotting factors, particularly fibrinogen.

Objectives

1. Understand that pleuritic chest pain and severe dyspnea are common presenting symptoms of pulmonary embolism.
2. Know that the pregnant woman is predisposed to deep venous thrombosis due to venous obstruction and a hypercoagulable state.
3. Understand that the ventilation-perfusion scan is an initial diagnostic test for pulmonary embolism.

APPROACH TO RESPIRATORY DISTRESS IN PREGNANCY

Definitions

Deep venous thrombosis: Blood clot involving the deep veins of the lower extremity, rather than just the superficial involvement of the saphenous system.
Pulmonary embolus: Blood clot that is lodged in the pulmonary arterial circulation, usually arising from a thrombus of the lower extremity or pelvis.
Ventilation-perfusion scan-imaging procedure: Using a small amount of intravenous radioactively tagged albumin, such as technetium, in conjunction with a ventilation imaging, with inhaled xenon or technetium, in an effort to find large ventilation-perfusion mismatches suggestive of pulmonary embolism.

Clinical Approach

Respiratory distress is an acute emergency and necessitates rapid assessment and therapy. Oxygen is the most important substrate for the human body, and even 5 or 10 min of hypoxemia can lead to devastating consequences. Hence, a quick evaluation of the patient's respiratory condition, including the respiratory rate and effort; use of accessory muscles, such as intercostal and supraclavicular muscles; anxiety; and cyanosis; may indicate mild or severe disease. (See Figure 22–1 for one

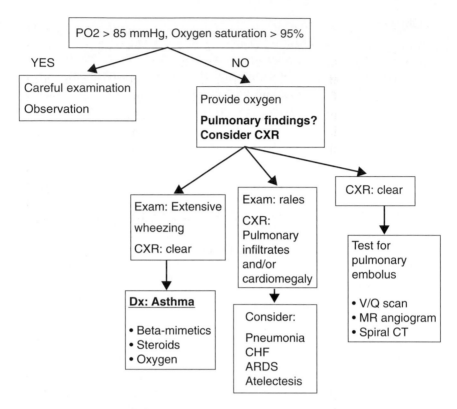

Figure 22–1.   Algorithm for evaluating dyspnea in pregnancy.

algorithm to evaluate dyspnea in pregnancy). **The highest priority is to identify impending respiratory failure,** since this condition would require immediate intubation and mechanical ventilation. Pulse oximetry and arterial blood gas studies should be ordered while information is gathered during the history and physical. A cursory and targeted history directed at the pulmonary or cardiac organs, such as a history of reactive airway disease, exposure to anaphylactoid stimuli such as penicillin or bee sting, chest trauma, cardiac valvular disease, chest pain, or palpitations, are important. Meanwhile, the physical examination should be directed at the heart and lung evaluation. The heart should be assessed for cardiomegaly and valvular disorders, and the lungs should be auscultated for wheezes, rhonchi, rales, or absent breath sounds. The abdomen, back, and skin should also be examined.

A pulse oximetry reading of less than 90% corresponds to an oxygen tension of less than 60 mm Hg. Supplemental oxygen should immediately be given. An arterial blood gas should be obtained to assess for hypoxemia, carbon dioxide retention, and acid–base status. A chest radiograph should be performed rather expeditiously to differentiate cardiac versus pulmonary causes of hypoxemia. A large cardiac silhouette may indicate peripartum cardiomyopathy, which is treated by diuretic and inotropic therapy; pulmonary infiltrates may indicate pneumonia or pulmonary edema. A clear chest radiograph in the face of hypoxemia suggests pulmonary embolism, although early in the course of pneumonia, the chest x-ray may appear normal.

The diagnosis of pulmonary embolism may be made presumptively on the basis of the clinical presentation, hypoxemia on arterial blood gas analysis, and a clear chest x-ray. Intravenous heparin may be initiated to stabilize the deep venous thrombosis, which is usually located in the pelvis or lower extremity. A ventilation-perfusion scan confirms the diagnosis. Once the diagnosis of acute thromboembolism is confirmed, the pregnant woman is usually placed on full intravenous anticoagulation therapy for 5 to 7 days. After, the therapy is generally switched to subcutaneous therapy to maintain the aPTT at 1.5 to 2.5 times control for at least 3 months after the acute event. Low-molecular-weight heparin can also be utilized. After 3 months, either full heparinization or "prophylactic heparinization" can be utilized for the remainder of the pregnancy and for 6 weeks postpartum. Newer imaging tests that are more sensitive for pulmonary embolism include magnetic resonance angiography and spiral computer tomographic evaluation.

Usually, the pregnant woman is placed on prophylactic low-dose heparin for the remainder of pregnancy and up to 6 weeks postpartum. Estrogen products, such as oral contraceptive agents, are relatively contraindicated. Prophylactic anticoagulation for future pregnancies is more controversial, but often is used. Although pregnancy itself may induce thrombosis, many experts advise obtaining tests for other causes of thrombosis such as Leiden factor V mutation, antiphospholipid syndrome, or other thrombophilias.

Comprehension Questions

[22.1] Which of the following is the most common presenting symptom of pulmonary embolism?

   A. Dyspnea
   B. Chest pain
   C. Palpitations
   D. Hemoptysis
   E. Sudden death

[22.2] Which of the following is the most common cause of maternal mortality?

   A. Hemorrhage
   B. Embolism
   C. Hypertensive disease
   D. Sepsis
   E. Ectopic pregnancy

[22.3] Which of the following is the most common ECG finding of pulmonary embolism?

   A. Tachycardia
   B. Right axis deviation
   C. Right bundle branch block
   D. S wave in lead III
   E. QT interval prolongation

[22.4] Each of the following is a risk factor for deep venous thrombosis except:

   A. Gynecologic surgery
   B. Bed rest
   C. Pregnancy
   D. Depomedroxyprogesterone acetate (Depoprovera)

[22.5] Which of the following arterial blood gas readings is most likely that of a pregnant woman at 22 weeks' gestation?

	pH	PO_2 (mm Hg)	PCO_2 (mm Hg)	HCO_3 (mEq/L)
A.	7.40	100	40	24
B.	7.45	100	30	21
C.	7.38	85	25	20
D.	7.55	95	35	22

Answers

[22.1] **A.** Dyspnea is the most common symptom of pulmonary embolus, whereas tachypnea is the most common sign.

[22.2] **B.** Including amniotic fluid embolism and thromboembolism.

[22.3] **A.** Although an S wave in lead I, Q wave in lead III, and right axis deviation may be seen, tachycardia is the most common electrocardiographic abnormality associated with pulmonary embolism.

[22.4] **D.** Depoprovera is a progestin and is not a major cause of deep venous thrombosis.

[22.5] **B.** The pregnant woman has a respiratory alkalosis with partial metabolic compensation.

CLINICAL PEARLS

 The diagnosis of pulmonary embolism is suspected in a patient with dyspnea, a clear chest radiograph, and hypoxemia. It is confirmed with imaging tests such as ventilation-perfusion scan or spiral CT scan.

 The most common presenting symptom of pulmonary embolism is dyspnea.

 The most common cause of maternal mortality is embolism (both thromboembolism and amniotic fluid embolism).

 A PO2 of less than 80 mm Hg in a pregnant woman is abnormal.

 Anticoagulation is the best treatment of deep venous thrombosis or pulmonary embolism.

REFERENCES

Cunningham FG, Gant NF, Leveno KJ, Gilstrap LC III, Hauth JC, Wenstrom KD. Pulmonary disorders. In: Williams obstetrics, 21st ed. New York: McGraw-Hill. 2001:1236–1240.

Nuwayhid B, Nguyen T, Khalife S. Medical complications of pregnancy. In: Hacker NF and Moore JG, eds. Essentials of obstetrics and gynecology, 3rd ed. Philadelphia: Saunders. 1998:237–239.

American College of Obstetricians and Gynecologists. Thromboembolism in pregnancy. Practice Bulletin No. 19, August 2000.

A 31-year-old G3 P2 woman at 39 weeks' gestation arrives at the labor and delivery area complaining of strong uterine contractions of 4-hr duration; her membranes ruptured 2 ago. She has a history of herpes simplex virus infections. She denies any blisters, and her last herpetic outbreak was 4 months ago. She notes a 1-day history of tingling in the perineal area. On examination, her BP is 110/60, temperature is 99°F, and HR is 80 bpm. Her lungs are clear to auscultation. Her abdomen reveals a fundal height of 40 cm. The fetal heart rate is 140 bpm, reactive, and without decelerations. The external genitalia are normal without evidence of lesions. The vagina, cervix, and perianal region are normal in appearance. The vaginal fluid is consistent with rupture of membranes.

◆ **What is your next step?**

◆ **What is the most likely diagnosis?**

ANSWERS TO CASE 23: Herpes Simplex Virus Infection in Labor

Summary: A 31-year-old G3 P2 woman at 39 weeks' gestation is in labor and her membranes ruptured 2 hours ago. She has a history of herpes simplex virus (HSV) infections. She has a 1-day history of tingling in the perineal area.

◆ **Next step:** Counsel patient about risks of neonatal HSV infection and offer a cesarean delivery.

◆ **Most likely diagnosis:** Herpes simplex virus recurrence with prodromal symptoms.

Analysis

Objectives

1. Understand the indications for cesarean delivery due to herpes simplex virus.
2. Know that herpes simplex virus may cause neonatal encephalitis.
3. Understand that symptoms of prodromal infection may indicate viral shedding.

Considerations

The patient is in labor and has experienced rupture of membranes. She has a history of herpes simplex virus infections. Although she has no lesions visible and is taking acyclovir suppressive therapy, she complains of tingling of the perineal region. These symptoms are sufficient to suggest an HSV outbreak. With herpes simplex virus shedding of the genital tract, there is risk of neonatal infection, especially encephalitis. The patient should be counseled about the neonatal risks, and offered cesarean delivery.

APPROACH TO HERPES SIMPLEX VIRUS IN PREGNANCY

Definitions

Herpes simplex virus prodromal symptoms: Prior to the outbreak of the classic vesicles, the patient may complain of burning, itching, or tingling.

Neonatal herpes infection: HSV can cause disseminated infection with major organ involvement; be confined to encephalitis, eyes, skin or mucosa; or be asymptomatic.

Clinical Approach

Herpes cultures are not useful in the acute management of pregnant women who present in labor or with rupture of membranes. They are helpful in making the diagnosis during the prenatal course, when the patient may develop lesions and the diagnosis is in question. **Once a woman has been diagnosed with herpes simplex virus, the practitioner uses his or her best clinical judgment to assess for the presence of HSV in the genital tract during the time of labor.** A meticulous inspection of the external genitalia, vagina, cervix (by speculum examination), and perianal area should be undertaken for the typical herpetic lesions, such as vesicles or ulcers (Figure 23–1). Additionally, the patient should be queried thoroughly about the presence of prodromal symptoms. When there are no lesions or prodromal symptoms, the patient should be counseled that she is at low risk for viral shedding and has an unknown risk of neonatal herpes infection. Almost always, the patient will opt for vaginal delivery under these circumstances. In contrast, **the presence of prodromal symptoms or genital lesions suspicious for HSV is sufficient to warrant a cesarean delivery** to prevent neonatal infection.

The use of suppressive acyclovir therapy is usually reserved for frequent outbreaks. Some practitioners advocate the use of oral suppressive acyclovir when the woman has her first episode of HSV infection during pregnancy. This therapy may decrease the symptoms during the time of labor, and decrease the need for cesarean delivery.

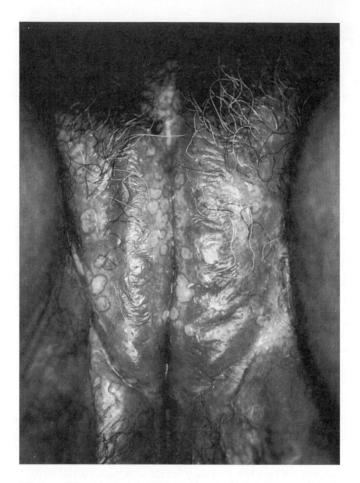

Figure 23–1.   First episode primary genital herpes simplex virus infection.

(Reproduced, with permission, from Cunningham FG et al. Williams obstetrics, 21st ed. New York: McGraw-Hill; 2001: 1495.)

Comprehension Questions

[23.1] Each of the following is an indication for cesarean section due to maternal herpes simplex virus except:

A. Lesions noted on the cervix
B. Lesions noted on the vagina

C. Lesions noted on the posterior thigh
D. Tingling of the perianal region

[23.2] In pregnant women with rupture of membranes, cesarean section is abandoned when the duration since rupture of membranes exceeds which of the following?

A. 2 hr
B. 4 hr
C. 12 hr
D. 24 hr
E. No limit

[23.3] Which of the following is the least likely fetal/neonatal sequelae of herpes simplex virus?

A. Transplacental infection
B. Encephalitis
C. Disseminated neonatal infection
D. Conjunctivitis
E. Gastrointestinal infection

[23.4] Which of the following is the most common cause of an infectious vulvar ulcer disease in the United States?

A. Syphilis
B. Herpes simplex virus
C. Chanchroid
D. Lymphogranuloma venereum
E. Bartholin gland abscess

Answers

[23.1] **C.** The posterior thigh is unlikely to inoculate the baby during delivery.

[23.2] **E.** With suspected active herpes, there is no time limit for duration since rupture of membranes that would cause a practitioner to chose not to perform a cesarean delivery.

[23.3] **A.** Generally, HSV infection inoculates the infant during the labor and delivery process and not via transplacental passage.

[23.4] **B.** HSV is the most common cause of infectious vulvar ulcers in the United States.

CLINICAL PEARLS

 Cesarean delivery should be offered to a woman with a history of HSV who has prodromal symptoms or suspicious lesions of the genital tract.

 Herpes simplex virus is the most common cause of infectious vulvar ulcers in the United States.

The cervix, vagina, and vulva must be inspected carefully for lesions in a laboring patient with a history of herpes simplex virus.

REFERENCES

Cunningham FG, Gant NF, Leveno KJ, Gilstrap LC III, Hauth JC, Wenstrom KD. Sexually transmitted diseases. In: Williams obstetrics, 21st ed. New York: McGraw-Hill. 2001:1494–1498.

Goodman RJ. AIDS and infectious diseases in pregnancy. In: Hacker NF and Moore JG, eds. Essentials of obstetrics and gynecology, 3rd ed. Philadelphia: Saunders. 1998:215–216.

American College of Obstetricians and Gynecologists. Management of herpes in pregnancy. Practice Bulletin No. 8, October 1999.

A 40-year-old G5 P5 woman complains of menorrhagia of 2-yr duration. She states that several years ago a doctor had told her that her
uterus was enlarged. Her records indicate that 1 yr ago she underwent
a uterine dilation and curettage, with the tissue showing benign pathology. She takes ibuprofen without relief of her vaginal bleeding. On examination, her BP is 135/80, HR 80 bpm, and temp is 98°F. The heart
and lung examinations are normal. The abdomen reveals a lower abdominal midline irregular mass. On pelvic examination, the cervix is
anteriorly displaced. An irregular midline mass approximately 18
weeks' size seems to move in conjunction with the cervix. No adnexal
masses are palpated. Her pregnancy test is negative. Her hemoglobin
level is 9.0 g/dL, leukocyte count is 10,000/ mm^3, and platelet count is
160,000/mm^3.

◆ **What is the most likely diagnosis?**

◆ **What is your next step?**

ANSWERS TO CASE 24: Uterine Leiomyomata

Summary: A 40-year-old G5 P5 woman with a history of an enlarged uterus complains of menorrhagia and anemia despite ibuprofen. A prior uterine dilation and curettage showed benign pathology. Examination reveals an irregular midline mass approximately 18 weeks' size that is seemingly contiguous with the cervix and there is an anteriorly displaced cervix.

◆ **Most likely diagnosis:** Symptomatic uterine leiomyomata.

◆ **Next step:** Hysterectomy.

Analysis

Objectives

1. Understand that the most common reason for hysterectomy in the United States is symptomatic uterine fibroids.
2. Know that hysterectomy is reserved for symptomatic uterine fibroids that are refractory to an adequate trial of medical therapy.
3. Know that menorrhagia is the most common symptom of uterine leiomyomata.

Considerations

This 40-year-old woman complains of menorrhagia. The physical examination is consistent with uterine fibroids, because of the enlarged midline mass that is irregular and contiguous with the cervix. If the mass were lateral or moved apart from the cervix, another type of pelvic mass, such as ovarian, would be suspected. This patient complains of **menorrhagia,** which is the most common symptom of uterine fibroids. If she had intermenstrual bleeding, the clinician would have to consider other diseases, such as endometrial hyperplasia, endometrial polyp, or uterine cancer, in addition to the uterine leiomyomata. The patient has anemia despite medical therapy, which constitutes the indication for hysterectomy. If the uterus were smaller, consideration may be given toward another medical agent, such as medroxyprogesterone acetate (Provera). Also, a gonadotropin-releasing hormone agonist (GnRHa) can be used to shrink the fibroids temporarily, to correct the anemia, or make the surgery easier. The maximum shrinkage of fibroids is usually seen after 3 months of GnRH agonist therapy.

APPROACH TO SUSPECTED UTERINE LEIOMYOMATA

Definitions

Leiomyomata: Smooth muscle, benign tumors, usually of the uterus.

Leiomyosarcoma: Malignant, smooth muscle tumor, with numerous mitoses.

Submucous fibroid: Leiomyomata that are primarily on the endometrial side of the uterus and impinge on the uterine cavity (Figure 24–1).

Intramural fibroid: Leiomyomata that are primarily in the uterine muscle.

Subserosal fibroid: Leiomyomata that are primarily on the outside of the uterus, on the serosal surface. Physical examination may reveal a "knobby" sensation.

Pedunculated fibroid: Leiomyoma that is on a stalk.

Carneous degeneration: Changes of the leiomyomata due to rapid growth; the center of the fibroid becomes red, causing pain.

Clinical Approach

Uterine leiomyomata are the most common tumors of the pelvis, and the leading indication for hysterectomy in the United States. They occur in up to 25% of women, and have a variety of clinical presentations. The most common clinical manifestation is **menorrhagia,** or excessive bleeding during menses. The exact mechanism is unclear and may be due to an increased endometrial surface area, or the disruption of

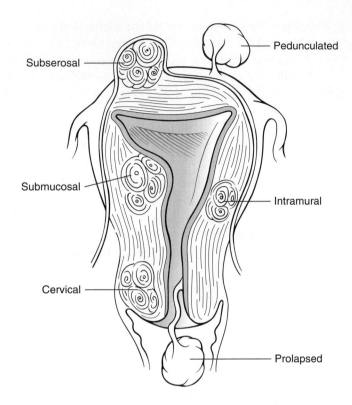

Figure 24–1.   Uterine leiomyomata. Various uterine leiomyomata are depicted based on their location in the uterus.

hemostatic mechanisms during menses by the fibroids. Another speculated explanation is ulceration of the submucosal fibroid surfaces.

Many uterine fibroids are asymptomatic and only need to be monitored. Very rarely, uterine leiomyomata degenerate into **leiomyosarcoma.** Some signs of this process include **rapid growth,** such as an increase of more than 6 weeks' gestational size in 1 yr. A **history of radiation** to the pelvis is a risk factor.

If the uterine leiomyomata is sufficiently large, patients may also complain of pressure to the pelvis, bladder, or rectum. Rarely, the uterine fibroid on a pedicle may twist, leading to necrosis and pain. Also, a **submucous leiomyomata can prolapse through the cervix, leading to labor-like uterine contraction pain.**

The physical examination typical of uterine leiomyomata is an **irregular, midline, firm, nontender mass that moves contiguous with the cervix.** This presentation is approximately 95% accurate. Most of the time, ultrasound examination is performed to confirm the diagnosis. Lateral, fixed, or fluctuant masses are not typical for fibroids.

The initial treatment of uterine fibroids is medical, such as with nonsteroidal anti-inflammatory agents or progestin therapy. **Gonadotropin-releasing hormone agonists** lead to a decrease in uterine fibroid size, reaching its **maximal effect in 3 months.** After the discontinuation of this agent, the leiomyomata usually regrow to the pretreatment size. Thus, GnRH agonist therapy is reserved for tumor shrinkage or correction of anemia prior to operative treatment. Uterine artery ligation and embolization techniques are currently being studied in the treatment of uterine fibroids. The indications for surgery are persistent symptoms despite medical therapy. Significant menorrhagia often leads to anemia.

Comprehension Questions

[24.1] Which of the following types of uterine fibroids would most likely lead to recurrent abortion?

    A. Submucosal
    B. Intramural
    C. Subserous
    D. Parasitic
    E. Pedunculated

[24.2] Which of the following is the most common clinical presentation of uterine leiomyomata?

    A. Infertility
    B. Menorrhagia
    C. Ureteral obstruction
    D. Pelvic pain
    E. Recurrent abortion

[24.3] A 29-year-old G2 P1 woman at 39 weeks' gestation had a myomectomy for infertility previously. While pushing during the
second stage of labor, she is noted to have fetal bradycardia associated with some vaginal bleeding. The fetal head, which was
previously at +2 station, is now noted to be –3 station. Which of
the following is the most likely diagnosis?

    A. Submucosal myomata
    B. Umbilical cord prolapse
    C. Uterine rupture
    D. Placental abruption
    E. Fetal congenital heart block

[24.4] A 65-year-old woman is noted to have suspected uterine fibroids on physical examination. Over the course of 1 yr, she is
noted to have enlargement of her uterus from approximately 12
weeks' size to 20 weeks' size. Which of the following is the best
management?

    A. Continued careful observation
    B. Monitoring with ultrasound examinations
    C. Exploratory laparotomy with hysterectomy
    D. Gonadotropin-releasing hormone agonist (GnRH)
    E. Progestin therapy

Answers

[24.1] **A.** Submucous fibroids are the ones most likely to be associated
with recurrent abortion due to their effect on the uterine cavity.

[24.2] **B.** Menorrhagia is the most common symptom of uterine fibroids.

[24.3] **C.** Extensive myomectomies sometimes necessitate cesarean
delivery because of the risk of uterine rupture. Most practitioners use the rule of thumb that if the endometrial cavity is entered
during myomectomy, a cesarean delivery should be performed
with pregnancy.

[24.4] **C.** The rapid growth suggests the concern of leiomyosarcoma; the diagnosis and treatment is surgical. Also, it is unusual for a postmenopausal women to experience substantial growth of uterine fibroids.

CLINICAL PEARLS

 The most common reason for hysterectomy is symptomatic uterine fibroids.

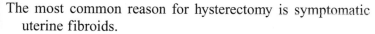 The most common symptom of uterine fibroids is menorrhagia.

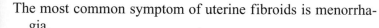 The physical examination consistent with uterine leiomyomata is an irregular pelvic mass that is mobile, midline, and moves contiguously with the cervix.

 Leiomyosarcoma rarely arises from leiomyoma; rapid growth or a history of prior pelvic irradiation should raise the index of suspicion.

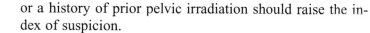 Significant growth in suspected uterine fibroids in a postmenopausal women is unusual and generally requires surgical evaluation.

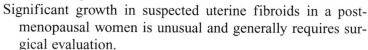

REFERENCES

Droegemueller W. Benign gynecologic lesions. In: Stenchever MA, Droegemueller W, Herbst AL, Mishell DR, eds. Comprehensive gynecology, 4th ed. St. Louis: Mosby-Year Book. 2001:479–530.

Moore GJ. Benign diseases of the uterine corpus. In: Hacker NF and Moore JG, eds. Essentials of obstetrics and gynecology, 3rd ed. Philadelphia: Saunders. 1998:412–418.

A 19-year-old G1 P0 woman at 29 weeks' gestation has severe preeclampsia, with several blood pressures of 160/110 and 4+ proteinuria. She denies headaches or visual abnormalities. She notes a 2-day history of severe unremitting epigastric tenderness. The patient's platelet count was 130,000/mL, hemoglobin level is 13 mg/dL, and SGOT is 2100 mIU/mL (nL<35). Shortly after admission, she received intravenous magnesium sulfate and was induced with oxytocin. She delivered vaginally. Two hr after delivery, the patient complains of the sudden onset of severe abdominal pain and has a syncopal episode. The patient is found to have a blood pressure of 80/60, a distended abdomen, and heart rate of 140 bpm with a thready pulse.

◆ **What is the most likely diagnosis?**

◆ **What is your next step?**

ANSWERS TO CASE 25: Preeclampsia and Hepatic Rupture

Summary: A 19-year-old G1 P0 woman who delivered at 29 weeks' gestation is noted to have severe preeclampsia, epigastric tenderness, and markedly elevated liver function tests. Shortly after delivery, she develops sudden, severe abdominal pain, abdominal distension, syncope, hypotension, and tachycardia.

◆ **Most likely diagnosis:** Hepatic rupture.

◆ **Next step:** Emergent exploratory laparotomy and blood product replacement.

Analysis

Objectives

1. Know the clinical presentation of preeclampsia.
2. Know the serious sequelae of severe preeclampsia, including hepatic rupture.
3. Understand that immediate laparotomy and massive blood product replacement are important in the management of hepatic rupture.

Considerations

The patient is nulliparous, which is a risk factor for preeclampsia. She has severe preeclampsia based on blood pressure criteria, proteinuria, epigastric tenderness, and elevated liver function tests. The epigastric tenderness occurs because of the ischemia to the liver. Rarely, a hepatic hematoma may form, and if rupture of the hematoma occurs, catastrophic hemorrhage can ensue, leading to rapid exsanguination if immediate exploratory laparotomy is not undertaken.

APPROACH TO PREECLAMPSIA

Definitions

Chronic hypertension: Blood pressure of 140/90 mm Hg before pregnancy or at less than 20 weeks' gestation.

Gestational hypertension: Hypertension without proteinuria at greater than 20 weeks' gestation.

Preeclampsia: Hypertension with proteinuria (greater than 300 mg over 24 hr) at a gestational age greater than 20 weeks, caused by vasospasm.

Eclampsia: Seizure disorder associated with preeclampsia.

Severe preeclampsia: Vasospasm associated with preeclampsia of such extent that maternal end organs are threatened, usually necessitating delivery of the baby regardless of gestational age.

Clinical Approach

Hypertensive disorders complicate 6% to 8% of pregnancies and can be organized into several categories: gestational hypertension, mild and severe preeclampsia, chronic hypertension, superimposed preeclampsia, and eclampsia. Gestational hypertensive patients have only increased blood pressures without proteinuria. Chronic hypertension includes pre-existing hypertension or hypertension that develops prior to 20 weeks' gestation. A patient with chronic hypertension is at risk for developing preeclampsia and, if this develops, her diagnosis is labeled superimposed preeclampsia. Eclampsia occurs when the patient with preeclampsia develops convulsions or seizures.

Preeclampsia is characterized by hypertension and proteinuria. Although not a criterium, nondependent edema is also usually present. An elevated blood pressure is diagnosed with a systolic blood pressure at or higher than 140 mm Hg or diastolic blood pressure at or higher than 90 mm Hg. Two elevated BPs, measured 6 hr apart (BP taken in the seated position), are needed for the diagnosis of preeclampsia. **Proteinuria** is usually based on a timed urine collection, defined as **equal to or greater than 300 mg of protein in 24 hr.** Facial and hand edema would be considered nondependent edema.

Preeclampsia is further categorized into mild and severe. Severe disease is diagnosed with a systolic BP at or higher than 160 mm Hg, diastolic BP of 110 mm Hg or higher, or a 24-hr urine protein level of more than 5 g. If there is no time for a 24-hr urine protein collection (i.e., while in labor), a urine dipstick helps estimate proteinuria, with 3 to 4+ consistent with severe disease and 1 to 2+ with mild disease. Patients may also be diagnosed with severe disease when symptoms of preeclampsia occur, such as headache, right upper quadrant or epigastric pain, and vision changes.

The **underlying pathophysiology of preeclampsia is vasospasm and "leaky vessels,"** but its origin is unclear. It is cured only by termination of the pregnancy, and the disease process almost always resolves after delivery. Vasospasm and endothelial damage result in leaking between the endothelial cells and cause local hypoxemia of tissue. Hypoxemia leads to hemolysis, necrosis, and other end organ damage. Patients are usually unaware of the hypertension and proteinuria, and typically the presence of symptoms indicates severe disease. Hence, one of the important roles of prenatal care is to identify patients with hypertension and proteinuria prior to severe disease. **Complications of preeclampsia include placenta abruption, eclampsia (with possible intracerebral hemorrhage), coagulopathies, renal failure, hepatic subcapsular hematoma, hepatic rupture, and uteroplacental insufficiency.**

Risk factors for preeclampsia include: nulliparity, extremes of age, African-American race, family history of preeclampsia, chronic hypertension, chronic renal disease, antiphospholipid syndrome, diabetes, and multifetal gestation. The history and physical examination is focused on end organ disease (Table 25–1). It is important to review and evaluate the blood pressures prior to 20 weeks' gestation (to assess for chronic hypertension), evaluate proteinuria, and to document any sudden increase in weight (indicating possible edema). On physical examination serial blood pressures should be checked along with a urinalysis.

Laboratory tests should include a CBC (check platelets and hemoconcentration), urinalysis and 24-hr urine protein collection if possible (check for proteinuria), liver function tests, LDH (elevated with hemolysis), and uric acid (usually increased with preeclamp-

Table 25–1

LISTING OF CRITERIA FOR SEVERE PREECLAMPSIA

END ORGAN (by system)	SIGNS AND SYMPTOMS OF PREECLAMPSIA
Neurologic	Headache
	Vision changes
	Seizures
	Hyper-reflexia
	Blindness
Renal	Decreased glomerular filtration rate
	Proteinuria
	Oliguria
Pulmonary	Pulmonary edema
Hematologic and vascular	Thrombocytopenia
	Microangiopathic anemia
	Coagulopathy
	Severe hypertension (160/110)
Fetal	Intrauterine growth restriction (IUGR)
	Oligohydramnios
	Decreased uterine perfusion (i.e., late decelerations)
Hepatic	Increased liver enzymes
	Subcapsular hematoma
	Hepatic rupture

sia). A nonstress test can also be performed to rule out uteroplacental insufficiency along with an ultrasound to evaluate amniotic fluid volume.

After the diagnosis is made, the management will depend on the gestational age of the fetus and the severity of the disease (see Figure 25–1 for one management scheme). Delivery is the definitive treatment and the risks of preeclampsia must be weighed against the risk of prematurity. When the pregnancy is at term, delivery is indicated. When the fetus is premature, severity of the disease needs to be assessed. When severe preeclampsia is diagnosed, delivery is usually indicated regardless of gestational age. In preterm patients, mild preeclampsia can be monitored closely for worsening disease until the risk of prematurity has decreased.

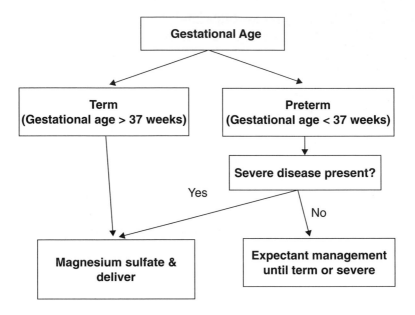

Figure 25–1.   Algorithm for the management of preeclampsia.

Eclampsia is one of the most feared complications of preeclampsia and the greatest risk for occurrence is just prior to delivery, during labor (intrapartum), and within the first 24 hr postpartum. During labor, the patient should be started on the anticonvulsant, magnesium sulfate. **Since magnesium is excreted by the kidneys, it is important to monitor urine output, respiratory depression, dyspnea (side effect of magnesium sulfate is pulmonary edema), and abolition of the deep tendon reflexes (toxicity first effects the reflexes).** Hypertension is not affected by the magnesium, but is used to prevent seizures. Severe hypertension needs to be controlled with antihypertensive medications, such as hydralazine or labetolol. After delivery, $MgSO_4$ is discontinued approximately 24 hr postpartum. The hypertension and proteinuria frequently will resolve. Occasionally, the patient's blood pressure remains high and an antihypertensive medication is needed after delivery. After discharge, the patient usually follows up in 1 to 2 weeks to check blood pressures and proteinuria.

Comprehension Questions

[25.1] Each of the following is a criteria for severe preeclampsia except:

   A. Elevated liver function tests
   B. 5 g of proteinuria excreted in a 24-hr period
   C. 4+ pedal edema
   D. Platelet count of 50,000/uL

[25.2] Which of the following is the best management of a 18-year-old G1 P0 woman at 28 weeks' gestation with a blood pressure of 160/110 mm Hg, elevated liver function tests, and a platelet count of 60,000/uL?

   A. Oral antihypertensive therapy
   B. Platelet transfusion
   C. Magnesium sulfate therapy and induction of labor
   D. Intravenous immunoglobulin therapy

[25.3] Which of the following is the most common mechanism whereby eclampsia leads to maternal mortality?

   A. Intracerebral hemorrhage
   B. Myocardial infarction
   C. Electrolyte abnormalities
   D. Aspiration

[25.4] A 33-year-old woman at 29 weeks' gestation is noted to have blood pressures of 150/90 and 2+ proteinuria. The platelet count and liver function tests were normal. Which of the following is the best management for this patient?

   A. Induction of labor
   B. Cesarean section
   C. Antihypertensive therapy
   D. Expectant management

Answers

[25.1] **C.** Pedal edema is not pathologic; nondependent edema, such as of the face and hands, is more concerning.

[25.2] **C.** Although the pregnancy is only 28 weeks, in light of the severe preeclampsia, the best treatment is delivery.

[25.3] **A.** The most common cause of maternal death due to eclampsia is intracerebral hemorrhage.

[25.4] **D.** In the preterm patient with mild preeclampsia, expectant management is employed.

CLINICAL PEARLS

In general, the treatment of preeclampsia at term is magnesium sulfate and delivery.

The management of preeclampsia in a preterm pregnancy is observation until severe criteria are noted, or term gestation is reached.

The most common cause of significant proteinuria in pregnancy is preeclampsia.

Magnesium sulfate is the best anticonvulsant to prevent eclampsia.

The first sign of magnesium toxicity is loss of deep tendon reflexes.

Chronic hypertension is diagnosed when a pregnant woman has hypertension prior to 20 weeks' gestation, or if the hypertension persists beyond 12 weeks postpartum.

REFERENCES

Castro LC. Hypertensive disorders of pregnancy. In: Hacker NF and Moore JG, eds. Essentials of obstetrics and gynecology, 3rd ed. Philadelphia: Saunders. 1998:196–207.

Cunningham FG, Gant NF, Leveno KJ, Gilstrap LC III, Hauth JC, Wenstrom KD. Hypertensive disorders in pregnancy. In: Williams obstetrics, 21st ed. New York: McGraw-Hill. 2001:567–618.

American College of Obstetricians and Gynecologists. Diagnosis and management of preeclampsia and eclampsia. Practice Bulletin No. 33, January 2002.

◈ CASE 26

A 1-cm breast mass is discovered during a routine physical examination of a 22-year-old woman. She has no family history of breast cancer. She denies breast leakage or prior irradiation. On examination, her BP is 100/60. Her physical examination is unremarkable except for the breast mass. Her neck is supple and the heart and lung examinations are normal. Palpation of her right breast reveals a firm mobile nontender rubbery 1-cm mass in the upper outer quadrant. No adenopathy is noted. The left breast is normal to palpation.

◆ **What is your next step?**

◆ **What is the most likely diagnosis?**

ANSWERS TO CASE 26: Fibroadenoma of the Breast

Summary: A 22-year-old woman is noted to have a 1-cm breast mass on routine physical examination. Palpation of her right breast reveals a firm, mobile, nontender, rubbery 1-cm mass in the upper outer quadrant. No adenopathy is noted.

◆ **Next step:** Biopsy of the mass (fine needle biopsy).

◆ **Most likely diagnosis:** Fibroadenoma of the breast.

Analysis

Objectives

1. Understand that any three-dimensional dominant mass needs a biopsy.
2. Know the characteristic presentation of fibroadenomas of the breast.
3. Understand that the greater the risk of breast cancer, the more tissue that is needed for biopsy.

Considerations

This woman is young and has a dominant breast mass. The firm, nontender, rubbery description is classic for a fibroadenoma. Fibroadenomas, as opposed to fibrocystic changes, do not change with the menstrual cycle. Although the most likely diagnosis is a fibroadenoma, this diagnosis needs to be confirmed by biopsy. A fine needle aspiration (FNA) is acceptable since the patient is at low risk for breast cancer. She has no family history of breast cancer, is of a young age, and her examination does not contain any worrisome features of breast cancer. If the mass were fixed, or if there were nipple retraction or bloody nipple discharge, the better method of biopsy would be excisional biopsy to remove the entire mass for histologic analysis.

APPROACH TO BREAST MASSES

Definitions

Fine needle aspiration (FNA): The use of a small-gauge needle with associated vacuum via a syringe to aspirate fluid or some cells from a breast mass and/or cyst.

Fibroadenoma: Benign, smooth muscle tumor of the breast, usually occurring in young women.

Clinical Approach

Fibrocystic changes, the most common of the benign breast conditions, are described as multiple, irregular, "lumpiness of the breast." It is not a disease per se, but rather an exaggerated response to ovarian hormones. **Fibrocystic changes are very common in premenopausal women, but rare following menopause.** The clinical presentation is cyclic, painful, engorged breasts, more pronounced just before menstruation, and occasionally associated with serous or green breast discharge. Fibrocystic changes can usually be differentiated from the three-dimensional dominant mass suggestive of cancer, but occasionally a fine-needle or core biopsy must be performed to establish the diagnosis. Treatment includes decreasing caffeine ingestion, and adding NSAIDs, a tight-fitting bra, oral contraceptives, or oral progestin therapy. With severe cases, danazol (a weak anti-estrogen and androgenic compound) or even mastectomy are considered.

In a woman in the adolescent years or in her 20s, the most common cause of a dominant breast mass is a fibroadenoma. These tumors **are firm, rubbery, mobile, and solid in consistency.** They typically do not respond to ovarian hormones and do not vary during the menstrual cycle. Since any three-dimensional dominant mass necessitates histologic confirmation, a biopsy should be performed. In a woman less than age 35 years, a fine needle aspiration is often chosen. If the histologic examination supports fibroadenoma (mature smooth muscle cells) and the mass is small and not growing, careful follow-up is possible. Nevertheless, many women choose to have excision of the mass. Most clinicians will excise any dominant three-dimensional mass occurring in a woman over the age of 35 years, or in those with an increased likelihood of mammary cancer (family history).

Comprehension Questions

Match the breast lesion (A–E) to the clinical presentation (1–4).

    A. Fibroadenoma
    B. Fibrocystic changes
    C. Intraductal papilloma
    D. Breast cancer
    E. Galactocele

[26.1] A 34-year-old woman complains of unilateral serosanguinous nipple discharge from the breast, expressed from one duct. No mass is palpated.

[26.2] A 27-year-old woman complains of breast pain, which increases with menses. The breast has a lumpy-bumpy sensation.

[26.3] A 47-year-old woman has a 1.5-cm right breast mass with nipple retraction and skin dimpling over the mass.

[26.4] An 18-year-old woman has an asymptomatic, 1-cm, nontender, mobile, right breast mass.

Answers

[26.1] **C.** The most common cause of bloody (serosanguinous) nipple discharge when only one duct is involved and in the absence of a breast mass is intraductal papilloma. Ductal exploration is required to rule out cancer.

[26.2] **B.** A diffuse "lumpy-bumpy" examination suggests fibrocystic changes.

[26.3] **D.** Nipple retraction or skin dimpling over a mass is very suggestive of malignancy.

[26.4] **A.** A young woman with a dominant nontender mass most likely
has a fibroadenoma.

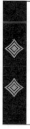

CLINICAL PEARLS

Rule #1: Any three-dimensional dominant mass of the breast
should be biopsied.

Rule #2: The greater the risk of cancer (such as age), the more
tissue should be taken for biopsy.

REFERENCES

Droegemuller W, Valea FA. Breast diseases. In: Stenchever MA, Droegemueller W,
Herbst AL, Mishell DR, eds. Comprehensive gynecology, 4th ed. St. Louis:
Mosby-Year Book. 2001:359–398.
Hacker NF. Breast disease: a gynecologic perspective. In: Hacker NF and Moore
JG, eds. Essentials of obstetrics and gynecology, 3rd ed. Philadelphia: Saunders.
1998:507–515.

CASE 27

A 23-year-old G1 P0 woman at 40 weeks' gestation is undergoing labor induction with oxytocin for oligohydramnios. She has been at 6-cm dilation for 3 hr. A significant amount of caput is noted on cervical examination. Her uterine contractions are every 2 to 3 min and palpate firm. Each contraction lasts for 60 sec. The estimated fetal weight is 7.5 lb, and the pelvis clinically seems adequate. The fetal heart tones are in the 145 to 150 bpm range without decelerations.

◆ **What is your next step?**

◆ **What is the most likely diagnosis?**

ANSWERS TO CASE 27: Labor, Arrest of Active Phase

Summary: A 23-year-old G1 P0 woman at 40 weeks' gestation is being induced. Her cervix has remained at 6-cm dilation for 3 hr, and a significant amount of caput is noted on examination. Her uterine contractions are every 2 to 3 min and palpate firm. Each contraction lasts for 60 sec. The estimated fetal weight is 7.5 lb, and the pelvis seems adequate.

◆ **Next step:** Cesarean delivery; some clinicians would consider the placement of an intrauterine pressure catheter to assess contraction pattern.

◆ **Most likely diagnosis:** Arrest of active phase.

Analysis

See also Case 6.

Objectives

1. Know the normal latent phase and active phase of labor.
2. Understand that when the labor is abnormal, then the 3 Ps need to be considered.
3. Understand the criteria for adequate uterine contractions.

Considerations

This 23-year-old woman is being induced for oligohydramnios at 40 weeks' gestation. She has not changed her cervix from 6 cm for 3 hr, which is arrest of active phase (2 hr of no change is sufficient for the diagnosis). When there is a labor abnormality, the next step is to consider the "3 Ps," which are pelvis, passenger, and powers. On examination, the pelvis seems clinically adequate and the estimated fetal weight is not excessive (7.5 lb). The assessment of the powers may be either clinical (contractions every 2 to 3 min, firm by palpation, and lasting for 40 to 60 sec) or by intrauterine pressure catheter. When the uterine contractions are judged to be adequate, with arrest of active phase, then cesarean section is the best treatment. If the uterine contractions are not adequate, oxytocin augmentation of labor would be appropriate. The caput on the fetal head, which is edema on the scalp, is indicative of the adequate uterine contractions.

APPROACH TO LABOR

See explanation for Case 6.

Comprehension Questions

[27.1] The cervix of a 19-year-old G1 P0 at 39 weeks' gestation is noted to change from 2 cm to 3 cm over 4 hr. Which of the following is the most likely diagnosis?

    A. Normal labor
    B. Prolonged latent phase
    C. Protracted active phase
    D. Arrest of active phase
    E. Arrest of descent

[27.2] A 25-year-old G2 P1001 woman at 41 weeks' gestation is noted to change her cervix from 6 cm to 9 cm over 2 hr. Which of the following is the most likely diagnosis?

    A. Normal labor
    B. Prolonged latent phase
    C. Protracted active phase
    D. Arrest of active phase
    E. Arrest of descent

[27.3] A 30-year-old G1 P0 at 39 week's gestation, who does not have an epidural catheter, is completely dilated, pushing for 2 hr at 0 station. Which of the following is the most likely diagnosis?

A. Normal labor
B. Prolonged latent phase
C. Protracted active phase
D. Arrest of active phase
E. Arrest of descent

[27.4] A 38-year-old G3 P2 woman at 38 weeks' gestation has changed
her cervix from 6 cm to 8 cm over 3 hr. Which of the following
is the most likely diagnosis?

A. Normal labor
B. Prolonged latent phase
C. Protracted active phase
D. Arrest of active phase
E. Arrest of descent

Answers

[27.1] **A.** This is a normal latent phase; upper limit of normal is 18 to
20 hr in a nullipara.

[27.2] **A.** This is normal labor, since a multiparous patient should dilate at or greater than 1.5 cm/hr in the active phase.

[27.3] **E.** In the second stage of labor, when there is no progress past 0
station for 2 hr, this is arrest of descent.

[27.4] **C.** Protracted labor means some progress but less than the lower
limits of normal. This patient is multiparous; thus, the expected
dilation is 1.5 cm/hr or greater. Her dilation rate is only 0.66
cm/hour.

CLINICAL PEARLS

◈ In general, cesarean delivery for labor abnormalities is reserved for arrest of active phase with adequate uterine contractions.

◈ Adequate uterine contractions may be established by intrauterine pressure monitoring of 200 Montevideo units, or contractions every 2 to 3 min that are firm and last for 40 to 60 sec.

◈ With a labor abnormality, the next step is to evaluate the 3 Ps: pelvis, passenger, and powers.

REFERENCES

Cunningham FG, Gant NF, Leveno KJ, Gilstrap LC III, Hauth JC, Wenstrom KD. Dystocia: abnormal labor and fetopelvic disproportion. In: Williams obstetrics, 21st ed. New York: McGraw-Hill. 2001:425–450.

Ross MG, Hobel CJ. In: Hacker NF and Moore JG, eds. Essentials of obstetrics and gynecology, 3rd ed. Philadelphia: Saunders. 1998:150–167.

American College of Obstetricians and Gynecologists. Dystocia and the augmentation of labor. Technical Bulletin No. 218, December 1995.

A 31-year-old G1 P1 woman presents with a history of infertility of 2-yr duration. She states that her menses began at age 12 years and occurs at 28-day intervals. A biphasic basal body temperature chart is recorded. She denies sexually transmitted diseases, and a hysterosalpingogram shows patent tubes and a normal uterine cavity. Her husband is 34 years old and his semen analysis is normal.

◆ **What is the most likely etiology?**

ANSWERS TO CASE 28: Infertility, Peritoneal Factor

Summary: An infertile couple is evaluated. Her menses are regular, and a biphasic basal body temperature chart is recorded. She denies sexually transmitted diseases, and a hysterosalpingogram shows patent tubes and a normal uterine cavity. The semen analysis is normal.

◆ **Most likely etiology:** Endometriosis (peritoneal factor).

Analysis

Objectives

1. Know the five basic etiologies of infertility.
2. Understand the history and laboratory tests for these five factors.
3. Understand that endometriosis is more common than cervical factor infertility.

Considerations

This 31-year-old woman has secondary infertility. In approaching infertility, there are **five basic factors to examine: 1) ovulatory, 2) uterine/tubal, 3) male factor, 4) cervical factor, and 5) peritoneal factor (endometriosis).** The patient has regular monthly menses. That by itself argues strongly for regular ovulation; the biphasic basal body temperature chart is further evidence for regular ovulation. The uterus/tubal factor is normal based on the normal hysterosalpingogram, which is a radiologic study in which dye is placed into the uterine cavity via a transcervical catheter. The male factor is not an issue, based on the normal semen analysis. Therefore the two remaining factors not addressed are the cervical factor and peritoneal factor. If the patient had prior cryotherapy to the cervix, the examiner might be directed to consider cervical factor; similarly, if the patient complained of the 3 Ds of endometriosis (dysmenorrhea, dyspareunia, and dyschezia), then the examiner would be pointed toward the peritoneal factor. Since there are no hints favoring one factor over another, the clinician must pick the most common condition, which is endometriosis.

APPROACH TO INFERTILITY

Definitions

Infertility: Inability to conceive after 1 year of unprotected intercourse.
Primary infertility: A woman has never been able to get pregnant.
Secondary infertility: A woman has been pregnant in the past, but has 1 year of inability to conceive.

Clinical Approach

Infertility affects approximately 10% to 15% of couples in the reproductive age group. Fecundability, defined as the probability of achieving a pregnancy within one menstrual cycle, has been estimated at 20% to 25% for a normal couple. On the basis of this estimate, approximately 90% of couples should conceive after 12 months. The physician's initial encounter with the couple is very important and sets the tone for further evaluation and treatment. It is extremely important that after the initial evaluation, a realistic plan be established and followed (Table 28–1). The five main causes of infertility are as follows.

1. **Ovulatory disorders (ovulatory factor).** Ovulatory disorders account for approximately 30% to 40% of all cases of female infertility. **A history of regularity or irregularity of the menses is fairly predictive of the regularity of ovulation.** The basal body temperature **(BBT)** chart is the easiest and least expensive method of detecting ovulation (Figure 28–1). The temperature should be determined orally, preferably with a basal body thermometer, before the patient arises out of bed, eats, or drinks. The chart documents the rise of temperature of about 0.5°F that

Table 28–1
APPROACH TO INFERTILITY

FACTOR	HISTORY	TEST	THERAPY
Ovulatory dysfunction	Irregular menses, obesity	Basal body temperature chart, or LH surge, or progesterone level	Clomiphene citrate
Uterine and tubal disorder	Chlamydial or gonococcal infection; pelvic inflammatory disease	Hysterosalpingogram (showing abnormal uterine cavity or no dye flowing through tubes)	Hysteroscopic procedure or laparoscopic procedure; in vitro fertilization
Male factor	Hernia; varicocele; mumps	Semen analysis	Repair of hernia or varicocele; in vitro fertilization
Cervical factor	Cone biopsy; cryotherapy to cervix	Postcoital test (assessing cervical mucus for motile sperm after intercourse)	Intrauterine insemination
Peritoneal factor (endometriosis)	3 Ds: dysmenorrhea, dyspareunia, dyschezia	Laparoscopy (Some advocate CA 125)	Ablation of endometriosis, medical therapy

occurs **after** ovulation due to the release of **progesterone** (a thermogenic hormone) by the ovary. The rise of temperature accounts for the biphasic pattern indicative of ovulation. Midluteal (day 21) serum progesterone level is an indirect method of documenting ovulation. Luteinizing hormone (LH) and, particularly the **LH surge,** can be detected with self-administered urine test kits. Ovulation occurs predictably about 36 hr after the onset of the LH surge. Other tests include the endometrial biopsy showing secretory tissue, or an ultrasound documenting a decrease in

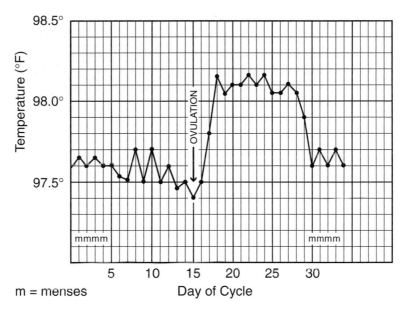

m = menses

Figure 28–1.   Basal body temperature chart. After ovulation, the temperature rises by 0.5°F for 10 to 12 days.

follicular size and presence of fluid in the cul-de-sac, suggesting ovulation.

2. **Uterine and tubal problems.** The **hysterosalpingogram** (HSG) is the initial test for intrauterine shape and tubal patency. It should be performed between days 6 and 10 of the cycle. It is fairly accurate but not perfect; hence, abnormal findings should be confirmed with laparoscopy, which is considered the "gold standard" for diagnosing tubal and peritoneal disease. In addition, operative laparoscopy can provide for the treatment of tubal and peritoneal disease through a minimally invasive technique. Hysteroscopy likewise provides direct visualization of the uterine cavity when the HSG suggests an intrauterine defect. Uterine abnormalities have been associated with recurrent pregnancy losses. Uterine myomata and, in particular, submucosal myomata may interfere with implantation and fertility.

3. **Abnormalities in the semen (male factor).** The semen analysis is a very basic and noninvasive test and should be one of the initial examinations. Even men who have fathered other children should have a semen analysis. The semen should be evaluated in terms of: volume (nl $\geq$ 2.0 mL), **sperm concentration (nl $\geq$ 20 million/mL),** motility (nl $\geq$ 50%), and morphology (nl $\geq$ 30% normal forms). An abstinence period of 2 to 3 days prior to semen collection is recommended. One abnormal test is not sufficient to establish the diagnosis of a male factor abnormality, and the test should be repeated after 2 to 3 months (the process of transforming spermatogonia into mature sperm cells requires 74 days).

4. **Cervical factor.** Cervical etiologies do not commonly cause infertility. The **postcoital test (PCT)** is the classical test in evaluating the cervical factor, usually performed 1 to 2 days prior to the anticipated time of ovulation. The time of intercourse has been a subject of controversy, with optimal being less than 2 hr and adequate within 24 hr. A small amount of cervical mucus is withdrawn with forceps or a small catheter. **It is evaluated for spinnbarkeit (stretchability), ferning, clarity, and the presence, number, and motility of sperm per high-power field.** The mucus should stretch 8 to 10 cm, demonstrate a ferning pattern, and should be clear and watery. The number of motile sperm should be counted; however, the normal count has not been established. In general, more than 20 sperm per high-power field is considered normal.

5. **Peritoneal factor (endometriosis).** Endometriosis, a common condition associated with infertility, should be suspected in any infertile woman. The suspicion should increase if she complains of dysmenorrhea and dyspareunia, but often is present even in asymptomatic women. Although not completely understood, endometriosis may cause infertility by inhibiting ovulation, inducing adhesions, and, perhaps, interfering with fertilization. **Laparoscopy is the gold standard for the diagnosis of endometriosis,** and can allow for surgical ablation of the lesions. Lesions can be of various appearances, from clear to red to the classic "powder burn" color.

Comprehension Questions

[28.1] A 22-year-old G0 P0 woman complains of irregular menses every 30 to 65 days. The semen analysis is normal. The hysterosalpingogram is normal. Which of the following is the most likely treatment for this patient?

A. Laparoscopy
B. Intrauterine insemination
C. In vitro fertilization
D. Clomiphene citrate

[28.2] A 26-year-old G0 P0 woman has regular menses every 28 days. The semen analysis is normal. The patient had a postcoital test revealing motile sperm and stretchy watery cervical mucus. She has been treated for chlamydial infection in the past. Which of the following is the most likely etiology of her infertility?

A. Peritoneal factor
B. Male factor
C. Cervical factor
D. Uterine and tubal factor
E. Ovulatory factor

[28.3] A 28-year-old G1 P1 woman complains of painful menses and pain with intercourse. She has menses every month and denies a history of sexually transmitted diseases. Which of the following tests would most likely identify the etiology of the infertility?

A. Semen analysis
B. Laparoscopy
C. Basal body temperature chart
D. Hysterosalpingogram
E. Progesterone assay

[28.4] A 34-year-old infertile woman is noted to have evidence of blocked fallopian tubes by hysterosalpingogram. Which of the following is the best next step for this patient?

A. FSH therapy
B. Clomiphene citrate therapy
C. Laparoscopy
D. Intrauterine insemination

Answers

[28.1] **D.** Clomiphene citrate is a treatment for anovulation, particularly polycystic ovarian syndrome (PCOS). The diagnosis of PCOS is a clinical one, with characteristics of obesity, anovulation, hirsutism, and possibly glucose intolerance.

[28.2] **D.** The history of chlamydial infection would strongly suggest tubal factor infertility.

[28.3] **B.** The history suggests endometriosis, which is best diagnosed by laparoscopy.

[28.4] **C.** The HSG is not specific, and should be followed up with laparoscopy. Dye is injected into the uterus and observed laparoscopically (chromotubation).

CLINICAL PEARLS

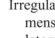

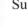

The five basic factors causing infertility are: ovulatory, uterine and tubal, male, cervical, and peritoneal.

Irregular menses usually means irregular ovulation; regular menses usually indicates regular ovulation. In general, ovulatory disorders are fairly amenable to therapy.

A history of salpingitis or chlamydial cervicitis suggests tubal factor infertility.

Laparoscopy is the "gold standard" in diagnosing endometriosis, and lesions may have a variety of appearances.

Surgery is the main therapy for endometrial or tubal abnormalities associated with infertility.

REFERENCES

Mishell DR. Infertility. In: Stenchever MA, Droegemueller W, Herbst AL, Mishell DR, eds. Comprehensive gynecology, 4th ed. St. Louis: Mosby-Year Book. 2001:1169–1216.

Meldrum DR. Infertility. In: Hacker NF and Moore JG, eds. Essentials of obstetrics and gynecology, 3rd ed. Philadelphia: Saunders. 1998:610–620.

CASE 29

A 23-year-old G2 P1 woman at 29 weeks' gestation complains of a
12-hr history of colicky right lower abdominal pain and nausea and
vomiting. She denies diarrhea or eating stale foods. She has a history
of an 8-cm ovarian cyst, and otherwise has been in good health. She denies dysuria or fever, and has had no surgeries. Her vital signs include
a BP of 100/70, HR 105 bpm, RR 12/minute, and temp 99°F. On abdominal examination, her bowel sounds are hypoactive. The abdomen
is tender in the right lower quadrant region with significant involuntary
guarding. The cervix is closed.

◆ **What is the most likely diagnosis?**

◆ **What is the best treatment for this condition?**

ANSWERS TO CASE 29: Abdominal Pain in Pregnancy (Ovarian Torsion)

Summary: A 23-year-old G2 P1 woman at 29 weeks' gestation with an 8-cm ovarian cyst complains of a 12-hr history of colicky right lower abdominal pain and nausea and vomiting. The abdomen is tender in the right lower quadrant region with significant involuntary guarding.

◆ **Most likely diagnosis:** Torsion of the ovary.

◆ **Best treatment for this condition:** Surgery (laparotomy due to the pregnancy).

Analysis

Objectives

1. Know the clinical presentation of some of the common causes of abdominal pain in pregnancy (acute appendicitis, acute cholecystitis, ovarian torsion, placental abruption, and ectopic pregnancy).
2. Understand that surgery is the best treatment for ovarian torsion.
3. Know that oophorectomy does not necessarily need to be performed in ovarian torsion.

Considerations

This woman, who is pregnant at 29 weeks' gestation, has a history of an 8-cm ovarian cyst. The ovarian mass is most likely a dermoid cyst in this young patient. The acute onset of colicky lower abdominal pain and nausea with vomiting are consistent with ovarian torsion, which is the twisting of the ovarian vessels leading to ischemia. Gastrointestinal complaints are common. The treatment for ovarian torsion is surgical. If this woman were not pregnant, laparoscopy would be an option. Sometimes, the size of the mass makes exploratory laparotomy the best choice. Upon opening the abdomen, the surgeon would examine the ovary for viability. Sometimes, untwisting of the ovarian pedicle can lead to reperfusion of the ovary. An ovarian cystectomy is the best treatment, that is, removing only the cyst and leaving the remainder of the normal ovarian tissue intact. This patient is somewhat atypical regarding the gestational age, since the majority of pregnant women with ovarian torsion present either at 14 weeks gestation when the uterus rises above the pelvic brim, or immediately postpartum when the uterus rapidly involutes.

APPROACH TO ABDOMINAL PAIN IN PREGNANCY

Diseases related to and unrelated to the pregnancy must be considered. Additionally, the pregnancy state may alter the risk factors for the different causes of abdominal pain, and change the presentation and symptoms. Common causes of abdominal pain in pregnant women include appendicitis, acute cholecystitis, ovarian torsion, placental abruption, and ectopic pregnancy. Often, it is difficult to differentiate from among these different etiologies, but a careful history and physical and reexamination are the most important steps (Table 29–1).

Acute Appendicitis

The diagnosis of appendicitis can be difficult to make because many of the presenting symptoms are common complaints in pregnancy. Furthermore, a delay in diagnosis (especially in the third trimester) frequently leads to maternal morbidity and perinatal problems, such as preterm labor and abortion. Patients typically present with nausea, emesis, fever, and anorexia. The location of the abdominal pain is not typically in the right lower quadrant (as is classic for nonpregnant patients), but instead is **superior and lateral to McBurney's point.** This is due to the effect of the enlarged uterus pushing on the appendix to move it upward and outward toward the flank, at times mimicking pyelonephritis. Diagnosis is made clinically, and because of the morbidity involved in a missed diagnosis, it is generally better to err on the side of overdiagnosing than underdiagnosing this disease. When appendicitis is suspected, the treatment is surgical regardless of gestational age, along with intravenous antibiotics.

Table 29–1

DIFFERENTIAL DIAGNOSIS OF ABDOMINAL
PAIN IN PREGNANCY

	TIME DURING PREGNANCY	LOCATION	ASSOCIATED SYMPTOMS	TREATMENT
Appendicitis	Any trimester	Right lower quadrant → Right flank	Nausea and vomiting Anorexia Leukocytosis Fever	Surgical
Cholecystitis	After first trimester	Right upper quadrant	Nausea and vomiting Anorexia Leukocytosis Fever	Surgical
Torsion	More commonly 14 weeks and after delivery	Unilateral abdominal or pelvic	Nausea and vomiting	Surgical
Placental abruption	Second and third trimester	Midline persistent uterine	Vaginal bleeding Abnormal fetal heart tracings	Delivery
Ectopic pregnancy	First trimester	Pelvic or abdominal pain, usually unilateral	Nausea and vomiting Syncope Spotting	Surgical or medical

Acute Cholecystitis

A common physiologic effect of pregnancy is an increase in gallbladder volume and biliary sludge (especially after the first trimester). The
biliary sludge then serves as a precursor to gallstones. While gallstones
are often asymptomatic, the most common symptoms are right upper
quadrant pain following a meal, nausea, a "bloated sensation," and, possibly, emesis. In the absence of infection or fever, this is called biliary

colic. Less commonly, when obstruction of the cystic or common bile duct occurs, the pain may be severe and unrelenting, and the patient may become icteric. When fever and leukocytosis are present, the patient with gallstones likely has cholecystitis. Other complications of gallstones include pancreatitis and ascending cholangitis, a serious life-threatening infection. The diagnosis of cholelithiasis is often established by an abdominal ultrasound revealing gallstones and dilation and thickening of the gallbladder wall. **Simple biliary colic in pregnancy is usually treated with a low-fat diet and observed until postpartum.** However, in the face of **cholecystitis, biliary obstruction, or pancreatitis** in pregnancy, **surgery** is the treatment of choice.

Ovarian Torsion

Patients with known or newly diagnosed large ovarian masses are at risk for ovarian torsion. Ovarian torsion is the most frequent and serious complication of a benign ovarian cyst. Pregnancy is a risk factor, especially around 14 weeks and after delivery. Symptoms include unilateral abdominal and pelvic colicky pain associated with nausea and vomiting. The **acute onset of colicky pain** is typical. Treatment is surgical with ovarian conservation if possible. If untwisting the adnexa results in reperfusion, an ovarian cystectomy may be performed. However, if perfusion can not be restored, oophorectomy is indicated.

Placental Abruption

Abruption is a common cause of third trimester bleeding and is usually associated with abdominal pain. Risk factors include a history of previous abruption, hypertensive disease in pregnancy, trauma, cocaine use, smoking, or preterm premature rupture of membranes. Patients typically present with vaginal bleeding with persistent crampy midline uterine tenderness and at times abnormal fetal heart tracings. Diagnosis is made clinically and ultrasound is not very reliable. The treatment is generally delivery, often by cesarean.

Ectopic Pregnancy

The leading cause of maternal mortality in the first and second trimesters is ectopic pregnancy. Patients usually have amenorrhea with some vaginal spotting and lower abdominal and pelvic pain. The pain is typically sharp and tearing and may be associated with nausea and vomiting. Physical findings include a slightly enlarged uterus and perhaps a palpable adnexal mass. If the ectopic ruptures, the patient may experience syncope or hypovolemia. Transvaginal sonography and serum hCG levels can help with the diagnosis of ectopic pregnancy in more than 90% of cases. Treatment options includes surgery (especially with hemodynamically unstable patients) and, in appropriately selected patients, methotrexate.

Comprehension Questions

[29.1] Which of the following describes the movement of the appendix in pregnancy as compared with a nonpregnant state?

A. Superior and lateral
B. Inferior and lateral
C. Superior and medial
D. Inferior and to the right

[29.2] Upon performing laparoscopy for a suspected ovarian torsion on an 18-year-old nulliparous woman, the surgeon sees that the ovarian vascular pedicle has twisted 1-1½ times and that the ovary appears somewhat bluish. Which of the following is the best management at this point?

A. Oophorectomy with excision close to the ovary
B. Oophorectomy with excision of the vascular pedicle to prevent possible embolization of the thrombosis
C. Unwind the vascular pedicle to assess the viability of the ovary
D. Bilateral salpingoophorectomy
E. Intravenous heparin therapy

[29.3] Each of the following describes the correct anatomic character-istics of the vessels in the infundibular pelvic ligament leading to the ovary except:

A. Right ovarian artery arises from the abdominal aorta
B. Right ovarian vein drains into the vena cava
C. Left ovarian artery arises from the left renal artery
D. Left ovarian vein drains into the left renal vein

[29.4] An 18-year-old G1 P0 woman complains of a 2-month history of colicky right abdominal pain when she eats. It is associated with nausea and emesis. She states the pain radiates to her right shoulder. The patient has a family history of diabetes. Which of the following is the most likely diagnosis?

A. Peptic ulcer disease
B. Cholelithiasis
C. Appendicitis
D. Ovarian torsion

Answers

[29.1] **A.** The growing uterus pushes the appendix superior and lateral.

[29.2] **C.** Unless the ovary appears necrotic, the ovarian pedicle can be untwisted and the ovary observed for viability. Embolization of the thrombus is exceedingly rare.

[29.3] **C.** Both ovarian arteries arise from the abdominal aorta.

[29.4] **B.** This is a typical history of cholelithiasis.

CLINICAL PEARLS

In pregnancy, the appendix moves superiorly and lateral from the normal location.

The acute onset of colicky abdominal pain is typical of ovarian torsion.

With ovarian torsion, the clinician can untwist the pedicle and observe the ovary for viability.

REFERENCES

Droegemuller W. Benign gynecologic lesions. In: Stenchever MA, Droegemueller W, Herbst AL, Mishell DR, eds. Comprehensive gynecology, 4th ed. St. Louis: Mosby-Year Book. 2001:479–530.

Moore GJ. Surgical conditions in pregnancy. In: Hacker NF and Moore JG, eds. Essentials of obstetrics and gynecology, 3rd ed. Philadelphia: Saunders. 1998:263–269.

A 19-year-old G2 Ab 1 woman at 7 weeks' gestation by LMP complains of vaginal spotting. She denies the passage of tissue per vagina,
any trauma, or recent intercourse. Her past medical history is significant for a pelvic infection approximately 3 yr ago. She had used an oral
contraceptive agent 1 yr previously. Her appetite is normal. On examination, her BP is 100/60, HR 90 bpm, and temp afebrile. The abdomen
is nontender with normoactive bowel sounds. On pelvic examination,
the external genitalia are normal. The cervix is closed and nontender.
The uterus is 4 weeks' size, and no adnexal tenderness is noted. The
quantitative beta-hCG is 2300 mIU/mL (Third International Standard).
A transvaginal sonogram reveals an empty uterus and no adnexal
masses.

◆ **What is your next step?**

◆ **What is the most likely diagnosis?**

ANSWERS TO CASE 30: Ectopic Pregnancy

Summary: A 19-year-old G2 Ab 1 woman at 7 weeks' gestation by LMP has vaginal spotting. Her history is significant for a prior pelvic infection. Her BP is 100/60, HR 90 bpm, and her abdomen is nontender. Pelvic examination shows a closed and nontender cervix, a uterus of 4 weeks' size, and no adnexal tenderness. The quantitative beta-hCG is 2300 mIU/mL (3rd IS). A transvaginal sonogram reveals an empty uterus and no adnexal masses.

◆ **Next step:** Laparoscopy.

◆ **Most likely diagnosis:** Ectopic pregnancy.

Analysis

Objectives

1. Understand that any woman with amenorrhea and vaginal spotting or lower abdominal pain should have a pregnancy test to evaluate the possibility of ectopic pregnancy.
2. Understand the role of the hCG level and the threshold for transvaginal sonogram.
3. Know that the lack of clinical or ultrasound signs of ectopic pregnancy does not exclude the disease.

Considerations

The woman is at 7 weeks' gestation by last menstrual period and presents with vaginal spotting. Any woman with amenorrhea and vaginal spotting should have a pregnancy test. The physical examination is normal. Notably, the uterus is slightly enlarged at 4 weeks' gestational size. The enlarged uterus does not exclude the diagnosis of an ectopic pregnancy, due to the human chorionic gonadotropin (hCG) effect on the uterus. The lack of adnexal mass or tenderness on physical examination likewise does not rule out an ectopic pregnancy. The hCG level and transvaginal ultrasound are key tests in the assessment of an extrauterine pregnancy. The ultrasound is primarily used to assess for the presence or absence of an intrauterine pregnancy (IUP), because a confirmed IUP would decrease the likelihood of an ectopic pregnancy significantly (risk 1:10,000 of both an intrauterine and ectopic pregnancy). Also, the presence of free fluid in the peritoneal cavity, or a complex adnexal mass, would make an extrauterine pregnancy more likely. This woman's hCG level of 2300 mIU/mL is greater than the threshold of 1500 mIU/mL (transvaginal sonography); thus, the patient has a high likelihood of an ectopic pregnancy. Although the risk of an extrauterine pregnancy is high, it is not 100%. Therefore, laparoscopy is indicated, and not methotrexate, since the latter would destroy any intrauterine gestation.

APPROACH TO POSSIBLE ECTOPIC PREGNANCY

Definitions

Ectopic pregnancy: A gestation that exists outside of the normal endometrial implantation sites.

Human chorionic gonadotropin: A glycoprotein produced by syncytiotrophoblasts, which is assayed in the standard pregnancy test.

Threshold hCG level: The serum level of hCG where a pregnancy should be seen on ultrasound examination. When the hCG exceeds the threshold and no pregnancy is seen on ultrasound, there is a high likelihood of an ectopic pregnancy.

Laparoscopy: Surgical technique to visualize the peritoneal cavity through a rigid telescopic instrument, known as a laparoscope.

Clinical Approach

See also Case 7.

The vast majority of ectopic pregnancies involve the fallopian tube (97%), but the cervix, abdominal cavity, and ovary have also been affected. In the United States, 2% of pregnancies are extrauterine.

Table 30–1
RISK FACTORS FOR ECTOPIC PREGNANCY

Salpingitis, particularly with *Chlamydia trachomatis*
Tubal adhesive disease
Infertility
Progesterone-secreting IUD
Tubal surgery
Prior ectopic pregnancy
Ovulation induction
Congenital abnormalities of the tube

Hemorrhage from ectopic gestation is the most common reason for maternal mortality in the first 20 weeks of pregnancy. Risk factors for ectopic pregnancy are summarized in Table 30–1.

A woman with an ectopic pregnancy typically complains of **abdominal pain, amenorrhea** of 4 to 6 weeks' duration, and **irregular vaginal spotting.** If the ectopic ruptures, the pain becomes acutely worse, and may lead to **syncope.** Shoulder pain can be a prominent complaint due to the blood irritating the diaphragm. An ectopic pregnancy can lead to tachycardia, hypotension, or orthostasis. Abdominal or adnexal tenderness is common. An adnexal mass is only palpable half the time; hence, the absence of a detectable mass does not exclude an ectopic pregnancy. The uterus may be normal in size, or slightly enlarged. A hemoperitoneum can be confirmed by the aspiration of nonclotting blood with a spinal needle piercing the posterior vaginal fornix into the cul-de-sac **(culdocentesis).**

The diagnosis of an ectopic pregnancy can be a clinical challenge. The differential diagnosis is noted in Table 30–2.

The usual strategy in ruling out an ectopic pregnancy is to try to prove whether an intrauterine pregnancy (IUP) exists. Because the likelihood of a coexisting intrauterine and extrauterine (heterotopic) gestation is so low, in the range of 1 in 10,000, if a definite IUP is demonstrated, the risk of ectopic pregnancy becomes very low. Transvaginal sonography is more sensitive than transabdominal sonography, and can detect pregnancies as early as 5.5 to 6 weeks' gestational age. Hence, the demonstration of a definite IUP by crown–rump length or

Table 30–2

DIFFERENTIAL DIAGNOSIS OF ECTOPIC PREGNANCY

Acute salpingitis
Abortion
Ruptured corpus luteum
Acute appendicitis
Dysfunctional uterine bleeding
Adnexal torsion
Degenerating leiomyomata
Endometriosis

---

yolk sac is reassuring. The "identification of a gestational sac" is sometimes misleading since an ectopic pregnancy can be associated with fluid in the uterus, a so-called "pseudogestational sac." **Other sonographic findings of an extrauterine gestation include an embryo seen outside the uterus, or a large amount of intra-abdominal free fluid, usually indicating blood.**

Often, the quantitative human chorionic gonadotropin (hCG) level is used in conjunction with transvaginal sonography. When the hCG level equals or exceeds 1500 to 2000 mIU/mL, an intrauterine gestational sac is usually seen on transvaginal ultrasound; in fact, **when the hCG level meets or exceeds this threshold and no gestational sac is seen, the patient has a high likelihood of an ectopic pregnancy.** Laparoscopy is usually performed in this situation. When the hCG level is less than the threshold, and the patient does not have severe abdominal pain, hypotension, or adnexal tenderness and/or mass, then a repeat hCG level in 48 hr is permissible. **A rise in the hCG of at least 66% above the initial level is good evidence of a normal pregnancy; in contrast, a lack of an appropriate rise of the hCG is indicative of an abnormal pregnancy, although the abnormal change does not identify whether the pregnancy is in the uterus or the tube.** Some practitioners will use a progesterone level instead of serial hCG levels to assess the health of the pregnancy. A progesterone level of greater than 25 ng/mL almost always correlates with a normal intrauterine pregnancy, whereas a level of less than 5 ng/mL almost always correlates with an abnormal pregnancy.

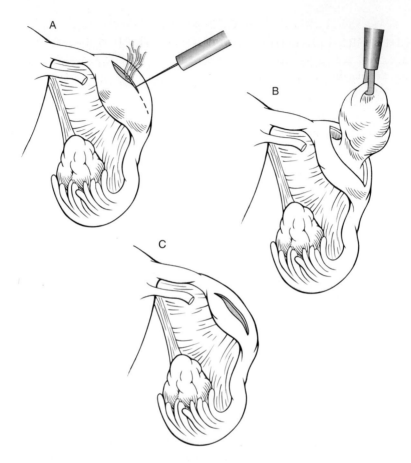

Figure 30–1.   Salpingostomy. Needle-point cautery is used to incise over the ectopic pregnancy (A). The pregnancy tissue is extracted (B), and heals without closure of the incision (C).

Treatment of an ectopic pregnancy may be surgical or medical. **Salpingectomy (removal of the affected tube)** is usually performed for those gestations too large for conservative therapy, when rupture has occurred, or for those women who do not want future fertility. For a woman who wants to preserve her fertility and has an unruptured tubal pregnancy, a **salpingostomy** can be performed (Figure 30–1). An incision is carried out along the long axis of the tube, and the pregnancy tissue is removed. The incision on the tube is not reapproximated, because suturing may lead to stricture formation. Conservative treatment of the tube is associated with a 10% to 15% chance of persistent ectopic pregnancy. Serial hCG levels are, therefore, required with conservative surgical therapy to identify this condition.

Methotrexate, a folic acid antagonist, is the principal form of medical therapy. It is usually given as a one-time, low dose, intramuscular injection, reserved for ectopic pregnancies less than 4 cm in diameter. Methotrexate is highly successful, leading to resolution of properly chosen ectopic pregnancies in 85% to 90% of cases. Occasionally, a second dose is required because the hCG level does not fall. Between 3 to 7 days following therapy, **a patient may complain of abdominal pain,** which is usually due to tubal abortion and, less commonly, rupture. Most women may be observed; however, hypotension, worsening or persistent pain, or a falling hematocrit may indicate tubal rupture and necessitate surgery. About 10% of women treated with medical therapy will require surgical intervention.

Rare types of ectopic gestations such as cervical, ovarian, abdominal, or cornual (involving the portion of the tube that traverses the uterine muscle) pregnancies usually require surgical therapy.

Comprehension Questions

[30.1] A 22-year-old woman at 8 weeks' gestation has vaginal spotting. Her physical examination reveals no adnexal masses. The hCG level is 400 mIU/mL and the transvaginal ultrasound shows no pregnancy in the uterus and no adnexal masses. Which of the following is the best next step?

A. Laparoscopy
B. Methotrexate
C. Repeat the hCG level in 48 hr
D. Dilatation and curettage

[30.2] A 26-year-old G2 P1 woman at 7 weeks' gestation was seen 1 week ago with crampy lower abdominal pain and vaginal spotting. Her hCG level was 1000 mIU/mL at that time. Today, the woman does not have abdominal pain or passage of tissue per vagina. Her repeat hCG level is 1100 mIU/mL. A transvaginal ultrasound examination today shows no clear pregnancy in the uterus and no adnexal masses. Which of the following can be concluded based on the information presented?

A. The woman has a spontaneous abortion and needs a dilation and curettage.
B. The woman has an ectopic pregnancy.
C. No clear conclusion can be drawn from this information, and the hCG needs to be repeated in 48 hr.
D. The woman has a nonviable pregnancy, but its location is unclear.

[30.3] A 17-year-old woman with lower abdominal pain and spotting comes into the emergency room. She is noted to have a hCG level of 1000 mIU/mL and a progesterone level of 26 ng/mL. Which of the following is the most likely diagnosis?

A. This is most likely a normal intrauterine pregnancy.
B. This is most likely an ectopic pregnancy.
C. This is most likely a nonviable intrauterine pregnancy.
D. No clear conclusion can be drawn form this information.

[30.4] Which of the following statements describes the primary utility of the transvaginal ultrasound in the assessment of an ectopic pregnancy?

A. Assessment of an intrauterine pregnancy
B. Assessment of adnexal masses
C. Assessment of fluid in the peritoneal cavity
D. Color Doppler flow in the adnexal region

[30.5] A 29-year-old woman complains of syncope. She is 6 weeks' pregnant and on examination has diffuse significant lower abdominal tenderness. The pelvic examination is difficult to accomplish due to guarding. Her hCG level is 400 mIU/mL and the transvaginal ultrasound shows no pregnancy in the uterus and no adnexal masses. Which of the following is the best next step?

A. Follow-up hCG level in 48 hr
B. Institution of methotrexate
C. Observation in the hospital
D. Surgical therapy

Answers

[30.1] **C.** When the hCG is below the threshold in an asymptomatic patient, the hCG level may be repeated in 48 hr to assess for viability.

[30.2] **D.** A plateau in hCG over 48 hr means it is a nonviable pregnancy; this finding does not identify the location of the pregnancy.

[30.3] **A.** A progesterone level of greater than 25 ng/mL reflects a normal intrauterine pregnancy.

[30.4] **A.** The best use of ultrasound for the assessment of an ectopic pregnancy is to diagnose an intrauterine pregnancy, since an IUP and coexisting ectopic pregnancy is very rare.

[30.5] **D.** Surgery is indicated. Although this woman has an hCG level lower than the threshold, she has an acute abdomen and this is most likely due a ruptured ectopic pregnancy.

CLINICAL PEARLS

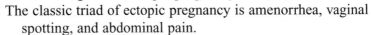

Levels of hCG that plateau in the first 8 weeks of pregnancy indicate an abnormal pregnancy, which may either be a miscarriage or an ectopic pregnancy.

The classic triad of ectopic pregnancy is amenorrhea, vaginal spotting, and abdominal pain.

When the quantitative hCG exceeds 1500 to 2000 mIU/mL and the transvaginal sonogram does not show an intrauterine gestational sac, then the risk of ectopic pregnancy is high.

REFERENCES

Mishell DR. Ectopic pregnancy. In: Stenchever MA, Droegemueller W, Herbst AL, Mishell DR, eds. Comprehensive gynecology, 4th ed. St. Louis: Mosby-Year Book. 2001:443–478.

Palmieri A, Moore GJ, DeCherney AH. Ectopic pregnancy. In: Hacker NF and Moore JG, eds. Essentials of obstetrics and gynecology, 3rd ed. Philadelphia: Saunders. 1998:487–488.

CASE 31

A 29-year-old woman G2 P1 at 28 weeks' gestation complains of fatigue of 1-week duration. Her antenatal history is unremarkable except for a urinary tract infection treated with an antibiotic 2 weeks ago. The patient also states that she has had dark-colored urine over the past week. On examination, her BP is 100/60, HR 80 bpm, and she is afebrile. The thyroid gland appears normal on palpation. The heart and lung examinations are unremarkable. The fundal height is 28 cm. The fetal heart tones are in the 140 to 150 bpm range. Her hemoglobin level is 7.0 g/dL.

◆ **What is the most likely diagnosis?**

◆ **What is the underlying mechanism?**

ANSWERS TO CASE 31: ANEMIA IN PREGNANCY (HEMOLYTIC)

Summary: A 29-year-old woman G2 P1 at 28 weeks' gestation complains of fatigue of 1-week duration. She took an antibiotic for a urinary tract infection 2 weeks ago, after which she noted dark-colored urine. On examination, her BP is 100/60, HR 80 bpm, and temperature is normal. Her hemoglobin level is 7.0 g/dL.

◆ **Most likely diagnosis:** Hemolysis due to glucose-6-phosphate dehydrogenase deficiency

◆ **Underlying mechanism:** Nitrofurantoin-induced hemolysis due to increased fragility of the erythrocytes.

Analysis

Objectives

1. Know that dark-colored urine and anemia are probably caused by hemolysis.
2. Understand that some medications may be associated with hemolysis.
3. Know some of the common causes of anemia in pregnancy.

Considerations

This 29-year-old woman at 28 weeks' gestation complains of fatigue. She took an antibiotic for a urinary tract infection and then developed dark-colored urine. She was also probably icteric. Currently, her hemoglobin level is low, reflecting an anemia. This constellation of symptoms likely reflects a hemolytic process. The dark urine suggests bilirubinuria. Other causes of hemolysis could include malaria, HELLP (hemolysis, elevated liver enzymes, low platelets) syndrome, autoimmune hemolytic anemia, or sickle cell crisis. In this case, the woman ingested an antibiotic, which likely was nitrofurantoin, a commonly prescribed medication for pregnant women. She does not have hypertension, symptoms of systemic lupus erythematosus or other autoimmune diseases, or pain suggestive of sickle cell disease.

APPROACH TO ANEMIA IN PREGNANCY

Definitions

Anemia: A hemoglobin level of less than 10.5 g/dL in the pregnant woman.

Iron deficiency anemia: A fall in hemoglobin level that is due to insufficient iron to meet the increased iron requirements in pregnancy.

Hemolytic anemia: An abnormally low hemoglobin level due to red blood cell destruction, which may be divided into congenital causes and acquired causes.

Glucose-6-phosphate dehydrogenase deficiency: An X-linked condition whereby the red blood cell may have a decreased capacity for anaerobic glucose metabolism. Certain oxidizing agents, such as nitrofurantoin, can lead to hemolysis.

Clinical Approach

Anemia is a common complication in the pregnant woman. It is **most often due to iron deficiency,** partially because of decreased iron stores prior to pregnancy, and increased demands for iron (due to fetus' need and expanded maternal blood volume). A hemoglobin level below 10.5 g/dL is usually considered a sign of anemia in the pregnant woman, with a mild anemia between 8 to 10 g/dL and severe as less than 7g/dL. A gravid woman who presents with mild anemia and no risk factors for hemoglobinopathies (African American, Southeast Asian, or Mediterranean descent) may be treated with supplemental iron and the hemoglobin level reassessed in 3 to 4 weeks. **Persistent anemia necessitates an evaluation for iron stores, such as ferritin level (low with iron deficiency) and hemoglobin electrophoresis.**

The size of the red blood cell may give a clue about the etiology. A **microcytic anemia** is most commonly due to **iron deficiency,** although **thalassemia** may also be causative. Macrocytic anemias may be due to vitamin B_{12} and folate deficiency. Because vitamin B_{12} stores last for many years, **megaloblastic anemias in pregnancy are much more likely to be caused by folate deficiency.**

Less commonly, a woman with glucose-6-phosphate dehydrogenase deficiency (G6PD) may develop hemolytic anemia triggered by various medications such as **sulfonamides, nitrofurantoin, and antimalarial agents.** Nitrofurantoin is one of the most common medications utilized for uncomplicated urinary tract infections. Affected women usually have dark-colored urine due to the bilirubinuria, jaundice, and fatigue due to the anemia. G6PD deficiency is more commonly seen in the African American population.

In the pregnant woman with anemia, jaundice, and thrombocytopenia, the examiner must also consider other hemolytic processes, such as **HELLP syndrome (hemolysis, elevated liver enzymes, low platelets),** which is a life-threatening condition best treated by delivery. In evaluating anemia, if other hematologic cell lines are also decreased, such as the white blood cell count or platelet count, a bone marrow process, such as leukemia or tuberculosis infection of the marrow, should be considered. Bone marrow biopsy may be indicated in these circumstances.

Comprehension Questions

[31.1] A 30-year-old woman G1 P0 complains of nausea and vomiting for the first 3 months of her pregnancy. She is noted to have a hemoglobin level of 9.0 g/dL and the mean corpuscular volume was increased above normal. Which of the following is the most likely etiology of the anemia?

   A. Iron deficiency
   B. Folate deficiency
   C. Vitamin B_{12} deficiency
   D. Physiologic anemia of pregnancy

[31.2] Each of the following is elevated with hemolysis except:

    A. Serum haptoglobin level
    B. Serum bilirubin level
    C. Reticulocyte count
    D. Serum lactate dehydrogenase level

[31.3] A 33-year-old African American woman G1 P0 at 16 weeks' gestation is diagnosed with sickle cell trait. Her husband also is a carrier for the sickle cell gene. Which of the following best describes the likelihood that their unborn baby will have sickle cell disease?

    A. 1/100
    B. 1/50
    C. 1/10
    D. 1/4

[31.4] A 36-year-old G2 P1 at 24 weeks' gestation is noted to have fatigue of 4 weeks' duration. Her hemoglobin level is 8.0 g/dL, leukocyte count is 2.0 cells/uL, and platelet count is 20,000/uL. Which of the following is the most likely diagnosis?

    A. Iron deficiency anemia
    B. HELLP syndrome
    C. Severe preeclampsia
    D. Acute leukemia

Answers

[31.1] **B.** Of the macrocytic causes of anemia, folate deficiency is more commonly seen than vitamin B_{12} deficiency.

[31.2] **A.** Haptoglobin levels are decreased with hemolysis due to hemoglobin binding to this protein.

[31.3] **D.** With autosomal recessive disorders, when both parents are heterozygous for the gene (gene carriers), then there is a 1 in 4 chance of the offspring being affected with the disease, or ho-mozygous for the gene.

[31.4] **D.** Pancytopenia suggests a bone marrow process.

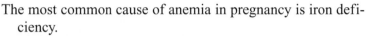

CLINICAL PEARLS

 The most common cause of anemia in pregnancy is iron defi-ciency.

 For mild anemias, it is acceptable to initiate a trial of iron sup-plementation and reassess the hemoglobin level.

 The most common cause of megaloblastic anemia in preg-nancy is folate deficiency.

 Hemolysis in individuals with glucose-6-phosphate dehydro-genase deficiency may be triggered by sulfonamides, nitro-furantoin, or antimalarial agents.

REFERENCES

Cunningham FG, Gant NF, Leveno KJ, Gilstrap LC III, Hauth JC, Wenstrom KD. Teratology, drugs, and medications. In: Williams obstetrics, 21st ed. New York: McGraw-Hill. 2001:1021.

Nuwayhid B, Nguyen T, Khalife S. In: Hacker NF and Moore JG, eds. Essentials of obstetrics and gynecology, 3rd ed. Philadelphia: Saunders. 1998:251–253.

A healthy 19-year-old G1 P0 at 29 weeks' gestation presents to the labor and delivery area complaining of intermittent abdominal pain. She denies leakage of fluid or bleeding per vagina. Her antenatal history has been unremarkable. She has been eating and drinking normally. On examination, her BP is 110/70, HR 90/min, and temperature 99°F. The fetal heart rate tracing reveals a baseline heart rate of 120 bpm and a reactive pattern. Uterine contractions are occurring every 3 to 5 min. On pelvic examination, her cervix is 3-cm dilated, 90% effaced and the fetal vertex is presenting at -1 station.

◆ **What is the most likely diagnosis?**

◆ **What is your next step in management?**

ANSWERS TO CASE 32: Preterm Labor

Summary: A healthy 19-year-old G1 P0 at 29 weeks' gestation complains of intermittent abdominal pain. Her vital signs are normal. The fetal heart rate tracing reveals a baseline heart rate of 120 bpm and is reactive. Uterine contractions are noted every 3 to 5 min. Her cervix is 3-cm dilated, 90% effaced, and the fetal vertex is presenting at -1 station.

◆ **Most likely diagnosis:** Preterm labor.

◆ **Next step in management:** Tocolysis, try to identify a cause of the preterm labor, antenatal steroids, and antibiotics for GBS prophylaxis.

Analysis

Objectives

1. Understand how to diagnose preterm labor.
2. Understand that the basic approach to preterm labor is tocolysis, identification of an etiology, and steroids (if appropriate).
3. Know the common causes of preterm delivery.

Considerations

This 19-year-old nulliparous woman is at 29 weeks' gestation and complains of intermittent abdominal pain. The monitor indicates uterine contractions every 3 to 5 min and her cervix is dilated at 3 cm, and effaced at 90%. This is sufficient to diagnose preterm labor in a nulliparous woman. If she had a previous vaginal delivery, the diagnosis may not be as clear-cut. Because of the significant prematurity, many practitioners may elect to treat for preterm labor. A single examination revealing 2-cm dilation and 80% effacement in a nulliparous woman would be sufficient to diagnose preterm labor. Tocolysis should be initiated, unless there is a contraindication (such as intra-amniotic infection or severe preeclampsia). Also, since the pregnancy is less than 34 weeks' gestation, intramuscular antenatal steroids should be given to enhance fetal pulmonary maturity. A careful search should also be undertaken to identify an underlying cause, such as urinary tract infection, cervical infection, bacterial vaginosis, generalized infection, trauma or abruption, hydramnios, or multiple gestation. Finally, intravenous antibiotics, such as penicillin, are helpful in case the tocolysis is unsuccessful, to reduce the likelihood of GBS sepsis in the neonate.

APPROACH TO PRETERM LABOR

Definitions

Preterm labor: Cervical change associated with uterine contractions prior to 37 completed weeks and after 20 weeks' gestation. In a nulliparous woman, uterine contractions and a single cervical examination revealing 2-cm dilation and 80% effacement or greater is sufficient to make the diagnosis.

Tocolysis: Pharmacologic agents used to delay delivery once preterm labor is diagnosed. The most commonly used agents are magnesium sulfate, terbutaline, ritodrine, and indomethacin.

Antenatal steroids: Betamethasone or dexamethasone given intramuscularly to the pregnant woman in an effort to decrease some of the complications of prematurity, particularly respiratory distress syndrome (intraventricular hemorrhage in the more extremely premature babies).

Clinical Approach

Preterm labor is defined as cervical change in the midst of regular uterine contractions occurring between 20 and 37 weeks' gestation. The incidence in the United States is approximately 11% of pregnancies, and it is the cause of significant perinatal morbidity and mortality. There are many risk factors associated with preterm delivery (Table 32–1).

The main symptoms of preterm labor are uterine contractions and abdominal tightening. Sometimes, pelvic pressure or increased vaginal

Table 32–1

RISK FACTORS FOR PRETERM LABOR

Preterm premature rupture of membranes
Multiple gestation
Previous preterm labor or birth
Hydramnios
Uterine anomaly
History of cervical cone biopsy
Cocaine abuse
African American race
Abdominal trauma
Pyelonephritis
Abdominal surgery in pregnancy

---

discharge may also be present. The diagnosis is established by confirming cervical change over time by the same examiner, if possible, or finding the cervix to be 2-cm dilated and 80% effaced in a nulliparous woman. Once the diagnosis has been made, then an etiology should be sought. Tocolysis is considered if the gestational age is less than 34 to 35 weeks, and **steroids are administered if the gestational age is less than 34 weeks.** The work-up for preterm labor is summarized in Table 32–2.

The most common tocolytic agent used in the United States is **magnesium sulfate.** Other medications include **terbutaline, ritodrine, nifedipine,** and **indomethacin.** The speculated mechanism of action of

Table 32–2

WORK-UP FOR PRETERM LABOR

History to assess for risk factors
Physical examination with speculum examination to assess for ruptured membranes
Serial digital cervical examinations
Complete blood count
Urine drug screen (especially for cocaine metabolites)
Urinalysis, urine culture and sensitivity
Cervical tests for gonorrhea (possibly *Chlamydia*)
Vaginal culture for group B streptococcus
Ultrasound examination for fetal weight and fetal presentation

---

magnesium is competitive inhibition of calcium to decrease its avail-ability for actin-myosin interaction, thus decreasing myometrial activity. Side effects include pulmonary edema, respiratory depression, neonatal depression, and if given long term, osteoporosis. **Pulmonary edema** is often the most serious side effect, and is seen more often with the beta-agonist agents. A complication of indomethacin is closure of the ductus arteriosus, leading to severe neonatal pulmonary hypertension.

Antenatal steroids are given between 24 and 34 weeks' gestation when there is no evidence of infection. Only one course of cortico-steroids is utilized. In other words, they are not repeated for recurrent threatened preterm delivery. In the early gestational ages, the effect is to lower the risk of intraventricular hemorrhage; at gestations greater than 28 weeks, the primary goal is to lower the incidence of respiratory distress syndrome.

Comprehension Questions

[32.1] Which of the following is least likely to be associated with preterm delivery?

    A. Incompetent cervix
    B. Hydramnios
    C. Uterine fibroids
    D. Abdominal pregnancy
    E. Hydrops fetalis

[32.2] Which one of the following is most likely to be a contraindica-tion for tocolysis at 28 weeks' gestation?

    A. Suspected abruption
    B. Group B streptococcal bacteriuria
    C. Recent laparotomy
    D. Uterine fibroid

[32.3] Which of the following is the first sign of magnesium sulfate toxicity?

A. Respiratory depression
B. Cardiac depression
C. Loss of deep tendon reflexes
D. Seizures

[32.4] Each of the following is a side effect of terbutaline except:

A. Tachycardia
B. Hyperglycemia
C. Hyperkalemia
D. Increased pulse pressure

Answers

[32.1] **D.** An abdominal pregnancy is associated with post-term gestation.

[32.2] **A.** Suspected abruption is a relative contraindication for tocolysis since the abruption may extend.

[32.3] **C.** Loss of deep tendon reflexes is one of the first signs of magnesium toxicity, and requires checking a serum magnesium level and/or reducing or stopping the infusion rate.

[32.4] **C.** Beta-agonist therapy is associated with an increased pulse pressure, hyperglycemia, **hypokalemia,** and tachycardia.

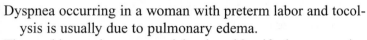

CLINICAL PEARLS

◆ Dyspnea occurring in a woman with preterm labor and tocolysis is usually due to pulmonary edema.

◆ The goal in treating preterm labor is to identify the cause, give steroids (if gestation is at 24 to 34 weeks), and tocolysis.

◆ The most common cause of neonatal morbidity in a preterm infant is respiratory distress syndrome.

◆ Beta-agonist therapy has multiple side effects including tachycardia, widened pulse pressure, hyperglycemia, and hypokalemia.

◆ A negative cervical fetal fibronectin assay virtually guarantees no delivery within one week.

REFERENCES

Cunningham FG, Gant NF, Leveno KJ, Gilstrap LC III, Hauth JC, Wenstrom KD. Preterm birth. In: Williams obstetrics, 21st ed. New York: McGraw-Hill. 2001:689–728.

Hobel CJ. Preterm labor and premature rupture of membranes. In: Hacker NF and Moore JG, eds. Essentials of obstetrics and gynecology, 3rd ed. Philadelphia: Saunders. 1998:312–323.

American College of Obstetricians and Gynecologists. Assessment of risk factors for preterm birth. Practice Bulletin 31, October 2001.

A 29-year-old woman complains of a 2-day history of dysuria, urgency, and urinary frequency. She denies the use of medications and has no significant past medical history. On examination, her BP is 100/70, HR 90/min, and temperature 98°F. The thyroid is normal on palpation. The heart and lung examinations are normal. She does not have back tenderness. The abdomen is nontender and without masses. The pelvic examination reveals normal female genitalia. There is no adnexal tenderness or masses.

✦ **What is the most likely diagnosis?**

✦ **What is the next step in the diagnosis?**

✦ **What is the most likely etiology of the condition?**

ANSWERS TO CASE 33: Urinary Tract Infection (Cystitis)

Summary: A 29-year-old woman complains of a 2-day history of dysuria, urgency, and urinary frequency. Her temperature is 98°F. She does not have back tenderness. The abdomen is nontender and without masses. The pelvic examination is normal

◆ **Most likely diagnosis:** Simple cystitis (bladder infection).

◆ **Next step in the diagnosis:** Urinalysis and/or urine culture.

◆ **Most likely etiology of the condition:** *Escherichia coli (E. coli).*

Analysis

Objectives

1. Know the symptoms of a urinary tract infection (cystitis).
2. Know that the most common bacteria causing cystitis is *Escherichia coli.*
3. Be familiar with some of the antibiotic therapies for cystitis.

Considerations

This 29-year-old woman has a 2-day history of urinary urgency, frequency, and dysuria, all which are very typical symptoms of a urinary tract infection. Because she does not have fever or flank tenderness, she most likely has a bladder infection or cystitis. Other symptoms of cystitis include hesitancy or hematuria (hemorrhagic cystitis). Urinalysis and/or urine culture and sensitivity would be the appropriate test to confirm the diagnosis. Since *E. coli* is the most common etiologic agent, the antibiotic treatment should be aimed at this organism. Sulfa agents, cephalosporins, quinolones, or nitrofurantoin are all acceptable. If the urine culture returns showing no organism and the patient still has symptoms, urethritis is a possibility (often caused by *Chlamydia tra-*

chomatis). In this setting, urethral swabbing for chlamydial testing is advisable. Another possibility is candidal vulvovaginitis. Finally, some women with symptoms of bladder discomfort with negative urine culture and urethral culture may have a chronic condition of urethral syndrome.

APPROACH TO URINARY TRACT INFECTIONS

Definitions

Cystitis: Bacterial infection of the bladder defined as having greater than 100,000 colony-forming units of a single pathogenic organism on a midstream voided specimen.

Urethritis: Infection of the urethra commonly caused by *Chlamydia trachomatis.*

Urethral syndrome: Urgency and dysuria caused by urethral inflammation of unknown etiology; urine cultures are negative.

Clinical Approach

Urinary tract infections (UTI) may involve the kidneys (pyelonephritis), bladder (cystitis), and urethra (urethritis). One in five women will acquire a UTI sometime in her life. The shorter urethra and its proximity to the rectum are the most commonly stated reasons for the increased incidence in women. Pregnancy further predisposes women to UTIs due to incomplete emptying of the bladder, ureteral obstruction, and immune suppression. Pathogenic bacteria include *E coli* (isolated 80% of the time), followed by *Enterobacter, Klebsiella, Pseudomonas, Proteus,* group B streptococcus, *Staphyloccoccus saprophyticus,* and *Chlamydia.*

The most common symptoms of lower tract infection (cystitis) are dysuria, urgency, and urinary frequency. Occasionally, the infection may induce a hemorrhagic cystitis and the patient will have gross hematuria. Nevertheless, **gross hematuria** should raise the suspicion of **nephrolithiasis.** Fever is uncommon unless there is kidney involvement, which is usually reflected by flank tenderness. The diagnosis of cystitis hinges on identification of pathogenic bacteria in the urine; bacteriuria is defined as greater than 100,000 colony-forming units per milliliter of a single uropathogen obtained from a midstream voided urine on culture. In symptomatic patients, as few as 1000 colony-forming units per milliliter may be significant. On a catheterized specimen, 10,000 colony-forming units per milliliter is considered bacteriuria. The presence of leukocytes in the urine is presumptive evidence of infection in a patient with symptoms.

Simple cystitis is the most common form of UTI and is diagnosed by the symptoms in the absence of fever or flank tenderness. Oral antimicrobial therapy is effective, and varies from one dose to 3 days, to 7 days, or even 10 days. Trimethroprim/sulfa (Bactrim), macrodantin, norfloxicin, ciprofloxicin, and cephalosporins, such as cephalothin, are effective. Ampicillin is generally not used due to the widespread resistance of *E. coli*. The utility of urine cultures in the first episode of simple cystitis is unclear. Some practitioners will routinely obtain cultures, whereas others will reserve these studies for recurrences, persistent symptoms, or in pregnancy. In the pregnant woman, asymptomatic bacteriuria (ASB) leads to acute infection in up to 25% of untreated women and thus it should always be treated.

A patient with urethritis has similar complaints to one with cystitis (i.e., urgency, frequency, and dysuria). Sometimes, the urethra may be tender on palpation and purulent drainage expressed on examination. The most commonly isolated organisms are ***Chlamydia, Gonococcus,*** and *Trichomonas*. Urethritis should be suspected in a woman with typical symptoms of UTI yet with sterile culture and no response to the standard antibiotics. Cultures of the urethra for *Gonococcus* and *Chlamydia* should be performed. Treatment may be initiated empirically for *Chlamydia* with doxycycline; if gonorrhea is suspected, intramuscular ceftriaxone with oral doxycycline is usually curative. Doxycycline should be avoided in pregnant women.

Women with pyelonephritis usually present with fever, chills, flank pain, and nausea and vomiting. Mild cases in the nonpregnant female may be treated with oral trimethroprim/sulfa or a fluoroquinolone for a 10- to 14-day course; these women should be reexamined within 48 hr. Sulfa agents are generally the most cost effective. Those who are more ill, unable to take oral medications, pregnant, or immunocompromised should be hospitalized and treated with intravenous antibiotics, such as ampicillin and gentamicin, or a cephalosporin, such as cefazolin, cefotetan, or ceftriaxone. Following resolution of fever and symptoms, pregnant women with acute pyelonephritis are often treated with suppressive antimicrobial therapy (such as nitrofurantoin macrocrystals 100 mg once daily) for the remainder of pregnancy.

Comprehension Questions

[33.1] Each of the following is a common causative organism of cystitis except:

    A. *E. coli*
    B. *Klebsiella* species
    C. *Proteus* species
    D. *Bacteroides* species

[33.2] For simple cystitis, which of the following are acceptable antibiotic treatment regimens?

    A. 3-day therapy
    B. 5-day therapy
    C. 7-day therapy
    D. All of the above

[33.3] Each of the following is a common manifestation of simple cystitis except:

    A. Fever
    B. Urgency
    C. Hesitancy
    D. Dysuria

[33.4] Which is least suggestive of a urinary tract infection?

    A. Urine showing presence of leukocyte esterase
    B. Urine microscopy showing leukocytes
    C. Urine microscopy showing crystals
    D. Urine microscopy showing bacteria

Answers

[33.1] **D.** Anaerobic bacteria, such as *Bacteroides* species, rarely cause cystitis.

[33.2] **D.** Various lengths of antibiotic therapy from a one-time dose to 7–10 days are used.

[33.3] **A.** Fever suggests an upper urinary tract infection, such as pyelonephritis.

[33.4] **C.** Crystals in the urine are usually not directly indicative of infection.

CLINICAL PEARLS

The most common cause of cystitis is *E. coli.*

Bacteriuria caused by group B streptococcus in pregnancy necessitates the use of intravenous penicillin or ampicillin in labor to decrease the risk of neonatal GBS sepsis.

Pyelonephritis presents with flank tenderness and fever.

Urethritis, commonly caused by *Chlamydia* or gonorrhea, should be suspected with negative urine cultures and symptoms of a UTI.

REFERENCES

Stenchever MA. Urogynecology. In: Stenchever MA, Droegemueller W, Herbst AL, Mishell DR, eds. Comprehensive gynecology, 4th ed. St. Louis: Mosby-Year Book. 2001:607–640.

Bhatia NN. Genitourinary dysfunction: pelvic organ prolapse, urinary incontinence, and infections. In: Hacker NF and Moore JG, eds. Essentials of obstetrics and gynecology, 3rd ed. Philadelphia: Saunders. 1998:470–476.

A 22-year-old nulliparous woman, whose last menstrual period was approximately 2 weeks ago, states that she had unprotected intercourse last night. She asks whether anything can be done to prevent her from getting pregnant. She usually uses a condom and foam for contraception. She is in good health. Her blood pressure is 120/70, HR 80/min, and temperature 99°F. Her heart and lung examinations are normal. The abdomen is nontender and without masses. The pelvic examination reveals a normal anteverted uterus. There are no adnexal masses. The pregnancy test is negative.

◆ **What is your next step?**

ANSWERS TO CASE 34: Emergency Contraception

Summary: A 22-year-old nulliparous woman, whose last menstrual period was approximately 2 weeks ago, states that she had unprotected intercourse last night. She asks whether anything can be done to prevent her from getting pregnant. She is in good health. Her physical examination is unremarkable. The pregnancy test is negative.

◆ **Next step:** Emergency contraception (EC; high-dose oral contraceptives or progestin).

Analysis

Objectives

1. Understand that emergency contraception may be used to help prevent an unwanted pregnancy after coitus.
2. Know that high-dose combination estrogen and progestin therapy or high-dose progestin therapy are methods of emergency contraception.

Considerations

This 22-year-old nulliparous woman is at approximately midcycle and had an episode of unprotected intercourse the night before. She is a candidate for emergency contraception, which is usually effective if given within 72 hr of coitus. Options include high-dose estrogen and progestin pills taken now and in 12 hr, or high-dose progestin-only therapy. The advantage of the progestin-only treatment is less nausea and vomiting. She does not have contraindications for this therapy (such as deep venous thrombosis, liver disease, or hypertension). Another potential treatment includes the insertion of an intrauterine contraceptive device.

APPROACH TO EMERGENCY CONTRACEPTION

Definitions

Emergency contraception (EC):   Use of an intervention shortly after coitus to prevent pregnancy.

Yuzpe regimen: The use of a specific oral contraceptive regimen first reported by Dr. Yuzpe, consisting of two tablets of Ovral oral contraceptives (total of 0.1 mg ethinyl estradiol and 0.5 mg levonorgestrel) at time zero and two tablets after 12 hr.

Plan B (progestin only):   Levonorgestrel 0.75 mg taken orally at time zero and the same dose after 12 hr.

Clinical Approach

Emergency contraception is the therapy for women who have had unprotected sexual intercourse, including victims of sexual assault. It is also known as the "morning after pill." The two most common regimens are the combination oral contraceptive method, known as the Yuzpe method, and the progestin-only regimen. The Yuzpe method consists of 0.1 mg of ethinyl estradiol and 0.5 mg of levonorgestrel in two doses, 12 hr apart, beginning within 72 hr of unprotected intercourse. The progestin-only (plan B) method consists of 0.75 mg of levonorgestrel in two doses taken 12 hr apart. The mechanisms of action may include inhibition of ovulation, decreased tubal motility, and, possibly, interruption of implantation.

The **efficacy of the combination method is accepted to be about a 75% reduction in pregnancy rate,** thus decreasing the risk of a midcycle coital pregnancy from 8 per 100 to about 2 per 100. The **progestin only** method appears to have slightly greater efficacy, with a pregnancy risk reduction of **about 85%.**

The **major side effect of emergency contraception is nausea and/or emesis,** which is more prominent with the combination method. An antiemetic is often prescribed with the Yuzpe regimen. Emergency contraception should not be used in patients with a suspected or known pregnancy, or those with abnormal vaginal bleeding. Those women who do not have onset on menses within 21 days following the emergency contraception should have a pregnancy test.

Comprehension Questions

[34.1] Which of the following describes the mechanism(s) whereby combination oral contraceptive therapy may act in emergency contraception?

    A. Inhibition of ovulation
    B. Decrease in tubal motility
    C. Inhibition of implantation
    D. All the of the above

[34.2] Which of the following is the most common side effect of the Yuzpe regimen?

    A. Vaginal spotting
    B. Nausea and/or vomiting
    C. Elevation of liver function enzymes
    D. Glucose intolerance
    E. Renal insufficiency

[34.3] Which of the following is the main effect of the progestin-only regimen as compared with the Yuzpe regimen in EC?

    A. Higher ectopic pregnancy rate
    B. Less effective prevention of pregnancy
    C. Less nausea
    D. More liver dysfunction

Answers

[34.1] **D.** The mechanisms whereby combination oral contraceptives may act in emergency contraception are ovulation inhibition, decreased tubal motility, and possibly interference with implantation.

[34.2] **B.** Because of the high dose of estrogens, nausea and vomiting are the most common side effect.

[34.3] **C.** The progestin-only method may have a better efficacy and fewer side effects (nausea).

CLINICAL PEARLS

◈ Emergency contraception consists of high-dose combination hormones or high-dose progestin.

◈ Emergency contraception is effective when initiated within 72 hr of intercourse.

◈ The main side effect of combination hormonal EC therapy are nausea and vomiting.

REFERENCES

Mishell DR. Family planning. In: Stenchever MA, Droegemueller W, Herbst AL, Mishell DR, eds. Comprehensive gynecology, 4th ed. St. Louis: Mosby-Year Book. 2001:295–368.

Moore GJ, DeCherney AH. Contraception and sterilization. In: Hacker NF and Moore JG, eds. Essentials of obstetrics and gynecology, 3rd ed. Philadelphia: Saunders. 1998:516–531.

A 16-year-old female comes into your office for a routine physical examination. She states that her menses began at age 12 years and occurs each month. She is sexually active and uses an oral contraceptive agent for birth control. She states that her aunt developed breast cancer at age 60 years. On examination, her BP is 100/70, HR 80/min, and temp is 99°F. Her thyroid gland is normal on palpation, as are her cardiac and pulmonary examinations. Her breasts and pubic hair are Tanner stage IV. She has a normal, nulliparous cervix on speculum examination. Bimanual examination reveals a normally sized uterus and no adnexal masses.

◆ **What is your next step?**

◆ **What is the most likely cause of mortality?**

ANSWERS TO CASE 35: Health Maintenance, Age 16 Years

Summary: A 16-year-old female comes into your office for a routine physical examination. Her menses occurs monthly. She is sexually active and uses an oral contraceptive. Her BP is 100/70. Examinations of her thyroid gland, heart, lungs, breasts, and pubic hair are within normal limits. The speculum and bimanual examinations are normal.

◆ **Next step:** Pap smear.

◆ **Most likely cause of mortality:** Motor vehicle accidents.

Analysis

Objectives

1. Understand that health maintenance of a 16-year-old female consists of cancer screening, immunizations, and counseling.
2. Know that motor vehicle accidents are the most common cause of mortality for someone of this age.
3. Know that eating disorders, depression, suicide, drug abuse, sexually transmitted diseases, and abuse are common conditions in adolescents.

Considerations

This 16-year-old adolescent is sexually active. Cervical cancer screening, by means of a Pap smear, should be initiated. Immunizations include hepatitis B vaccination and, possibly, a tetanus booster if indicated. Also, she should receive counseling about motor vehicle accident prevention, such as use of seat belts and avoiding intoxication while driving. Questions should be directed toward self-image, sexual or physical abuse, and eating disorders. Women who are bulimic will usually be forthright, but those with anorexia nervosa will usually deny their disorder. The stability of the sexual relationships should also be queried and counseling about pregnancy and disease prevention should be broached. In adolescent males, homicide is a leading cause of death.

APPROACH TO ADOLESCENT HEALTH MAINTENANCE

Also see Case 2.

Definitions

Anorexia nervosa: Eating disorder usually affecting adolescent females in which the affected person has a distorted body image thinking of herself as overweight, when in reality her weight is less than her ideal body weight.

Bulimia: Eating disorder where the affected individual will go through binges of eating and then induce emesis, use laxatives, or reduce calories.

Clinical Approach

Health risks to adolescents are more likely behavioral rather than caused by illnesses. Three-quarters of deaths in the age group 13 to 19 years are due to four preventable causes: 1) motor vehicle accidents, 2) homicide, 3) suicide, and 4) other unintentional injuries. Hence, one of the main focuses of the annual visit should be on injury prevention, such as avoiding alcohol intoxication, using seat belts, and avoiding the use of weapons. Other important issues to address include dietary habits, benefits of physical activity, and counseling about sexual behavior.

All teenagers should be screened for eating disorders by use of a body mass index table. They should be queried about laxative use and induction of emesis. Drug use and depression should be questioned in a nonjudgmental fashion. Cancer screening in this age group consists of annual Pap smears for those who have engaged in sexual activity or have reached the age of 18 years.

Immunizations include the bivalent tetanus-diphtheria booster administered between the ages of 11 and 12 years if not vaccinated within the past 5 yr. Hepatitis B vaccination may be considered if the individual is susceptible. Varicella immunization is also recommended for those at age 11 to 12 years who are nonimmune. The hepatitis A vaccine is usually given to patients traveling to countries with high endemic rates or for those with chronic liver disease or intravenous drug use.

Comprehension Questions

[35.1] Which of the following describes when cervical cancer screening be initiated?

    A. Only when sexually active, and does not need to be performed if never sexually active
    B. At age 18 years regardless of sexual activity
    C. At age 18 years or when sexually active, whichever comes first
    D. At age 16 years

[35.2] A 17-year-old woman is noted to have swollen, nontender cheeks and malodorous breath and dental caries. Which of the following is the most likely etiology?

    A. Acute mump infection
    B. Bulimia
    C. Anorexia nervosa
    D. Parotid gland infections
    E. Esophageal reflux

[35.3] Which of the following statements best describes the effect of oral contraceptive agents on adolescents?

    A. Use of oral contraceptive agents will lead to delayed maturation of the hypothalamic-pituitary axis.
    B. Use of oral contraceptive agents in adolescents will not affect the maturation of the hypothalamic-pituitary axis.

C. Oral contraceptive use may lead to sexual promiscuity.

D. Oral contraceptive use enhances the development of salpingitis.

[35.4] Each of the following vaccines is indicated in a 16-year-old female except:

A. Tetanus booster
B. Hepatitis B
C. Hepatitis A
D. Influenza

Answers

[35.1] **C.** Cervical cancer screening (Pap smear) should be started at age 18 years or when sexually active.

[35.2] **B.** With bulimia, patients may have malodorous breath, rotting teeth, swollen parotid glands, and callouses on the knuckles of their hands from inducing emesis.

[35.3] **B.** The combination oral contraceptive has not been shown to delay the maturation of the hypothalamic-pituitary-ovarian axis when used in teenagers.

[35.4] **D.** Influenza vaccine is not indicated until age 50 to 55 years, unless there are other coexisting conditions.

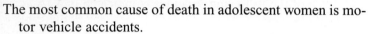

CLINICAL PEARLS

❖ Pap smear screening should be initiated when sexually active or at age 18 years, whichever occurs earlier.

❖ The most common cause of death in adolescent women is motor vehicle accidents.

❖ Eating disorders, depression, and abuse are common problems in adolescents.

REFERENCES

Seltzer VL. Preventive health care and screening during the stages of a woman's life. In: Seltzer VL and Pearse WH, eds. Women's primary health care, 2nd ed. New York: McGraw-Hill. 2000:23–32.

Peterson HB. Principles of screening. In: Holzman GB, Rinehart RD, Dunn LJ, eds. Precis: primary and preventive care. Washington, DC: ACOG. 1999:15–21.

American College of Obstetricians and Gynecologists. Primary and preventive care: periodic assessments. ACOG Committee Opinion 246. Washington, DC; 1999.

A 20-year-old G1 P0 woman at 29 weeks' gestation is hospitalized for acute pyelonephritis. She has no history of pyelonephritis in the past. She has been receiving intravenous ampicillin and gentamicin for 48 hr. She complains of acute shortness of breath. On examination, her HR is 100 bpm, RR 45/min and labored, and BP is 120/70. Right costovertebral tenderness is noted. Her abdominal examination reveals no masses or tenderness. The fetal heart tones are in the 140 to 150 bpm range. The urine culture revealed *Escherichia coli* sensitive to ampicillin.

◆ **What is the most likely diagnosis?**

ANSWERS TO CASE 36: Pyelonephritis, Unresponsive

Summary: A 20-year-old G1 P0 woman at 29 weeks' gestation has received intravenous ampicillin and gentamicin for 48 hr for acute pyelonephritis. She complains of acute shortness of breath. On examination, her HR is 100 bpm, RR 45/min, and BP is 120/70. Right costovertebral tenderness is noted. The urine culture revealed *E. coli* sensitive to ampicillin.

◆ **Most likely diagnosis:** Acute respiratory distress syndrome (ARDS).

Analysis

Objectives

1. Understand the clinical presentation of pyelonephritis.
2. Know that the primary treatment of pyelonephritis is intravenous antibiotic therapy.
3. Understand that endotoxins can cause pulmonary damage, leading to acute respiratory distress syndrome (ARDS).

Considerations

This patient is 20 years old at 29 weeks' gestation. She presented with pyelonephritis. She had been treated with intravenous ampicillin and gentamicin. The diagnosis is confirmed since *E. coli* has been cultured from the urine. She is now presenting with dyspnea and tachypnea. The most likely etiology for her respiratory symptoms is ARDS, with pulmonary injury due to the endotoxin release. This typically occurs after antibiotics have begun to lyse the bacteria, leading to endotoxemia. The endotoxins can induce damage to the myocardium, liver, and kidneys, as well as the lungs. The mechanism is leaky capillaries, which allows fluid from the intravascular space to permeate into the alveolar areas. A chest film may show patchy infiltrates; however, if the disease process is early, the chest radiograph may be normal. Treatment would include oxygen supplementation, careful monitoring of fluids (not to overload), and supportive measures. Occasionally, a patient may require intubation, but usually the condition stabilizes and improves.

APPROACH TO PYELONEPHRITIS IN PREGNANCY

Definitions

Pyelonephritis: Kidney parenchymal infection most commonly caused by gram-negative aerobic bacteria, such as *E. coli.*

Endotoxin: A lipopolysaccharide that is released upon lysis of the cell wall of bacteria, especially gram-negative bacteria.

Acute respiratory distress syndrome (ARDS): Alveolar and endothelial injury leading to leaky pulmonary capillaries, clinically causing hypoxemia, large alveolar-arterial gradient, and loss of lung volume.

Clinical Approach

Pyelonephritis in pregnancy can be a very serious medical condition, with an incidence of 1% to 2% of all pregnancies. It is the most common cause of sepsis in pregnant women. The patient generally complains of dysuria, urgency, frequency, costovertebral tenderness, fever and chills, and nausea and vomiting. The urinalysis usually will reveal pyuria and bacteriuria; a urine culture revealing greater than 100,000 colony-forming units/mL of a single uropathogen is diagnostic. The most common organism is *E. coli,* seen in about 80% of cases. *Klebsiella pneumoniae, Staphyloccoccus aureus,* and *Proteus mirabilis* may also be isolated.

Pregnant women with acute pyelonephritis should be hospitalized and given intravenous hydration and antibiotics. Cephalosporins, such as cefotetan or ceftriaxone, or the combination of ampicillin and gentamicin are usually effective. The patient should be treated until the fever and flank tenderness have substantially improved and then switched to oral antimicrobial suppressive therapy for the remainder of the pregnancy. Up to one-third of pregnant women with pyelonephritis

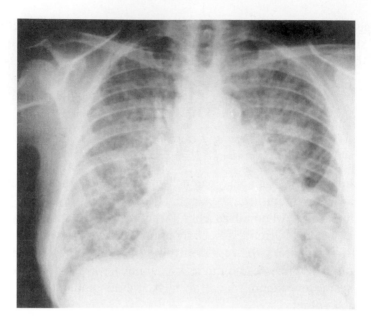

Figure 36–1. Acute respiratory distress syndrome. Chest radiograph depicts acute respiratory distress syndrome with diffuse pulmonary infiltrates.

(Reproduced, with permission, from Braunwald E et al. Harrison's principles of internal medicine, 15th ed. New York: McGraw-Hill; 2001: 1524.

will develop a recurrent UTI if suppressive therapy is not utilized. A repeat urine culture should be obtained to ensure eradication of the infection. If clinical improvement has not occurred after 48 to 72 hr of appropriate antibiotic therapy, a urinary tract obstruction (i.e., ureterolithiasis) or a perinephric abscess should be suspected.

Approximately 2% to 5% of pregnant women with pyelonephritis will develop acute respiratory distress syndrome (ARDS), which is defined as pulmonary injury due to sepsis, usually endotoxin related. The endotoxins derived from the gram-negative bacterial cell wall enter the blood stream, especially after antibiotic therapy, and may induce transient elevation of the serum creatinine as well as liver enzymes. Also, the endotoxemia may cause uterine contractions and place a patient into preterm labor. Diffuse bilateral or interstitial infiltrates are typically seen on chest radiograph (Figure 36–1). The treatment of ARDS is supportive, with priorities on oxygenation and careful fluid management. In severe cases, mechanical ventilation may be required to maintain adequate oxygen levels.

Comprehension Questions

[36.1] Which of the following is the most commonly isolated etiologic agent causing pyelonephritis in pregnancy?

A. *Proteus* species
B. Candidal species
C. *E. coli*
D. *Klebsiella* species

[36.2] Which of the following is the most common cause of septic shock in pregnancy?

A. Pelvic inflammatory disease
B. Pyelonephritis
C. Wound infection
D. Mastitis

[36.3] When a pregnant woman with pyelonephritis does not improve on adequate antibiotic therapy for 48 hr and experiences continued severe flank tenderness and fever, each of the following should be considered except:

A. Obstruction of the urinary tract, such as by nephrolithiasis
B. Perinephric abscess
C. Resistant organism
D. Consider drug fever and stop antibiotic therapy and observe

[36.4] Asymptomatic bacteriuria is best identified by which of the following?

A. Careful questioning for dysuria or urinary frequency
B. Urine culture on the first prenatal visit
C. Urine culture at 35 weeks' gestation
D. Urinalysis for any patient with family history of UTI

Answers

[36.1] **C.** *E. coli* is the most commonly bacteria in pyelonephritis.

[36.2] **B.** Pyelonephritis is the most common cause of septic shock in pregnancy.

[36.3] **D.** Each of the other answers is a cause of continued fever and flank tenderness; flank tenderness would not be noted with a drug fever.

[36.4] **B.** Urine culture for every patient at the first prenatal visit helps to identify asymptomatic bacteriuria. Treatment prevents sequelae such as preterm labor or pyelonephritis during pregnancy.

CLINICAL PEARLS

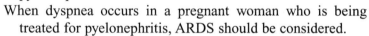

The most common cause of septic shock in pregnancy is pyelonephritis.

When dyspnea occurs in a pregnant woman who is being treated for pyelonephritis, ARDS should be considered.

Endotoxin release from gram-negative bacteria is the cause of acute respiratory distress syndrome associated with pyelonephritis.

REFERENCES

Cunningham FG, Gant NF, Leveno KJ, Gilstrap LC III, Hauth JC, Wenstrom KD. Renal and urinary tract disorders. In: Williams obstetrics, 21st ed. New York: McGraw-Hill. 2001:1255–1258.

Goodman JR. AIDS and infectious diseases in pregnancy. In: Hacker NF and Moore JG, eds. Essentials of obstetrics and gynecology, 3rd ed. Philadelphia: Saunders. 1998:335–37.

A 31-year-old G1 P0 woman at 24 weeks' gestation complains of a 2-day history of soreness of the right calf. She states that she has been walking slightly more over the past several days. She denies a history of medical illnesses or trauma to her legs. Her family history is unremarkable. On examination, her BP is 100/60, HR 100 bpm, RR 12/min, and she is afebrile. The neck is supple. Her heart and lung examinations are normal. The abdomen is nontender and without masses. The fundal height is 23 cm and the fetal heart tones are in the range of 140 to 150 bpm. The right calf is somewhat tender and slightly swollen. No palpable cords are present. The Homan's sign is negative.

◆ **What is your next step?**

ANSWERS TO CASE 37: Deep Venous Thrombosis In Pregnancy

Summary: A 31-year-old G1 P0 woman at 24 weeks' gestation, who has been walking slightly more than usual, complains of a 2-day history of right calf soreness. On examination, her HR is 100 bpm and RR 12/min. Her heart and lung examinations are normal. The right calf is somewhat tender and slightly swollen. No palpable cords are present, and the Homan's sign is negative.

◆ **Next step:** Noninvasive assessment for a deep venous thrombosis of the right leg.

Analysis

Objectives

1. Know that pregnancy is a hypercoagulable state and predisposes to thrombosis.
2. Know that the physical examination is not an accurate method to diagnose deep venous thrombosis.
3. Know the diagnostic and therapeutic measures for deep venous thrombosis.

Considerations

This 31-year-old woman at 24 weeks' gestation has been walking slightly more than usual and complains of calf tenderness. The right calf is mildly tender and swollen. These subtle findings are sufficient to warrant investigations for a deep venous thrombosis. Because of the increased levels of clotting factors (predominantly fibrinogen) and the venous stasis, pregnancy produces a hypercoagulable state. **The physical examination is not very sensitive or specific** in the assessment of deep venous thrombosis. The **Homan's sign,** that is, dorsiflexion of the foot to attempt to elicit tenderness in the patient is a **poor test,** and theoretically may itself cause embolization of clots. For these reasons, many experts advise against the performance of this test. Instead, a noninvasive test, such as **Doppler flow studies** of the venous system of the affected lower extremity, is an appropriate method to assess for deep venous thrombosis. If the Doppler flow test confirms a thrombosis, anticoagulation with an agent such as heparin should be initiated. In a **nonpregnant woman, venography** would be an option, that is, injecting radiopaque dye into a vein of the foot and taking radiographic images of the venous system.

APPROACH TO DEEP VENOUS THROMBOSIS IN PREGNANCY

Definitions

Deep venous thrombosis: Deposit of a thrombus, platelet and fibrin, in the deep veins, usually of the lower extremity or pelvis.

Duplex ultrasound flow study: Ultrasound technique using both real-time sonography and Doppler flow to assess for deep venous thrombosis.

Pulmonary embolism: When a fragment of the thrombus is dislodged and migrates into the pulmonary arterial circulation.

Clinical Approach

Deep venous thrombosis occurs in slightly less than 1% of pregnancies. The pregnant state increases the risk fivefold due to the **venous stasis with the large gravid uterus** pressing on the vena cava and **the hypercoagulable state due to the increase in clotting factors. Cesarean delivery** further increases the risk of DVT. Whereas clots involving the superficial venous system pose virtually no danger and may be treated with analgesia, deep venous thrombosis is associated with pulmonary embolism in 40% of untreated cases. The risk of death is increased tenfold when pulmonary embolism is unrecognized and untreated. Therefore, early diagnosis and anticoagulation treatment are crucial.

Signs and symptoms of DVT include "muscle pain," deep linear cords of the calf, and tenderness and swelling of the lower extremity. A 2-cm difference in leg circumferences is also sometimes helpful.

Unfortunately, none of these findings are very specific for DVT, and in fact, the **examination is normal in half of the cases of DVT**. Hence, imaging tests are necessary for confirmation.

In **pregnancy, the diagnostic test of choice is Doppler ultrasound imaging,** which usually employs a 5 to 7.5 MHz Doppler transducer to measure venous blood flow with and without compression of the deep veins. This modality is nearly as sensitive and specific as the time-honored method of contrast venography.

Management of deep venous thrombosis is primarily anticoagulation with bed rest and extremity elevation. During pregnancy, **heparin** is usually preferable over coumadin, since **coumadin** may cause **congenital abnormalities and is more difficult to reverse.** Heparin, which is a potent thrombin inhibitor that blocks conversion of fibrinogen to fibrin, combines with antithrombin III. It stabilizes the clot and inhibits its propagation. After full intravenous anticoagulation therapy for 5 to 7 days, the therapy is generally switched to subcutaneous therapy to maintain the aPTT at 1.5 to 2.5 times control for at least 3 months after the acute event. After 3 months, either full heparinization or "prophylactic heparinization" can be utilized for the remainder of the pregnancy and for 6 weeks postpartum (see Case 22).

Comprehension Questions

[37.1] Which of the following is a reason for the hypercoagulable state in pregnancy?

  A. Venous stasis
  B. Deceased clotting factors levels
  C. Elevated platelet count
  D. Endothelial damage

[37.2] Long-term heparin therapy may lead to each of the following except:

  A. Osteoporosis
  B. Thrombocytopenia

C. Fetal intracranial hemorrhage
D. Maternal bleeding

[37.3] Which of the following is the most common location of a deep venous thrombosis after gynecologic surgery?

A. Inferior vena cava
B. Lower extremities
C. Ovarian vein
D. Superior vena cava
E. Subclavian vein

[37.4] After a woman develops a deep venous thrombosis during pregnancy, which of the following agents is most likely to be contraindicated?

A. Medroxyprogesterone acetate depot (Depoprovera) contraception
B. Intrauterine contraceptive device (IUD)
C. Combination oral contraceptive
D. Levonorgestrel silastic implants (Norplant)
E. Prostaglandin compounds

Answers

[37.1] **A.** Venous stasis is present due to the uterus compressing the vena cava. Usually, the platelet count is slightly lower in the pregnant state. The lower limit of normal in the nonpregnant patient is 150,000/uL, and 120,000 in the pregnant woman.

[37.2] **C.** Heparin is a large, charged glycoprotein that does not cross the placenta very well.

[37.3] **B.** The most common locations of a deep venous thrombosis associated with gynecologic surgery are the lower extremities and the pelvic veins.

[37.4] **C.** The estrogen in the combination oral contraceptive is slightly
thrombogenic, and may be contraindicated in a women with a
prior DVT.

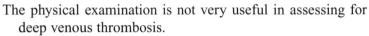

CLINICAL PEARLS

❖ The physical examination is not very useful in assessing for
deep venous thrombosis.

❖ Venous duplex Doppler sonography is an accurate method to
diagnose deep venous thrombosis.

❖ After a deep venous thrombosis or pulmonary embolus is diagnosed, anticoagulation is indicated.

❖ The most common locations for deep venous thrombosis after
gynecologic surgery are the lower extremities and the
pelvic veins.

REFERENCES

Cunningham FG, Gant NF, Leveno KJ, Gilstrap LC III, Hauth JC, Wenstrom KD.
Pulmonary disorders. In: Williams obstetrics, 21st ed. New York: McGraw-Hill.
2001:1237–1240.
Nuwayhid B, Nguyen T, Khalife S. Medical complications in pregnancy. In: Hacker
NF and Moore JG, eds. Essentials of obstetrics and gynecology, 3rd ed. Philadel-
phia: Saunders. 1998:237–239.
American College of Obstetricians and Gynecologists. Thromboembolism in preg-
nancy. Practice Bulletin No. 19, August 2000.

A 50-year-old G4 P4 woman comes in for a well-woman examination. She had used the contraceptive diaphragm for birth control until she went into menopause 1 yr ago. Her family history is unremarkable for cancer. Her surgical history includes a myomectomy for symptomatic uterine fibroids 10 yr ago. On examination, her BP is 120/74, HR 80 bpm, and she is afebrile. Her thyroid is normal on palpation. Her heart and lung examinations are normal. The breast examination shows a 1.5-cm, mobile, nontender mass of the upper outer quadrant of the right breast. No adenopathy or skin changes are appreciated. Mammography and ultrasound examinations of the breasts are normal.

◆ **What is your next step?**

ANSWERS TO CASE 38: Dominant Breast Mass

Summary: A 50-year-old postmenopausal woman comes in for a well-woman examination. The breast examination shows a 1.5-cm, mobile, nontender mass of the upper outer quadrant of the right breast. No adenopathy or skin changes are appreciated. Mammography and ultrasound examinations of the breasts are normal.

◆ **Next step:** Excisional biopsy of the breast mass.

Analysis

Objectives

1. Understand that any three-dimensional dominant breast mass requires tissue for histologic analysis.
2. Understand that the age of the patient is usually the biggest risk factor for breast cancer.
3. Understand that normal imaging of a palpable breast mass does not rule out cancer.

Considerations

This 50-year-old woman came in for a well-woman examination. The physical examination is aimed at screening for common and/or serious conditions, such as hypertension, thyroid disease, cervical cancer (Pap smear), colon cancer (stool for occult blood), and breast cancer. A single 1.5-cm breast mass is palpated, but there are no associated skin changes, such as nipple retraction or dimpling of the skin. There is no associated adenopathy. Furthermore, the imaging tests (mammography and ultrasonography) are normal. Despite the normal imaging, there is a possibility that the breast mass is malignant. Therefore, biopsy of the mass is indicated. Because of the patient's age, removal of the entire mass (excisional biopsy) is preferable over fine needle aspiration. Fine needle aspiration may miss a malignancy, and at this patient's age, leaving a mass in the breast would make future examinations more difficult.

APPROACH TO BREAST MASSES

Definitions

Dominant breast mass: A three-dimensional mass that, on palpation, is felt to be separate from the remainder of the breast tissue.
Excisional biopsy: Surgical procedure removing the entire mass.
Skin dimpling: Retraction of the skin, which is suspicious for an underlying malignancy, due to the cancer being fixed to the skin.

Clinical Approach

Breast cancer is the most common cancer in women. It is the second leading cause of female cancer deaths, exceeded only by lung cancer. The prevalence of breast cancer is age specific and **age is the most important risk factor.** One in 2500 women will develop breast cancer at the age of 20 years; whereas 1 in 30 women will develop breast cancer at the age of 60 years, giving an overall lifetime risk of 1 in 8. **Other risk factors include a family history of mammary cancer, especially of premenopausal onset.**

Early diagnosis improves survival. The most common way that breast cancer is first discovered is a mass palpated by the patient. Unfortunately, this frequently occurs at an advanced stage. Routine screening is preferable. Monthly self-breast examination and clinical breast examination every 3 yr should be performed for women ages 20 to 39 years. Women over the age of 40 years should perform a monthly self-breast examination, and have a yearly clinical breast examination; some experts advocate mammography every 2 yrs between the ages of 40 to 49 years. **Annual mammography should be initiated at age 50 years, but may be performed sooner if risk factors warrant the need.**

Mammograms carry a false negative rate of up to 10%. Thus, **any palpable dominant mass, regardless of mammographic findings, requires histologic diagnosis.** The type of biopsy will vary depending on the risk of cancer. For example, a young woman with a clinical examination consistent with a fibroadenoma may have a fine needle aspiration; in contrast, a woman aged 50 years, at greater risk for malignancy due to age, will usually have an excisional biopsy. **The greater the risk for cancer, the more tissue that should be sampled.**

If a mammogram detects a suspicious lesion, a biopsy is usually performed. For nonpalpable lesions, the biopsy requires needle-localization excisional biopsy or stereotactic core needle biopsy.

Comprehension Questions

Match the best diagnostic approach (A–F) to the following situations (38.1–38.4).

    A. Mammography
    B. Ultrasound examination
    C. Fine needle aspiration
    D. Excisional biopsy
    E. Thermographic examination
    F. Bilateral mastectomy

[38.1] A 17-year-old woman with an ill-defined, mobile,1-cm cyst of the right breast.

[38.2] A 50-year-old woman with no breast masses whose mother died of breast cancer.

[38.3] A 60-year-old woman with a 1.7-cm, mobile breast mass of the left breast.

[38.4] A 52-year-old woman with bilateral saline breast implants.

Answers

[38.1] Both **B** and **C** are correct answers. Ultrasound can help to delineate the mass and differentiate a cyst versus solid mass. Fine needle aspiration may be chosen and if fluid is aspirated and the mass disappears, then no further therapy is needed.

[38.2] **A.** Mammography should be initiated at a minimum by age 50 years.

[38.3] **D.** Excisional biopsy should be performed on a dominant mass in an older patient.

[38.4] **A.** Mammography is still the best test in women with saline implants, although some of the breast architecture may be obscured.

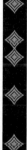

CLINICAL PEARLS

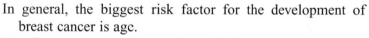

A three-dimensional dominant breast mass must be biopsied, regardless of the imaging results.

Early detection of breast cancer leads to better survival.

In general, the biggest risk factor for the development of breast cancer is age.

Two first-degree family members with breast cancer suggests a familial syndrome, such as mediated by the BRCA-1 or BRCA-2 gene.

The most common cause of unilateral serosanguinous nipple discharge from a single duct is intraductal papilloma.

REFERENCES

Droegemuller W, Valea FA. Breast diseases. In: Stenchever MA, Droegemueller W, Herbst AL, Mishell DR, eds. Comprehensive gynecology, 4th ed. St. Louis: Mosby-Year Book. 2001:359–398.

Hacker NF. Breast disease: a gynecologic perspective. In: Hacker NF and Moore JG, eds. Essentials of obstetrics and gynecology, 3rd ed. Philadelphia: Saunders. 1998:507–515.

A 22-year-old parous woman complains of a 3-month history of weight loss, nervousness, palpitations, and sweating. She denies a history of thyroid disease, and is not taking any weight loss medications. She denies abdominal pain, nausea or vomiting, fever, or prior irradiation. On examination, her BP is 110/60, HR is 110 bpm, and she is afebrile. Her thyroid gland is normal to palpation. She does not have proptosis or lid lag. Her abdomen is nontender and with normal bowel sounds. She is noted to have a fine tremor. Her uterus is normal in size. A mobile, nontender, 9-cm mass is palpated on the right side of the pelvis, which on sonography has the appearance of an adnexal mass with solid and cystic components.

⬥ **What is the most likely diagnosis?**

⬥ **What is your management of this patient?**

ANSWERS TO CASE 39: Ovarian Tumor (Struma Ovarii)

Summary: A 22-year-old parous woman without a history of thyroid disease complains of a 3-month history of weight loss, nervousness, palpitations, and sweating. She has tachycardia, but her thyroid gland is normal to palpation. She does not have proptosis or lid lag. She is noted to have a mobile, nontender, 9-cm mass, which on sonography has solid and cystic components.

◆ **Most likely diagnosis:** Hyperthyroidism caused by a benign cystic teratoma containing thyroid tissue (struma ovarii).

◆ **Management of this patient:** Exploratory laparotomy with ovarian cystectomy.

Analysis

Objectives

1. Know that benign cystic teratomas (dermoid cysts) are the most common ovarian tumors in women younger than 30 years.
2. Understand that dermoid cysts sometimes contain thyroid tissue and cause hyperthyroidism.
3. Know that surgical therapy is the treatment of choice for ovarian tumors.
4. Understand how to evaluate and manage adnexal masses in the various age groups.

Considerations

This 22-year-old woman has symptoms of hyperthyroidism with weight loss, palpitations, and nervousness. **The most common cause of hyperthyroidism in the United States is Graves' disease,** but the patient has no history of thyroid disease and her thyroid is normal to palpation. A patient with Graves' disease usually will have a nontender goiter, and many times eye-related symptoms (proptosis or lid lag). She has an ovarian mass, which on sonography is noted to be complex, that is, to have both solid and cystic components. There is no mention of ascites in the maternal abdomen; the presence of **ascites would be consistent with ovarian cancer.** In a young woman (less than 30 years of age) with a unilateral complex ovarian mass, the most likely diagnosis is a cystic teratoma, or dermoid cyst. These tumors sometimes contain thyroid tissue and may cause hyperthyroidism. The treatment of choice for ovarian neoplasms is exploratory laparotomy with ovarian cystectomy, if benign, or more extensive surgery if malignant. At the time of surgery, the excised cyst is sent for frozen section to determine if it is benign (no further surgery needed) or malignant (surgical staging needed).

APPROACH TO ADNEXAL MASSES

Definitions

Cystic teratoma: A benign germ cell tumor that may contain all three germ cell layers.

Struma ovarii: Benign cystic teratoma containing thyroid tissue, which can cause symptoms of hyperthyroidism.

Ovarian neoplasm: An abnormal growth (either benign or malignant) of the ovary; most will not regress.

Epithelial ovarian tumor: Neoplasm arising from the outer layer of the ovary, which can imitate the other epithelium of the gynecologic or urologic system. This is the most common type of ovarian malignancy, usually occurring in older women.

Functional ovarian cyst: Physiologic cysts of the ovary, which occur in reproductive-aged women, of follicular, corpus luteal, or theca lutein in origin.

Dermoid Cysts

Germ cell tumors (Table 39–1) represent about one-quarter of all ovarian tumors, and are the second most frequent type of ovarian neoplasms. They are found mainly in young women, usually in the second

Table 39–1
GERM CELL CLASSIFICATION

Dysgerminoma
Endodermal sinus tumor
Embryonal carcinoma
Polyembryoma
Choriocarcinoma
Teratoma

and third decade of life. **The most common tumor is the benign cystic teratoma (dermoid).** A germ cell tumor usually presents as a pelvic mass and causes pain due to its rapidly enlarging size. Because of these symptoms, 60% to 70% of patients present at stage I, limited to one or both ovaries.

Teratomas

Mature benign cystic teratomas (dermoid cysts) constitute over 95% of all ovarian teratomas. They make up 15% to 25% of all ovarian tumors, especially in the second and third decades of life. The most common elements are ectodermal derivatives such as skin, hair follicles, and sebaceous or sweat glands. However, they can also contain tissues of the three embryonic layers, including mesoderm and endoderm. They are usually multicystic and contain hair intermixed with foul-smelling, sticky, keratinaceous, and sebaceous debris. Although most are unilateral, they can appear **bilaterally 10% to 15%** of the time. Ultrasound features of dermoid cysts include a hypoechoic area or echoic band-like strand in a hypoechoic medium or the appearance of a cystic structure with a fat fluid level. **Torsion is the most frequent complication, with severe acute abdominal pain** as the typical initial symptom. This is more commonly seen during pregnancy and the puerperium. Torsion is also more common in children and younger patients. Rupture is an uncommon complication and presents as shock or hemorrhage. A chemical peritonitis can be caused by the spill of the contents of the tumor into the peritoneal cavity. The treatment is usually a

cystectomy or unilateral oophorectomy with inspection of the contralateral ovary.

Immature teratomas contain all three germ layers as well as immature or embryonal structures. They are uncommon and comprise less than 1% of ovarian cancers. They occur primarily in the first and second decades of life and are basically unknown after menopause. Malignant teratomas contain immature neural elements and that quantity alone determines the grade. They are almost always unilateral. The prognosis is directly related to the stage and the cellular immaturity. The treatment is a unilateral salpingo-oophorectomy with wide sampling of peritoneal implants. If the primary tumor is grade 1 and all peritoneal implants are grade 0, no further treatment is warranted. However, if the primary tumor is grade 2 or 3 and if there are implants or recurrences, combination chemotherapy is usually effective.

Struma Ovarii

Struma ovarii is a teratoma in which **thyroid tissue** has overgrown the other elements. They are usually unilateral, occurring more frequently in the right adnexa, and generally measure less than 10 cm in diameter. Preoperative clinical or radiologic diagnosis is very difficult. Only rarely will patients develop thyrotoxicosis. On MRI, these tumors appear as complex multilobulated masses with thick septa, thought to represent multiple large thyroid follicles. Most of these tumors are benign, but about 10% can have malignant changes. They will rarely produce sufficient thyroid hormone to induce hyperthyroidism. The treatment is usually cystectomy or salpingo-oophorectomy.

Epithelial Tumors

The most common ovarian tumors in women **over the age of 30 years** are of epithelial origin (Table 39–2). The serous subtype is most common and more often bilateral. **Mucinous tumors** are characterized by their **large size,** and if ruptured may lead to **pseudomyxoma peritoneii,** in which the mucinous material spills out into the intraabdominal cavity. Endometrioid tumors of the ovary may coexist with

Table 39–2
EPITHELIAL OVARIAN TUMORS

Serous
Mucinous
Endometriod
Brenner
Clear cell

a primary endometrial carcinoma of the uterus. The treatment of epithelial tumors is surgical, and if malignancy is confirmed, cancer staging is indicated. **Malignant ascites** is common with cancer, as is spread to the small bowel and omentum. Lymphatic extension may also be seen. The **tumor marker CA-125** is elevated in most epithelial ovarian tumors, and is more specific in postmenopausal women, since a variety of diseases during the reproductive years can elevate the CA-125 level.

Adnexal Masses

The evaluation of adnexal masses is guided by the suspicion of neoplasm (benign or malignant). At the extremes of ages, there are few functional ovarian cysts and the management is straightforward (Table 39–3). During the reproductive years, functional ovarian cysts, such as follicular and corpus luteal cysts, sometimes make the evaluation difficult. In general, any adnexal mass greater than 8 cm in size is likely to be a tumor and should be explored. Any adnexal mass less than 5 cm in size suggests a functional cyst. Between 5 and 8 cm, the sonographic features may help to distinguish functional versus neoplasm. Septations, solid components, or excrescences (growth on surface or inner lining) are consistent with a neoplastic process, whereas a simple cyst is more suggestive of a functional cyst. Sometimes, a practitioner will choose to observe an adnexal mass that is between 5 and 8 cm in size for 1 month and operate if it is persistent.

Table 39–3
EVALUATION OF ADNEXAL MASSES BASED ON AGE

AGE GROUP	OVARIAN SIZE	PLAN
Prepubertal	> 2 cm	Operate
Reproductive age	< 5 cm 5–8 cm > 8 cm	Observe Sonogram; if septations, solid components or excrescences, then operate; otherwise observe for 1 month Operate
Menopausal	> 4–5 cm	Operate

Comprehension Questions

[39.1] Each of the following is a germ cell tumor of the ovary except:

    A. Benign cystic teratoma (dermoid)
    B. Endodermal sinus tumor
    C. Brenner tumor
    D. Choriocarcinoma

[39.2] Benign cystic teratomas of the ovary may contain each the following except:

    A. Ectoderm
    B. Endoderm
    C. Mesoderm
    D. All the above may be found.

[39.3] Which of the following is the best treatment for a suspected dermoid cyst found in an 18-year-old nulliparous woman?

    A. Total abdominal hysterectomy
    B. Unilateral salpingo-oophrectomy
    C. Ovarian cystectomy
    D. Observation

Match the following sonographic findings (A–D) to the ovarian tumor type [39.4–39.6].

    A. Completely solid
    B. Simple cyst
    C. Complex
    D. Ascites is commonly seen

[39.4] Granulosa cell tumor

[39.5] Benign cystic teratoma (dermoid cyst)

[39.6] Follicular cyst

[39.7] A 44-year-old woman is noted to have a 30-cm tumor of the ovary. Which of the following is the most likely cell type?

    A. Dermoid cyst
    B. Granulosa cell tumor
    C. Serous tumor
    D. Mucinous tumor

Answers

[39.1] **C.** A Brenner tumor is an epithelial type of ovarian neoplasm.

[39.2] **D.** All cell lines may be found in a dermoid cyst of the ovary.

[39.3] **C.** Ovarian cystectomy is the best treatment for benign cystic teratomas.

[39.4] **A.** Granulosa cell tumors and Sertoli-Leydig cell tumors are usually solid on ultrasound, and may secrete sex hormones. Typically, granulosa-theca cell tumors produce estrogens, whereas Sertoli-Leydig cell tumors make androgens.

[39.5] **C.** Dermoids usually have both solid and cystic components.

[39.6] **B.** Follicular cysts are generally simple cysts without septations or solid parts.

[39.7] **D.** Mucinous tumors are characterized by their large size.

CLINICAL PEARLS

❖ The most common ovarian tumor in a woman younger than 30 years is a benign cystic teratoma (dermoid cyst). The best treatment of a dermoid in a young woman is ovarian cystectomy.

❖ The most common ovarian tumor in a woman older than 30 years is epithelial in origin, most commonly serous cystadenoma.

❖ An ovarian mass larger than 5 cm in a postmenopausal woman most likely represents an ovarian tumor and should generally be removed. An ovarian mass that is larger than 2 to 3 cm in a prepubertal girl likewise should be investigated and many times requires removal.

❖ During the reproductive years, functional ovarian cysts are common and are usually smaller than 5 cm in diameter. Any ovarian cyst larger than 8 cm in a reproductive-aged woman is probably a neoplasm and should be excised.

❖ The tumor marker CA 125 is most specific for ovarian cancer in postmenopausal women.

❖ Mucinous tumors of the ovary can grow to be very large. If they rupture intra-abdominally, they may cause pseudomyxoma peritoneii, which leads to repeated bouts of bowel obstruction.

❖ Ascites is a common sign of ovarian malignancy.

❖ Ovarian cancer staging consists of total abdominal hysterectomy, bilateral salpingo-oophrectomy, omentectomy, peritoneal biopsies, peritoneal washings or sampling of ascitic fluid, and lymphadenectomy.

REFERENCES

Herbst AL. Neoplastic diseases of the ovary. In: Stenchever MA, Droegemueller W, Herbst AL, Mishell DR, eds. Comprehensive gynecology, 4th ed. St. Louis: Mosby-Year Book. 2001:955–998.

Moore GJ. Benign tumors of the ovaries and fallopian tubes. In: Hacker NF and Moore JG, eds. Essentials of obstetrics and gynecology, 3rd ed. Philadelphia: Saunders. 1998:421–431.

A 45-year-old woman complains of profuse serosanguinous drainage from her abdominal incision site that has persisted over 4 hr and has soaked several large towels. She had staging surgery for ovarian cancer 7 days previously. Her past medical history is unremarkable. She denies the passage of blood clots or foul smelling lochia. She states that her vaginal bleeding was scant. Her past medical and surgical histories are unremarkable. On examination, her weight is 270 lb, BP is 100/70, HR 80/min, RR 12/min, and she is afebrile. The thyroid is normal to palpation. The heart and lung examinations are normal. The remainder of the physical examination is unremarkable except for the abdominal incision.

◆ **What is the most likely diagnosis?**

◆ **What is the most appropriate therapy?**

ANSWERS TO CASE 40: Fascial Dehiscence

Summary: A 45-year-old obese woman complains of a 4-hr history of profuse serosanguinous drainage from her abdominal incision site. She had undergone staging surgery for ovarian cancer 7 days previously.

◆ **Most likely diagnosis:** Fascial dehiscence.

◆ **Most appropriate therapy:** Immediate surgical closure and broad-spectrum antibiotic therapy.

Analysis

Objectives

1. Know the classic presentation of fascial dehiscence.
2. Understand that both fascial dehiscence and fascial evisceration are surgical emergencies.
3. Know the risk factors for wound disruptions.

Considerations

This 45-year-old woman underwent ovarian cancer staging surgery 7 days previously. She now complains of 4 hr of profuse and continuous serosanguinous drainage from her abdominal incision. This is the typical presentation for fascial dehiscence. Because the rectus fascia is interrupted, the peritoneal fluid escapes through the wound. If this were only a superficial fascial separation, caused by a seroma or other small fluid collection in the subcutaneous fat tissue, then the patient would have only complained of a limited amount of drainage. The patient does not have **intestinal contents penetrating through the incision;** thus, an **evisceration is not suspected.** Nevertheless, **fascial dehiscence is a surgical emergency,** requiring immediate surgical repair. Broad-spectrum antibiotic therapy is usually administered. This patient has numerous risk factors for fascial dehiscence including obesity, cancer, and a probable vertical incision. The time frame from the surgery is fairly typical, which is usually 7 to 10 days following surgery.

APPROACH TO WOUND DISRUPTIONS

Definitions

Wound dehiscence: A separation of part of the surgical incision, but with an intact peritoneum.
Fascial dehiscence: Separation of the fascial layer, usually leading to a communication of the peritoneal cavity with the skin.
Serosanguinous: Blood-tinged drainage.
Evisceration: A disruption of all layers of the incision with omentum or bowel protruding through the incision.

Approach to Wound Disorders

Wound complications include superficial separation, dehiscence, and evisceration. Separations of the subcutaneous tissue anterior to the fascia are usually associated with **infection or hematoma.** They affect about 3% to 5% of abdominal hysterectomy incisions. The affected patient usually presents with a red, tender, indurated incision, and fever 4 to 10 days postoperatively. The **treatment is opening the wound** and draining the purulence. A broad-spectrum antimicrobial agent is recommended, with wet-to-dry dressing changes. The wound may be allowed to close secondarily, or be approximated after several days.

   Fascial dehiscence, separation of the fascia but not the peritoneum, occurs in about 0.5% of abdominal incisions. It is **more common with vertical incisions, obesity, intra-abdominal distension, diabetes, corticosteroid use, infection, coughing, and malnutrition.** This condition often presents as profuse drainage from the incision 5 to 14 days after surgery. Fascial dehiscence requires **repair** as soon as possible with the initiation of broad-spectrum antibiotics.

   Evisceration is defined as protrusion of bowel or omentum through the incision, which connotes complete separation of all layers of the wound. This condition carries a **significant mortality due to sepsis, and is considered a surgical emergency.** When encountered, a sterile sponge wet with saline should be placed over the bowel, and the patient taken to the operating room. Antibiotics should be immediately started. The presentation is similar to that of wound dehiscence.

Comprehension Questions

[40.1] Each of the following is a risk for wound dehiscence except:

    A. Diabetes mellitus
    B. Chronic obstructive pulmonary disease
    C. Horizontal incision
    D. Obesity

[40.2] Which of the following is the most common reason for fascial dehiscence?

    A. Suture becomes untied
    B. Suture breakage
    C. Suture tear through fascia
    D. Defective suture material
    E. Suture hydrolytic process

[40.3] A 59-year-old woman who had staging surgery for ovarian cancer is noted to have clear serous drainage from her incision. The surgeon is concerned that it may represent lymphatic drainage versus a fistula from the urinary tract. Which of the following studies of the fluid would most likely help to differentiate between these two entities?

    A. Creatinine level
    B. Leukocyte count
    C. pH
    D. Hemoglobin level
    E. CA-125 level

[40.4] A 38-year-old woman had an abdominal hysterectomy for symptomatic uterine fibroids, namely menorrhagia that had failed to respond to medical therapy. One week later, she complains of low-grade fever and lower abdominal pain. On examination, she is noted to have a temperature of 100.8°F and the Pfannenstiel (low transverse) incision is red, indurated, and tender. Which of the following is the best therapy for this condition?

A. Oral antibiotic therapy
B. Observation
C. Opening the incision and draining the infection
D. Antibiotic ointment to the affected area
E. Interferon therapy

Answers

[40.1] **C.** A vertical incision as opposed to a transverse incision is associated with a greater risk of fascial dehiscence.

[40.2] **C.** Fascial breakdown is not usually due to suture breakage or knot slippage, but rather to the suture tearing through the fascia.

[40.3] **A.** A creatinine level may distinguish between urine and lymphatic fluid. The creatinine level would be significantly more elevated in urine.

[40.4] **C.** This is the presentation of a superficial wound infection, and best treated by opening of the incision.

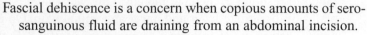

CLINICAL PEARLS

◈ Fascial dehiscence is a concern when copious amounts of serosanguinous fluid are draining from an abdominal incision.

◈ Fascial dehiscence or evisceration should be immediately repaired.

◈ The most common time period in which fascial dehiscence or evisceration occurs is 5 to 14 days postoperatively.

◈ A superficial wound separation usually occurs due to infection or hematoma, and is treated by opening the wound and using wet-to-dry dressing changes.

REFERENCES

Droegemuller W. Preoperative counseling and management. In: Stenchever MA, Droegemueller W, Herbst AL, Mishell DR, eds. Comprehensive gynecology, 4th ed. St. Louis: Mosby-Year Book. 2001:771–825.

Gallup DG. Incisions for gynecologic surgery. In: Rock JA and Thomson JD, eds. Telinde's operative gynecology, 8th ed. Philadelphia: Lippincott-Raven. 1997:308–311.

A 25-year-old woman at 10 weeks' gestation complains of severe abdominal pain and feeling faint for the last hour. She had moderately heavy vaginal bleeding that began yesterday morning, and noted that some tissue possibly passed vaginally. The tissue brought into the office floats when placed in saline with a "frond" pattern. Currently, she denies vaginal bleeding but feels lightheaded. On examination, her BP is 90/60, HR 120 bpm, and temperature 99°F. Her abdomen is diffusely tender, distended, with rebound tenderness, and a fluid wave is present. The cervix is closed.

◆ **What is the most likely diagnosis?**

◆ **What is your next step in the management?**

ANSWERS TO CASE 41: Abdominal Pain in Pregnancy (Ruptured Corpus Luteum)

Summary: A 25-year-old woman at 10 weeks' gestation complains of severe abdominal pain and lightheadedness. Yesterday, she had moderately heavy vaginal bleeding and passed some tissue, which floats with a "frond" pattern. Her BP is 90/60, HR 120 bpm, and temperature 99°F. Her abdomen is diffusely tender, distended, with rebound tenderness, and a fluid wave is present. The cervix is closed.

◆ **Most likely diagnosis:** Ruptured corpus luteum cyst with hemoperitoneum.

◆ **Next step in the management:** Admission to the hospital with surgical intervention (laparoscopy or laparotomy).

Analysis

Objectives

1. Know the symptoms and signs of hypovolemic shock.
2. Know that a hemoperitoneum in pregnancy is usually caused by a ruptured ectopic pregnancy and, less commonly, by a ruptured corpus luteum.
3. Understand that endometrial tissue that floats with a "frond pattern" is almost always diagnostic for an intrauterine pregnancy.

Considerations

This 25-year-old woman is at 10 weeks' gestation and complains of symptoms of hypovolemia. She feels faint, is hypotensive, and has tachycardia. This symptom complex is consistent with **hemorrhagic shock.** Furthermore, she has severe abdominal pain, abdominal distension, rebound tenderness, and a positive fluid wave. The most likely cause is a hemoperitoneum. The blood in the abdomen causes irritation of the peritoneal lining, causing the rebound tenderness. In nine out of ten cases, a pregnant woman with a hemoperitoneum has an **ectopic pregnancy.** However, in this case, the patient passed some tissue, which floated in a "frond pattern" when placed in saline. This is very good evidence of products of conception; in fact, the float test is more than 95% accurate for the presence of chorionic villi. An ectopic pregnancy coexisting with an intrauterine pregnancy is exceedingly rare (1 in 10,000). Thus, the hemoperitoneum is likely caused by a ruptured corpus luteum. Another less common possibility includes splenic injury or rupture.

APPROACH TO HYPOVOLEMIA IN PREGNANCY

Definitions

Corpus luteum: A physiologic ovarian cyst formed from mature graafian follicles following ovulation, which secretes progesterone.

Hemorrhagic corpus luteum: Bleeding occurring in a corpus luteum, which may cause a hemoperitoneum or cyst enlargement.

Hemoperitoneum: A collection of blood in the peritoneal cavity. The blood initially clots and then lyses, so that there may be a combination of clots and hemorrhagic fluid that will not clot.

Ruptured Corpus Luteum

Corpus luteum cysts develop from mature graafian follicles and are associated with normal endocrine function or prolonged secretion of progesterone. They are usually less than 3 cm in diameter. There can be intrafollicular bleeding because of thin-walled capillaries that invade the granulosa cells from the theca interna. When the hemorrhage is excessive, the cyst can enlarge and there is an increased risk of rupture. **Cysts tend to rupture more during pregnancy,** probably due to the increased incidence and friability of corpus lutea in pregnancy. **Anticoagulation therapy** also predisposes to cyst rupture, and these women should receive medication to prevent ovulation. Patients with hemorrhagic corpus lutea usually present with the **sudden onset of severe**

lower abdominal pain. This presentation is especially common in women with a hemoperitoneum. Some women will complain of unilateral cramping and lower abdominal pain for 1 to 2 weeks before overt rupture. Corpus luteum cysts rupture more commonly between days 20 and 26 of the menstrual cycle.

The **differential diagnosis of a suspected hemorrhagic corpus luteum should include ectopic pregnancy, ruptured endometrioma, adnexal torsion, appendicitis, and splenic injury or rupture.** Ultrasound examination may show free intraperitoneal fluid, and perhaps fluid around an ovary. The diagnosis is confirmed by **laparoscopy.** The first step in the treatment of a ruptured corpus luteal cyst is to secure hemostasis. Once the bleeding stops, no further therapy is required; if the bleeding continues, however, a cystectomy should be performed with preservation of the remaining normal portion of ovary.

Progesterone is largely produced by the corpus luteum until about 10 weeks' gestation. Until approximately the seventh week, the pregnancy is dependent on the progesterone secreted by the corpus luteum. Human chorionic gonadotropin serves to maintain the luteal function until placental steroidogenesis is established. There is shared function between the placenta and corpus luteum from the seventh to tenth week; after 10 weeks, the placenta emerges as the major source of progesterone. Therefore, **if the corpus luteum is removed surgically prior to 10 weeks' gestation, exogenous progesterone is needed to sustain the pregnancy**. If the corpus luteum is excised after 10 weeks' gestation, no supplemental progesterone is required.

Comprehension Questions

[41.1] A culdocentesis is performed in a 19-year-old G1 P0 woman with lower abdominal pain and vaginal spotting. A total of 3 cc of clotted blood is aspirated. Which one of the following is the best interpretation?

    A. A hemoperitoneum is present.
    B. No hemoperitoneum is present.
    C. The blood probably came from a blood vessel.
    D. The patient probably has an ectopic pregnancy.

[41.2] A 25-year-old woman G1 P0 is noted to have vaginal spotting
and beta-hCG levels have plateaued in the 1800 mIU/mL range.
A uterine curettage is performed and no chorionic villi are seen
on histologic examination. Which of the following describes the
most likely diagnosis for this patient?

A. Complete molar pregnancy
B. Intrauterine pregnancy
C. Incomplete molar pregnancy
D. Ectopic pregnancy
E. Spontaneous abortion

[41.3] Which of the following is the earliest indicator of hypovolemia
in a young healthy patient?

A. Tachycardia
B. Hypotension
C. Positive tilt
D. Lethargy and confusion
E. Decreased urine output

[41.4] A 20-year-old woman is brought into the emergency room with
a blood pressure of 70/40 and heart rate of 130 bpm, and a history of heavy vaginal bleeding. Which of the following describes the first step in treatment?

A. Intravenous isotonic fluids
B. Aggressive oral fluids
C. Immediate blood transfusion
D. Immediate uterine curettage
E. Intravenous dobutamine therapy

Answers

[41.1] **C.** A culdocentesis involves placing a needle into the cul-de-sac
transvaginally, in an effort to aspirate intraperitoneal fluid. Intraperitoneal blood would be nonclotting (due to the consumption

of clotting factors within the peritoneal cavity); whereas clotted blood most likely arises from a vaginal vessel.

[41.2] **D.** With no chorionic villi on uterine curettage and the hCG level being 1800 mIU/mL, the most likely diagnosis is an ectopic pregnancy.

[41.3] **E.** Renal blood flow is decreased with early hypovolemia as reflected by a decreased urine output.

[41.4] **A.** Isotonic intravenous fluid infusion is the first step to resuscitation of the patient with hypovolemia.

CLINICAL PEARLS

The most common cause of hemoperitoneum in early pregnancy is ectopic pregnancy.

A ruptured corpus luteum can mimic an ectopic pregnancy.
Non-clotted blood obtained from culdocentesis is consistent with intra-abdominal hemorrhage.
When the corpus luteum is excised in a pregnancy of less than 8 weeks gestation, progesterone should be supplemented.

REFERENCES

Droegemuller W. Benign gynecologic lesions. In: Stenchever MA, Droegemueller W, Herbst AL, Mishell DR, eds. Comprehensive gynecology, 4th ed. St. Louis: Mosby-Year Book. 2001:479–530.

Moore GJ. Benign tumors of the ovaries and fallopian tubes. In: Hacker NF and Moore JG, eds. Essentials of obstetrics and gynecology, 3rd ed. Philadelphia: Saunders. 1998:421–423.

CASE 42

A 33-year-old woman complains of 7 months of amenorrhea following a spontaneous abortion. She had a dilation and curettage at that time. Her past medical and surgical histories are unremarkable. She experienced menarche at age 11 years and notes that her menses have been every 28 to 31 days until recently. Her general physical examination is unremarkable. The thyroid is normal to palpation, and breasts are without discharge. The abdomen is nontender. The pelvic examination shows a normal uterus, closed and normal appearing cervix, and no adnexal masses. A pregnancy test is negative.

◆ **What is the most likely diagnosis?**

◆ **What is the next diagnostic test?**

ANSWERS TO CASE 42: Amenorrhea (Intrauterine Adhesions)

Summary: A 33-year-old woman complains of 7 months of amenorrhea after she had a D&C for a spontaneous abortion. Her menstrual history was normal previously. The thyroid, pelvic, and breast examinations are normal. The pregnancy test is negative.

◆ **Most likely diagnosis:** Intrauterine adhesions (Asherman's syndrome).

◆ **Next diagnostic test:** Hysterosalpingogram (or hysteroscopy).

Analysis

Objectives

1. Know the definition of secondary amenorrhea.
2. Understand how uterine curettage can cause endometrial adhesions and amenorrhea.
3. Know how to diagnose intrauterine adhesive disease (Asherman's syndrome).

Considerations

This 33-year-old woman has had 7 months of amenorrhea since experiencing a miscarriage. She had undergone a uterine dilation and curettage at that time. Her menstrual history was unremarkable previously; hence, she meets the definition of secondary amenorrhea (6 months of no menses in a woman with previously normal menses). Pregnancy should be the first condition to be ruled out. Secondary amenorrhea may be caused by hypothalamic etiologies (such as hypothyroidism or hyperprolactinemia), pituitary conditions (such as Sheehan's syndrome), or ovarian causes (such as premature ovarian failure). The patient does not have symptoms of hypothyroidism or galactorrhea, postpartum hemorrhage, or hot flushes. Additionally, her history suggests a proximate relationship to the miscarriage. Hence, the most likely diagnosis is intrauterine adhesions, arising from the curettage of the uterus. With this condition, the hypothalamus, pituitary, and ovary are working normally, but the endometrial tissue is not responsive to the hormonal changes. A hysterosalpingogram, a radiologic study where radiopaque dye is injected into the uterine cavity via a transcervical catheter, showing obliteration of the endometrial cavity would establish the diagnosis.

APPROACH TO SUSPECTED INTRAUTERINE ADHESIONS

Definitions

Secondary amenorrhea: Absence of menses for a period of 6 months or more in a woman who has had spontaneous menses.
Intrauterine adhesions (IUA): Condition when scar tissue or synechiae form to obliterate the endometrial cavity, usually occurring because of uterine curettage following a pregnancy.
Hysterosalpingogram: A radiologic study in which radiopaque dye is injected into the endometrial cavity via a transcervical catheter, used to evaluate the endometrial cavity and/or the patency of the fallopian tubes.
Hysteroscopy: Procedure of direct visualization of the endometrial cavity with a endoscope, a light source, and a distension media.

Intrauterine Adhesions (Asherman's Syndrome)

Intrauterine scarring leading to an unresponsive endometrium is most commonly due to injury to the pregnant or recently pregnant uterus. However, any mechanical, infectious, or radiation factor can produce endometrial sclerosis and adhesion formation. **The sine qua non for the development of intrauterine adhesions is endometrial trauma, especially to the basalis layer.** The adhesions are usually strands of avascular fibrous tissue but they may also consist of inactive endometrium or myometrium. Myometrial adhesions are usually dense and vascular carrying a poor prognosis. Women with atrophic and sclerotic endometrium without adhesions carry the worst prognosis. This is usually found after radiation or tuberculous endometritis and is not amenable to any therapy. **Postpartum curettage** performed between the second and fourth weeks after delivery, along with hypoestrogenic states such as breast-feeding or hypogonadotropic hypogonadism, is associated with extensive intrauterine scar formation. Uterine curettage performed after a missed abortion is associated with a higher incidence of intrauterine synechiae than curettage performed after an incomplete abortion. Adhesions may also form after a diagnostic D&C. In general, the routine use of uterine curettage at the time of a diagnostic laparoscopy is unwarranted and may damage the endometrium.

Intrauterine adhesions should be suspected if a woman presents with secondary amenorrhea, a negative pregnancy test, and does not have progestin-induced withdrawal bleeding. There is no consistent correlation between the menstrual bleeding patterns and the extent of intrauterine adhesions. The diagnosis of IUA should be **suspected on every patient with infertility, recurrent abortions, uterine trauma, and menstrual abnormalities.** The most common method of diagnosing IUA is by **hysterosalpingogram.** In cases of severe intrauterine adhesions, the cavity cannot be sounded, making the procedure very difficult to perform. Vaginal ultrasound can be used in the diagnosis of IUA; however, it lacks specificity. Sonohysterography is an excellent complement to the vaginal ultrasound and can allow for the evaluation of the uterine cavity. Magnetic resonance imaging (MRI) is expensive and does not offer a greater advantage over the other diagnostic modalities. **Hysteroscopy** allows for direct visualization of the uterine cavity and is considered the **"gold standard"** for the establishment of the diagnosis and extent of the IUA.

Operative hysteroscopy is the ideal treatment for IUA. The postoperative management may include the insertion of a loop IUD or a pediatric Foley catheter to prevent the recently lysed adhesions from reforming. In addition, the administration of conjugated estrogens and progesterone (medroxyprogesterone acetate) should be considered. The uterine cavity should be reevaluated prior to attempting conception.

Comprehension Questions

[42.1] A 34-year-old woman states that she has had no menses since she had a uterine curettage and cone biopsy of the cervix 1 yr previously. Since those surgeries, she complains of severe, crampy lower abdominal pain "similar to labor pain" for 5 days of each month. Her basal body temperature chart is biphasic, rising one-degree Fahrenheit for 2 weeks of every month. Which of the following is the most likely etiology of secondary amenorrhea?

A. Hypothalamic etiology
B. Pituitary etiology
C. Uterine etiology
D. Cervical condition

[42.2] Each of the following statements about Asherman's syndrome (intrauterine adhesions) is true except:

A. Usually occurs after uterine curettage for a pregnancy-related process
B. Best diagnosed by laparoscopy
C. Unusual to be associated with cramping pain every month
D. Treatment includes lysis of adhesions

[42.3] In which of the following circumstances is the sequential administration of estrogen and progestin (estrogen alone for 15 days, then estrogen and progestin together for 10 days, then nothing) *least* likely to cause endometrial bleeding?

A. A 52-year-old woman who is 9 months postmenopausal
B. A 10-year-old girl prior to puberty
C. A 23-year-old woman who has polycystic ovarian syndrome
D. A 25-year-old woman with intrauterine adhesions

[42.4] A 41-year-old woman is suspected of having intrauterine adhesions because she has had irregular menses since a spontaneous abortion 18 months previously. Which historical or laboratory pieces of information would support this diagnosis?

A. Presence of hot flushes
B. FSH level too low to be measurable
C. Normal estradiol levels for a reproductive-aged woman
D. Monophasic basal body temperature chart

Answers

[42.1] **D.** This patient has two potential causes for amenorrhea: IUA caused by the uterine curettage and cervical stenosis due to the cervical conization. The biphasic basal body temperature chart suggests normal functioning of the hypothalamus-pituitary-ovarian axis. The crampy abdominal pain most likely is due to retrograde menstruation; thus, this is most likely due to a cervical process, cervical stenosis. If untreated, this patient would likely develop severe endometriosis.

[42.2] **B.** It is not laparoscopy (which visualizes the intraperitoneal cavity), but hysteroscopy that is the best test.

[42.3] **D.** One of the methods of diagnosis of a uterine and/or cervical problem is the absence of menstrual bleeding with the use of cyclical hormonal therapy. If the endometrium has the capacity to respond to hormonal therapy, and the cervix is patent, menstrual blood should be seen. With IUA, the endometrium is not responsive to hormonal therapy.

[42.4] **C.** With IUA, the hormonal status of the woman should be normal. Hot flushes connote ovarian failure, leading to decreased levels of estradiol.

CLINICAL PEARLS

 The most common cause of secondary amenorrhea after uterine curettage is intrauterine adhesions.

Intrauterine adhesions are diagnosed by hysterosalpingogram and confirmed by hysteroscopy.

 Hysteroscopic resection is the best treatment of intrauterine adhesions.

Uterine curettage, especially associated with pregnancy, is a risk factor for intrauterine adhesions.

REFERENCES

Mishell DR. Primary and secondary amenorrhea. In: Stenchever MA, Droegemueller W, Herbst AL, Mishell DR, eds. Comprehensive gynecology, 4th ed. St. Louis: Mosby-Year Book. 2001:1099–1124.

Schlaff WD, Kletzky OA. Amenorrhea, hyperprolactinemia, and chronic anovulation. In: Hacker NF and Moore JG, eds. Essentials of obstetrics and gynecology, 3rd ed. Philadelphia: Saunders. 1998:580–593.

A 59-year-old woman comes into the doctor's office for a health maintenance examination. Her past medical history is remarkable for mild hypertension controlled with an oral thiazide diuretic agent. Her surgical history is unremarkable. On examination, her BP is 140/84, HR 70 bpm, and she is afebrile. The thyroid is normal to palpation. The breasts are nontender and without masses. The pelvic examination is unremarkable. Mammography revealed a small cluster of calcifications around a small mass.

◆ **What is your next step?**

ANSWERS TO CASE 43: Breast, Abnormal Mammogram

Summary: A 59-year-old woman comes into the doctor's office for a health maintenance examination. The breasts are nontender and without masses. Mammography revealed a small cluster of calcifications around a small mass.

◆ **Next step:** Stereotactic biopsy or needle-localization excisional biopsy of the breast.

Analysis

Objectives

1. Understand the role of mammography in screening for breast cancer.
2. Know that mammography is not perfect in identifying breast cancer.
3. Know the typical mammographic findings that are suspicious for cancer.

Considerations

This 59-year-old woman is going to her doctor for routine health maintenance. She is taking a thiazide diuretic for mild hypertension. Her blood pressure is mildly elevated. The mammogram reveals a **small cluster of calcifications around a small mass, which is one of the classic findings of breast cancer.** With this mammographic finding, it is of paramount importance to obtain tissue for histologic diagnosis. Because of the high risk of malignancy, a stereotactic-directed core biopsy, or surgical excisional biopsy, is preferable to a fine needle aspiration. For needle localization, mammographic guidance is employed so that the end of the needle is placed in the center of the suspicious area. The surgeon may then perform a breast biopsy using the needle as a guide. Because the mass is not palpable, a needle-localized approach is needed. The other option is a stereotactic core biopsy guided by computer-assisted imaging techniques.

APPROACH TO THE ABNORMAL MAMMOGRAM

Definitions

Suspicious mammographic findings: A small cluster of calcifications, or masses with ill-defined borders.

Needle localization: Procedure in which a sterile needle is placed via mammographic guidance such that the end of the needle is placed in the center of the suspicious area. The surgeon uses this guide to assist in excising breast tissue.

Stereotactic core biopsy: Procedure in which the patient is prone on the mammographic table and biopsies are taken as directed with computer-assisted techniques.

Clinical Approach

Although a clinical history and proper clinical breast examinations are important in detecting breast cancer, mammography remains the best method of detecting breast cancer at an early stage.

A mammogram is an x-ray of the breast tissue. Current radiation levels from mammography have been shown to be safe and cause no increased risk in developing breast cancer. The radiation exposure is less than 10 rads per lifetime if annual mammograms begin at age 40 years and continue up to age 90. **Both false positives and false negatives of up to 10%** have been noted. Hence, **a palpable breast mass in the face of a normal mammogram still requires a biopsy.** Breast implants can diminish the accuracy of a mammogram, particularly if the implants are in front of the chest muscles.

Mammographic findings strongly suggestive of breast cancer include **a mass, often with spiculating and invasive borders, or an architectural distortion, or an asymmetric increased tissue density** when compared with prior studies or a corresponding area in the

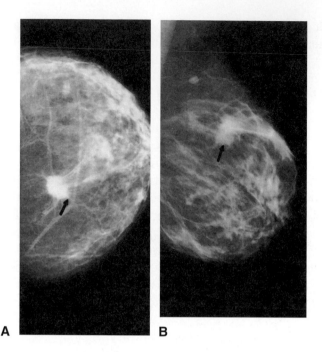

A   **B**

Figure 43–1.   Mammogram showing spiculated mass. Early invasive ductal carcinoma of the right breast. Craniocaudal (A) and oblique mediolateral (B) views of the right breast shows a spiculated mass in the upper outer quadrant.

(Reproduced, with permission, from Schwartz SI, Shires GT, Spencer FL et al, eds. Principles of surgery, 7th ed. New York: McGraw-Hill; 1999: 545.)

opposite breast (Figure 43–1). An **isolated cluster of tiny, irregular calcifications,** especially if linear and wispy, is an important sign of breast cancer. Skin thickening is also an important prognostic indicator.

If a breast cancer is suspected, biopsy is warranted. A stereotactic biopsy may be used to localize and sample the lesion. This method employs a computerized, digital, three-dimensional view of the breast and allows the physician to direct the needle to the biopsy site. The procedure carries a 2% to 4% "miss rate." Needle-localization biopsies employ multiple mammographic views of the breast and allow the surgeon to localize the lesion for evaluation. The latter procedure is more time consuming, carries a comparable 3% to 5% miss rate, but excises more tissue, which is helpful in "borderline" histologic conditions, such as ductal carcinoma-in-situ.

Comprehension Questions

[43.1] Which of the following imaging modalities has been shown to be cost-effective in screening for breast cancer?

A. Mammography only
B. Mammography and ultrasound
C. Mammography and CT scan
D. Mammography and thermography

[43.2] Which of the following describes the radiation risk with modern mammography given once annually?

A. Increased risk for thyroid cancer
B. No increased risks
C. Increased risk for lung cancer
D. Increased risk of skin cancer in the chest area

[43.3] A 55-year-old woman has several coarse calcifications found on mammography that are suspicious for breast cancer. She has no family history of breast cancer and no mass is palpable. Which of the following is the most accurate statement?

A. The best diagnostic method for this patient is fine needle aspiration.
B. The lesion is definitely cancer.
C. Since there is no palpable mass on physical examination, the patient may be observed for changes on mammography in 3 months.
D. One option for this patient is a core tissue biopsy by stereotactic means.

Answers

[43.1] **A.** Only mammography has been shown to be cost-effective in diagnosing breast cancer at an early stage, at a size less than 1 cm, which is the threshold for feeling a mass in a physical examination.

[43.2] **B.** Modern mammography has very low radiation and no increased risk.

[43.3] **D.** Mammographic findings that are suspicious for cancer must be addressed. Two viable methods include core biopsy via stereotactic guidance and needle-localization excision. Fine needle aspiration is not sensitive enough, and no mass is palpable to be able to serve for localizing.

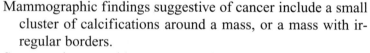

CLINICAL PEARLS

 Mammographic findings suggestive of cancer include a small cluster of calcifications around a mass, or a mass with irregular borders.

 Stereotactic core biopsy or needle-localization excisional biopsy are two accepted methods of assessing suspicious, mammographic, nonpalpable masses.

 The amount of radiation from mammography is negligible and has no significant sequalae.

 Trauma to the breast may lead to fat necrosis and produce mammographic findings similar to that seen in breast cancer. These lesions should be excised to confirm the diagnosis.

REFERENCES

Droegemuller W, Valea FA. Breast diseases. In: Stenchever MA, Droegemueller W, Herbst AL, Mishell DR, eds. Comprehensive gynecology, 4th ed. St. Louis: Mosby-Year Book. 2001:359–398.

Hacker NF. Breast disease: a gynecologic perspective. In: Hacker NF and Moore JG, eds. Essentials of obstetrics and gynecology, 3rd ed. Philadelphia: Saunders. 1998:507–515.

A 22-year-old woman G1 Ab1 complains of secondary infertility for 1 year. She states that her menarche was at age 12 years, and that her menses occur every 28 to 30 days. She denies dysmenorrhea or dyspareunia. She had a chlamydial infection treated at age 18 years, and no other infections. The family history is significant for hypothyroidism in a maternal aunt. She denies other significant medical or surgical history. The semen analysis is normal.

◆ **What is the most likely diagnosis?**

◆ **What is your next step in diagnosis?**

ANSWERS TO CASE 44: Infertility, Tubal Factor

Summary: A 22-year-old woman G1 Ab 1 has secondary infertility. Her menses occur every 28 to 30 days. She denies dysmenorrhea or dyspareunia. She had a chlamydial infection treated at age 16 years, but no other significant medical or surgical history. The semen analysis is normal.

- **Most likely diagnosis:** Tubal factor infertility.

- **Next step in diagnosis:** A hysterosalpingogram.

Analysis

Objectives

1. Understand the five basic causative factors in the approach to infertility.
2. Know that a prior chlamydial infection predisposes to tubal factor infertility.
3. Understand that the hysterosalpingogram is a method to diagnose tubal disease.

Considerations

This 22-year-old woman has had difficulty getting pregnant for 1 year. She had a pregnancy previously, so she has secondary infertility. Her menses are every 28 days, which speaks against an ovulation disorder; regular monthly menses almost always indicates regular ovulation. She denies dysmenorrhea or dyspareunia, which makes endometriosis less likely, but the **absence of symptoms does not rule out endometriosis.** The semen analysis is normal, so a male factor is unlikely. The history of chlamydial infection in the past definitely points toward tubal factor disease. *Chlamydia trachomatis* is particularly associated with tubal problems, leading to infertility or ectopic pregnancy. One method of evaluating tubal patency is with the hysterosalpingogram, assessing whether the radiopaque dye will spill through the fallopian tubes and out into the peritoneal cavity.

APPROACH TO TUBAL FACTOR INFERTILITY

See also Case 28.

Definitions

Salpingitis isthmic nodosa (tubal diverticuli): A condition in which the tubal epithelium penetrates into the muscularis or even the serosa, commonly associated with tubal infection.

Tubal factor infertility: Tube damage or disease leading to inability to conceive, usually divided into proximal blockage and distal blockage.

Chromotubation: A procedure whereby dye is injected into the uterus via a transcervical catheter and tubal patency is assessed by laparoscopy or laparotomy.

Tubal reconstructive surgery: Operative techniques for repairing tube damage in an attempt to enhance conception rates, which may or may not include microsurgery. Microsurgery uses magnification and fine suture material.

Tubal Factor Infertility

Tubal infertility is due to damage or obstruction of the fallopian tubes. The changes or obstruction are associated with previous pelvic inflammatory disease **(PID),** previous pelvic or tubal surgery, and peritoneal factors. Tubal and peritoneal factor infertility often occur concurrently and their treatments are often similar. Tubal and peritoneal factors account for 30% to 40% of the cases of female infertility. Salpingitis is the most important etiologic factor in tubal infertility. The risk of infertility is high after a single bout of PID. In addition, PID increases the incidence of ectopic pregnancy, which can also contribute to infertility. The incidence of infertility doubles with successive bouts of salpingitis, reported to be 12%, 23%, and 54% after one, two, and three episodes of PID respectively.

A common test used to assess tubal factor is the hysterosalpingogram **(HSG),** which has a 76% sensitivity and a 83% specificity. In general, an abnormal hysterosalpingogram should be confirmed by **laparoscopy,** which complements the HSG since it allows for direct visualization of the fallopian tubes, ovaries, and peritoneal surface. Operative laparoscopy is a therapeutic option for both tubal and peritoneal factors, thus avoiding the need for a laparotomy. Falloposcopy, which is a technique that allows for the direct visualization of the tubal lumen, can give additional information to laparoscopy and may offer prognostic information about the damaged fallopian tube.

The outcome of surgical management of tubal factor infertility is dependent on the following factors: 1) the severity of the disease process that affected the pelvis, 2) the extent of the tubal damage caused by previous disease or surgery, 3) the length of the reconstructed tube, 4) other fertility factors, and 5) the surgical technique.

Proximal tubal obstruction can be treated with tubocornual anastomosis. The procedure is associated with a success rate of 44%; however, it requires a laparotomy. In recent years, proximal tubal obstruction has been approached transcervically with the aid of ultrasound, fluoroscopy, or hysteroscopy, and either catheters or balloons. **Distal tubal obstruction can be treated with fimbrioplasty** or neosalpingoplasty. Both procedures can be performed via laparotomy or laparoscopy. A large hydrosalpinx (fluid-filled tube), abnormal fimbriae, and extensive pelvic or adnexal adhesions are associated with a poor prognosis. Patients who present with a combined proximal and distal obstruction or segmental tubal obstruction (as seen in salpingitis isthmica nodosa) usually have a poor prognosis. These women should be given the option of in vitro fertilization (IVF). Tubal surgery is associated with an increased incidence of ectopic pregnancy.

Comprehension Questions

[44.1] Which of the following infections is most likely to be associated with tubal disease?

A. *Trichomonas vaginalis*
B. *Bacteroides* species
C. *Chlamydia trachomatis*
D. *Proteus* species
E. *Treponema pallidum*

[44.2] Each of the following statements about tubal factor infertility in the United States is true except:

A. Proximal disease is more common than distal disease.
B. When both proximal and distal disease are present, in vitro fertilization should probably be recommended rather than tubal reconstruction.
C. Ovulatory dysfunction usually has a better success rate of treatment rather than tubal factor.
D. Lack of dye in the tube during hysterosalpingogram does not definitively establish tubal blockage.

[44.3] Which of the following characteristics describes the single most important factor in pregnancy success rate after tubal recon-structive surgery?

A. Microsurgical technique
B. Use of adhesion barrier during surgery
C. Meticulous tissue handling and nonreactive suture material
D. Extent of tubal disease prior to surgery
E. Length of surgical procedure

Answers

[44.1] **C.** *Chlamydia* is the most commonly isolated organism causing tubal damage, and because of its indolent course, affected women often do not seek medical treatment.

[44.2] **A.** In the United States, distal tubal damage is more common than proximal tubal damage.

[44.3] **D.** The extent of preoperative tubal damage is the single most
important prognostic factor in fertility success. In general, distal tubal disease is easier to treat surgically rather than proximal
tubal disease.

CLINICAL PEARLS

 Tubal factor infertility should be suspected when a patient
has a history of salpingitis, especially caused by chlamydial
infection.

 The hysterosalpingogram is the initial test to assess tubal patency.

 In general, an abnormal hysterosalpingogram is confirmed by
laparoscopy.

 Distal tubal disease may be treated surgically with frimbrio-
plasty.

REFERENCES

Mishell DR. Infertility. In: Stenchever MA, Droegemueller W, Herbst AL, Mishell
DR, eds. Comprehensive gynecology, 4th ed. St. Louis: Mosby-Year Book.
2001:1169–1216.
Meldrum DR. Infertility. In: Hacker NF and Moore JG, eds. Essentials of obstetrics
and gynecology, 3rd ed. Philadelphia: Saunders. 1998:610–620.

A 17-year-old nulliparous female complains that she has not yet started menstruating. She denies weight loss or excessive exercise. Each of her sisters achieved menarche by 13 years of age. The patient's mother recalls a doctor mentioning that her daughter had a missing right kidney on an abdominal x-ray film. On examination, she is 5 feet 6 in. tall and weighs 140 lb. Her blood pressure is 110/60. Her thyroid gland is normal on palpation. She has Tanner stage IV breast development and female external genitalia. She has Tanner stage IV axillary and pubic hair. There are no skin lesions.

◆ **What is the most likely diagnosis?**

◆ **What is the next step in diagnosis?**

ANSWERS TO CASE 45: Amenorrhea (Primary),
Müllerian Agenesis

Summary: A 17-year-old nulliparous female, who may have only one kidney, presents with primary amenorrhea. She denies weight loss or excessive exercise. On examination, she is 5 ft 6 in. tall and weighs 140 lb. Her blood pressure is 110/60. Her thyroid gland is normal. She has appropriate Tanner stage IV breast development, axillary and pubic hair, and female external genitalia.

◆ **Most likely diagnosis:** Müllerian (or vaginal) agenesis.

◆ **Next step in diagnosis:** Serum testosterone, or karyotype.

Analysis

Objectives

1. Know the definition of primary amenorrhea, that is, no menses by age 16 years.
2. Know that the two most common causes of primary amenorrhea when there is normal breast development are müllerian agenesis and androgen insensitivity.
3. Understand that a serum testosterone level or karyotype would differentiate the two conditions.

Considerations

This 17-year-old female has never had a menstrual period; therefore, she has primary amenorrhea. She has normal Tanner stage IV breast development, as well as normal axillary and pubic hair. Breast development connotes the presence of estrogen, and axillary and pubic hair suggests the presence of androgens. She also has a history of only one kidney. The most likely diagnosis is **müllerian agenesis,** because a significant fraction of these patients will have a **urinary tract abnormality.** Also, with **androgen insensitivity,** there is typically **scant axillary**

and pubic hair since there is a defective androgen receptor. The diagnosis can be confirmed with a serum **testosterone,** which would be normal in müllerian agenesis, and elevated (in the normal male range) in androgen insensitivity. A **karyotype** would also help to distinguish the two conditions.

APPROACH TO PRIMARY AMENORRHEA

Definitions

Primary amenorrhea: No menarche by the age of 16 years.

Androgen insensitivity: An androgen receptor defect in which 46,XY individuals are phenotypically female with normal breast development.

Müllerian agenesis: Congenital absence of development of the uterus, cervix, and fallopian tubes in a 46,XX female, leading to primary amenorrhea.

Clinical Approach

When a young woman presents with primary amenorrhea, the differential diagnosis can be narrowed based on **whether or not normal breast tissue is present,** and whether a uterus is present or absent. After pregnancy is excluded, the two most common etiologies that cause primary amenorrhea associated with **normal breast development and an absent uterus are androgen insensitivity syndrome and müllerian agenesis** (Table 45–1).

An individual with **androgen insensitivity syndrome,** also known as testicular feminization, has a **46,XY** karyotype with **normally functioning male gonads** that produce **normal male levels of testosterone.** However, due to **a defect of the androgen receptor** synthesis or action, there is no formation of male internal or external genitalia. The external genitalia remain female, as occurs in the absence of sex steroids. There are no internal female reproductive organs and the vagina is short or absent. Without androgenic opposition to the small circulating levels

Table 45–1
MÜLLERIAN AGENESIS VERSUS ANDROGEN
INSENSITIVITY

	MÜLLERIAN AGENESIS	ANDROGEN INSENSITIVITY
Breast tissue	Normal breast development	Normal breast development
Axillary and pubic hair	Normal	Scant or absent
Uterus and vagina	Absent uterus and blind vagina	Absent uterus and blind vagina
Testosterone level	Normal testosterone	High testosterone (male range)
Karyotype	46,XX	46,XY
Complications	Renal anomalies	Need gonadectomy

of estrogen secreted by the gonads and adrenals and produced by peripheral conversion of androstenedione, breast development is normal or enhanced. Pubic and axillary hair is absent or scant due to defective androgen receptors. Therefore, these individuals are genotypically male (46,XY karyotype) but phenotypically female (look like a woman). The abnormal intra-abdominal gonads are at increased risk for malignancy, but this rarely occurs before puberty. Thus, gonadectomy is not performed until after puberty is completed to allow full breast development and linear growth to occur. After these events take place, usually around age 16 to 18 years, the gonads should be removed. The diagnosis of androgen insensitivity syndrome should be suspected when a patient has primary amenorrhea, an absent uterus, normal breast development, and **scant or absent** pubic and axillary hair. The diagnosis can be confirmed with a karyotype evaluation and/or elevated testosterone levels (male normal range).

Women with **müllerian agenesis have a 46,XX** karyotype, have **no uterus or fallopian tubes, and have a short or absent vagina.** Externally, they resemble individuals with androgen insensitivity. They do, however, have normally functioning ovaries since the ovaries are not müllerian structures, and have normal breast development. They also have **normal pubic and axillary hair** growth because there is no defect in their androgen receptors. Congenital renal abnormalities occur in about one third of these individuals. These women are genotypically female (46,XX) and phenotypically female. The diagnosis of müllerian agenesis should be suspected when a patient has primary amenorrhea, an absent uterus, normal breast development, and **normal** pubic and axillary hair. The presence of normal pubic and axillary hair is what differentiates them from individuals with androgen insensitivity syndrome, and laboratory confirmation can be accomplished with a karyotype examination and/or testosterone level.

Comprehension Questions

[45.1] An 18-year-old nulliparous female complains of not having started her menses. Her breast development is Tanner stage V. She has a blind vaginal pouch and no cervix. Which of the following describes the most likely diagnosis?

    A. Müllerian agenesis
    B. Androgen insensitivity
    C. Both of the above
    D. Neither of the above

[45.2] A 20-year-old G0 P0 woman is told by her doctor that there is a strong probability that her gonads will turn malignant. She has not had a menses yet. Which of the following describes the most likely diagnosis?

    A. Müllerian agenesis
    B. Androgen insensitivity
    C. Both of the above
    D. Neither of the above

[45.3] A 19-year-old girl has primary amenorrhea and a pelvic kidney. Which of the following describes the correct diagnosis?

   A. Müllerian agenesis
   B. Androgen insensitivity
   C. Both of the above
   D. Neither of the above

[45.4] Which of the following is the best explanation for breast development in a patient with androgen insensitivity?

   A. Gonadal production of estrogens
   B. Adrenal production of estrogen
   C. Breast tissue sensitivity to progesterone
   D. Peripheral conversion of androgens
   E. Autonomous production of breast-specific estrogen

Answers

[45.1] **C.** Normal breast development, no cervix, and a blind vaginal pouch may be caused by either müllerian agenesis or androgen insensitivity.

[45.2] **B.** The Y-chromosome gonad may become malignant, which is present with androgen insensitivity.

[45.3] **A.** A pelvic kidney most likely is associated with a müllerian abnormality.

[45.4] **D.** Individuals with androgen insensitivity usually have full breast development due to the peripheral conversion of androgens to estrogens. Also, because of the defective androgen receptor, the high endogenous androgens do not inhibit breast development as in a normal male.

CLINICAL PEARLS

A pregnancy test should be the first test for any female with primary or secondary amenorrhea.

The two most common causes of primary amenorrhea in a woman with normal breast development are androgen insensitivity and müllerian agenesis.

Scant axillary and pubic hair suggest androgen insensitivity.

A karyotype and testosterone level help to differentiate between müllerian agenesis and androgen insensitivity.

Renal anomalies are common with müllerian abnormalities.

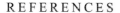

REFERENCES

Mishell DR. Primary and secondary amenorrhea. In: Stenchever MA, Droege-mueller W, Herbst AL, Mishell DR, eds. Comprehensive gynecology, 4th ed. St. Louis: Mosby-Year Book. 2001:1099–1124.

Growdon WA. Embryology and congenital anomalies of the female genital system. In: Hacker NF and Moore JG, eds. Essentials of obstetrics and gynecology, 3rd ed. Philadelphia: Saunders. 1998:363–374.

CASE 46

A 23-year-old woman underwent a dilation and curettage (D&C) for an incomplete abortion 3 days previously. She complains of continued vaginal bleeding and lower abdominal cramping. Over the last 24 hr, she notes significant fever and chills. On examination, her temperature is 102.5°F, BP 90/40, and HR 120 bpm. The cardiac examination reveals tachycardia and the lungs are clear. There is moderately severe lower abdominal tenderness. The pelvic examination shows the cervix to be open to 1.5 cm, and there is uterine tenderness. The leukocyte count is 20,000/mm^3 and the hemoglobin level is 12 g/dL. The urinalysis shows 2 wbc/hpf.

◆ **What is the most likely diagnosis?**

◆ **What is the next step in management?**

ANSWERS TO CASE 46: Abortion, Septic

Summary: A 23-year-old woman, who had undergone a D&C 3 days ago for an incomplete abortion, complains of continued vaginal bleeding, lower abdominal cramping, and fever and chills. Her temperature is 102.5°F, BP 90/40, and HR 120 bpm. The lungs are clear. There is moderately severe lower abdominal tenderness. The cervix is open, and there is uterine tenderness. The laboratory studies are significant for leukocytosis and a normal urinalysis.

◆ **Most likely diagnosis:** Septic abortion (with retained products of conception).

◆ **Next step in management:** Broad-spectrum antibiotics followed by dilatation and curettage of the uterus.

Analysis

Objectives

1. Understand the clinical presentation of septic abortion.
2. Know that the treatment of septic abortion involves both antibiotic therapy and uterine curettage.

Considerations

This 23-year-old woman underwent a D&C procedure for an incomplete abortion 3 days previously and now presents with lower abdominal cramping, vaginal bleeding, fever, and chills. The open cervical os, lower abdominal cramping, and vaginal bleeding suggest retained products of conception (POC). The retained POC may lead to ongoing bleeding or infection. In this case, the fever, chills, and leukocytosis point toward infection. The retained tissue serves as a nidus for infection. The most common source of the bacteria is the vagina, via an ascending infection. The best treatment is broad-spectrum antibiotics with anaerobic coverage and a uterine curettage. Usually, the surgery is delayed until antimicrobial agents are infused for 4 hr to allow for tissue levels to increase. Hemorrhage may occur with the curettage procedure. Also, the patient should be monitored for septic shock.

APPROACH TO SEPTIC ABORTION

Definitions

Septic abortion: Any type of abortion associated with a uterine infection.

Septic shock: The *septic* portion refers to the presence of an infection (usually bacterial), and the *shock* describes a process whereby the patient's cells, organs, and/or tissues are not being sufficiently supplied with nutrients and/or oxygen.

Clinical Approach

Septic abortion occurs in approximately 1% of all spontaneous abortions and about 0.5% of induced abortions. This risk is increased if an abortion is performed with nonsterile instrumentation. This condition is potentially fatal in 0.4 to 0.6/100,000 spontaneous abortions.

Signs and symptoms of septic abortion are **uterine bleeding and/or spotting in the first trimester with clinical signs of infection.** The mechanism is ascending infection from the vagina or cervix to the endometrium to myometrium to parametrium, and, eventually, the peritoneum. Affected women generally will have fever and leukocyte counts of greater than 10,500 cells/uL. There is usually lower abdominal tenderness, cervical motion tenderness, and a foul-smelling vaginal discharge. **The infection is almost always polymicrobial,** involving anaerobic streptococci, *Bacteroides* species, *Escherichia coli* and other gram-negative rods, and group B beta-hemolytic streptococci. Rarely, *Clostridium perfringens, Hemophilus influenzae,* and *Campylobacter jejuni* may be isolated.

When patients present with signs and symptoms of septic abortion, a **CBC with differential, urinalysis, and blood chemistries including**

electrolytes should be obtained. A specimen of cervical discharge should be sent for **Gram's stain,** as well as for culture and sensitivity. If the patient appears seriously ill or is **hypotensive, blood cultures, a chest x-ray, and blood coagulability studies** should be done. The **blood pressure, oxygen saturation, heart rate, and urine output should be monitored.**

The **treatment has four general parts: 1) maintain the blood pressure; 2) monitor the blood pressure, oxygenation, and urine output, 3) start antibiotic therapy; and 4) perform a uterine curettage.** Immediate therapeutic steps include intravenous isotonic fluid replacement, especially in the face of hypotension. Concurrently, intravenous broad-spectrum antibiotics with particular attention to anaerobic coverage should be infused. The combination of gentamicin and clindamycin has a favorable response 95% of the time. Alternatives include beta-lactam antimicrobials (cephalosporins and extended-spectrum penicillins) or those with beta-lactamase inhibitors. Another regimen includes metronidazole plus ampicillin and an aminoglycoside. Because retained POC are common in these situations, becoming a nidus for infection to develop, evacuation of the uterine contents is important. Uterine curettage is usually performed approximately 4 hr after antibiotics are begun, allowing serum levels to be achieved.

Because oliguria is an early sign of septic shock, the **urine output** should be carefully observed. Also, for women in shock, a central venous pressure catheter may be warranted. **Aggressive intravenous fluids** are usually effective in maintaining the blood pressure; however, at times, vasopressor agents, such as a **dopamine** infusion, may be required. Other therapies include oxygen, digitalis, and steroids.

Comprehension Questions

[46.1] Which of the following is the most likely mechanism of septic abortion following an induced abortion?

A. Instrumental contamination
B. Ascending infection
C. Skin organisms

    D. Urinary tract penetration
    E. Hematogenous infection

[46.2] Which of the following is the best treatment for septic abortion?

    A. Intravenous antibiotic therapy
    B. Uterine curettage
    C. Both A and B
    D. Neither A nor B

Answers

[46.1] **B.** Ascending infection is the most likely mechanism.

[46.2] **C.** Both IV antibiotics and uterine curettage are needed to treat septic abortion.

CLINICAL PEARLS

The bacteria involved in septic abortion are usually polymicrobial, particularly anaerobes that have ascended from the lower genital tract.

Hemorrhage often complicates the curettage for septic abortion.

Treatment of septic abortion consists of maintaining blood pressure; monitoring the blood pressure, oxygenation, and urine output; antibiotics; and uterine evacuation.

REFERENCES

Mishell DR. Spontaneous and recurrent abortion. In: Stenchever MA, Droege-mueller W, Herbst AL, Mishell DR, eds. Comprehensive gynecology, 4th ed. St. Louis: Mosby-Year Book. 2001:413–442.

Bennett MJ. Abortion. In: Hacker NF and Moore JG, eds. Essentials of obstetrics and gynecology, 3rd ed. Philadelphia: Saunders. 1998:477–486.

A 29-year-old parous (G5 P4) woman at 39 weeks' gestation with preeclampsia delivers vaginally. Her prenatal course has been uncomplicated except for asymptomatic bacteriuria caused by *E. coli* in the first trimester treated with oral cephalexin. She denies a family history of bleeding diathesis. After the placenta is delivered, there is appreciable vaginal bleeding estimated at 1000 cc.

◆ **What is the most likely diagnosis?**

◆ **What is the next step in therapy?**

ANSWERS TO CASE 47: Postpartum Hemorrhage

Summary: A 29-year-old parous (G5 P4) woman at 39 weeks' gestation with preeclampsia delivers vaginally. She denies a family history of a bleeding diathesis. After the placenta is delivered, there is appreciable vaginal bleeding, estimated at 1000 cc.

◆ **Most likely diagnosis:** Uterine atony.

◆ **Next step in therapy:** Dilute intravenous oxytocin, and if this is ineffective, then intramuscular prostaglandin F$_2$-alpha.

Analysis

Objectives

1. Know the definition of postpartum hemorrhage.
2. Understand that the most common cause of postpartum hemorrhage is uterine atony.
3. Know the treatment for uterine atony, and the contraindications for the various agents.

Considerations

This 29-year-old woman delivers at 39 weeks' gestation and has an estimated blood loss of 1000 cc after the placenta delivers. This meets the **definition of postpartum hemorrhage, which is a loss of 500 mL or more after a vaginal delivery.** The most common etiology is **uterine atony,** in which the myometrium has not contracted to cut off the uterine spiral arteries that are supplying the placental bed. Uterine massage and dilute oxytocin are the first therapies. If these are ineffective, then prostaglandin F$_2$-alpha is the next agent to be used in this patient. Because she is hypertensive, methyleronovine maleate (methergine) is contraindicated. It should be noted that if the uterus is palpated and found to be firm and yet bleeding continues, a laceration to the genital tract should be suspected. Her risk factors for uterine atony include preeclampsia, since she is likely to be treated with magnesium sulfate.

APPROACH TO POSTPARTUM HEMORRHAGE (PPH)

Definitions

Postpartum hemorrhage: Classically defined as greater than 500 mL blood loss at a vaginal delivery and greater than 1000 mL during a cesarean delivery. Practically speaking, it means significant bleeding that may result in hemodynamic instability if unabated.

Uterine atony: Lack of myometrial contraction, clinically manifested by a boggy uterus.

Methylergonovine maleate (methergine):   An ergot alkyloid agent that induces myometrial contraction as a treatment of uterine atony, contraindicated in hypertension.

Prostaglandin F$_2$-alpha: A prostaglandin compound that causes smooth muscle contraction, contraindicated in asthmatic patients.

Clinical Approach

Postpartum hemorrhage (PPH) is defined as early and late, according to whether it occurs within the first 24 hr or after that period. The **most common cause of early PPH is uterine atony, with bleeding arising from the placental implantation site.** (See Table 47–1 for risk factors.) The physical examination reveals a **boggy uterus.** The initial management should be **uterine massage,** best accomplished by bimanual compression with an abdominal hand as well as vaginal hand. Concurrently, **intravenous dilute oxytocin** is given. If these maneuvers are ineffective, intramuscular **methyl ergonovine (methergine) is given;** intramuscular **prostaglandin F$_2$-alpha** may also be given. Ergot alkyloids **should not be given in women with hypertensive disease** because of the risk of stroke. **Prostaglandin F$_2$-alpha should not be administered in those with asthma** due to the potential for brochoconstriction. If medical therapy is ineffective, then two large-

Table 47–1
RISK FACTORS FOR UTERINE ATONY

Magnesium sulfate
Pitocin use during labor
Rapid labor and/or delivery
Overdistension of the uterus (macrosomia, multifetal pregnancy, hydramnios)
Intraamniotic infection (chorioamnionitis)
Prolonged labor
High parity

---

bore intravenous lines should be placed, the blood bank should be notified, and anesthesiologist alerted. **Surgical therapy may include exploratory laparotomy, with interruption of the blood vessels to the uterus such as uterine artery ligation or internal iliac artery ligation. If these fail, then hysterectomy** may be life-saving.

Other causes of early PPH include **genital tract lacerations,** which should be suspected with a **firm contracted uterus.** The vaginal side walls and cervix should be especially carefully inspected. Repair of the complete extent of the laceration is important. **Uterine inversion,** whether partial or complete, must also be considered. Placental causes include **accreta or retained placenta.** If the uterus is firm and there are no lacerations, one must also consider **coagulopathy.**

Late PPH, defined as occurring after the first 24 hr, may be caused by subinvolution of the placental site, usually occurring at **10 to 14 days after delivery.** In this disorder, the eschar over the placental bed usually falls off and the lack of myometrial contraction at the site leads to bleeding. Classically, the patient will not have bleeding until about 2 weeks after delivery, and is not significantly anemic. **Oral ergot alkyloid** and careful follow-up is the standard treatment; other options include intravenous dilute oxytocin or intramuscular prostaglandin F_2-alpha compounds.

Another causative process is **retained products of conception.** Women with retained POC generally have **uterine cramping and bleeding, and may have fever and/or foul-smelling lochia.** Ultrasound examination helps to confirm the diagnosis. The treatment includes **uterine curettage and broad-spectrum antibiotics.**

Comprehension Questions

[47.1] Which of the following is the most common cause of postpartum hemorrhage after a cesarean delivery?

    A. Uterine atony
    B. Uterine laceration
    C. Coagulopathy
    D. Uterine inversion
    E. Retained placenta

[47.2] Which of the following is the most common etiology for PPH in light of a well-contracted uterus?

    A. Retained placenta
    B. Genital tract laceration
    C. Uterine atony
    D. Coagulopathy
    E. Endometrial ulceration

[47.3] A 32-year-old woman has severe postpartum hemorrhage that does not respond to medical therapy. Which of the following methods is least likely to enable uterine conservation?

    A. Utero-ovarian ligament ligation
    B. Hypogastric artery ligation
    C. Surgical ligation of the cardinal ligaments
    D. Surgical ligation of the ascending branch of the uterine artery

[47.4] A 34-year-old woman is noted to have significant uterine bleeding after a vaginal delivery complicated by placenta abruption. She is noted to be bleeding from multiple venipuncture sites. Which of the following is the best therapy?

    A. Immediate hysterectomy
    B. Packing of the uterus
    C. Hypogastric artery ligation
    D. Ligation of utero-ovarian ligaments
    E. Correction of coagulopathy

Answers

[47.1] **A.** Uterine atony is the most common cause of PPH, even after cesarean delivery.

[47.2] **B.** Genital tract laceration is the most common cause of PPH in a well-contracted uterus.

[47.3] **C.** Ligation of the cardinal ligaments leads to interruption of the uterine arteries, which usually means that a hysterectomy needs to be performed.

[47.4] **E.** Bleeding from multiple venipuncture sites together with abruption suggests a coagulopathy.

CLINICAL PEARLS

♦ The most common cause of postpartum hemorrhage is uterine atony.

♦ The most common cause of early PPH with a firm well-contracted uterus is a genital tract laceration.

♦ The most common cause of late postpartum hemorrhage (after the first 24 hr) is subinvolution of the uterus.

♦ Hypertensive disease is a contraindication for ergot alkyloids, and asthma is a contraindication for prostaglandin F_2-alpha.

REFERENCES

Cunningham FG, Gant NF, Leveno KJ, Gilstrap LC III, Hauth JC, Wenstrom KD. Obstetrical hemorrhage. In: Williams obstetrics, 21st ed. New York: McGraw-Hill. 2001:619–670.

Hayashi RH. Postpartum hemorrhage and puerperal sepsis. In: Hacker NF and Moore JG, eds. Essentials of obstetrics and gynecology, 3rd ed. Philadelphia: Saunders. 1998:333–342.

CASE 48

A 16-year-old female is referred for never having menstruated. She is otherwise in good health. She has an older sister who experienced menarche at age 12 years. She denies excessive exercise or having an eating aversion. There is no family history of depression. On examination, she is 50 in. tall and weighs 100 lb. The neck is supple and without masses. Her breasts appear to be Tanner stage I, and her pubic hair pattern is also consistent with Tanner stage I. Abdominal examination reveals no masses. The external genitalia are normal for a prepubescent female. A normal-appearing small cervix is seen on speculum examination. On bimanual examination, a small uterus and no adnexal masses are palpated.

◆ **What is the most likely diagnosis?**

◆ **What is the next step in diagnosis?**

ANSWERS TO CASE 48: Pubertal Delay, Gonadal Dysgenesis

Summary: A healthy 16-year-old female is referred for never having menstruated. She denies excessive exercise or an eating aversion. On examination, she is 50 in. tall and weighs 100 lb. The neck is supple and without masses. Her breasts and pubic hair are both Tanner stage I. The abdominal examination reveals no masses. The pelvic examination is consistent with a prepubescent female.

◆ **Most likely diagnosis:** Gonadal dysgenesis (Turner's syndrome).

◆ **Next step in diagnosis:** Serum follicle-stimulating hormone (FSH).

Analysis

Objectives

1. Know that absence of secondary sexual characteristics by age 14 years constitutes delayed puberty.
2. Know that the most common cause of sexually infantile delayed puberty, gonadal dysgenesis, is usually associated with a chromosomal abnormality.
3. Understand that the FSH level can help to determine whether the delayed puberty is due to a CNS problem or an ovarian problem.

Considerations

This 16-year-old female has never menstruated and, therefore, has primary amenorrhea. Furthermore, she has not yet experienced breast development (which should occur by age 14 years) and thus has delayed puberty. The lack of breast development means a lack of estrogen, which may be caused by either a central nervous system problem (low gonadotropin levels) or an ovarian problem (elevated gonadotropins). She is also of short stature, confirming the lack of estrogen. The absent pubic and axillary hair is consistent with delayed puberty. The most likely diagnosis without further information would be gonadal dysgenesis, such as Turner's syndrome. An elevated FSH level would be confirmatory.

APPROACH TO PUBERTAL DELAY

See also Case 45.

Definitions

Delayed puberty: Lack of secondary sexual characteristics by age 14 years.

Gonadal dysgenesis: Failure of development of ovaries, usually associated with a karyotypic abnormality (such as 45,X) and often associated with streaked gonads.

Clinical Approach

Maturation of the hypothalamic–pituitary–ovarian axis leads to the onset of puberty. There are **four stages of pubertal development: 1) thelarche, 2) pubarche/adrenarche, 3) growth spurt, and 4) menarche.** The first sign of puberty is the appearance of breast budding (thelarche), which occurs at a mean age of 10.8 years. This is followed by the appearance of pubic and axillary hair (pubarche/adrenarche), usually at 11 years. The growth spurt typically occurs 1 year after thelarche. The onset of menses (menarche) is the final event of puberty, occurring approximately 2.3 years after thelarche, at a mean age of 12.9 years. Normal puberty takes place between the ages of 8 to14 years, with an average duration of 4.5 years. **Delayed puberty is the absence of secondary sexual characteristics by age 14 years.**

Thelarche   → Adrenarche   → Growth spurt → Menarche
Breast bud   Axillary & Pubic   Menses
                 Hair

Delayed puberty can be subdivided based on two factors: the **gonadotropic and the gonadal state. The FSH level** defines the gonadotropic state. The **ovarian production of estrogen** refers to **the gonadal state.** The FSH level differentiates between brain and ovarian causes of delayed puberty. Central nervous system defects result in low FSH levels secondary to disruption of the hypothalamic–pituitary axis. With ovarian failure, the negative feedback of estrogen on the properly functioning hypothalamic–pituitary axis is not present, resulting in high FSH levels.

Hypergonadotropic hypogonadism (high FSH, low estrogen) is due to gonadal deficiency. The most common cause of this type of delayed puberty is **Turner's syndrome.** These individuals have an abnormality in or absence of one of the X chromosomes leading to gonadal dysgenesis and a 45,X karyotype. They do not have true ovaries, but rather a fibrous band of tissue referred to as **gonadal streaks.** Thus, they lack ovarian estrogen production and, as a result, secondary sexual characteristics. The internal and external genitalia are that of a normal female, but remain infantile even into adult life. Other characteristic physical findings are short stature, webbed neck, shield chest, and increased carrying angle at the elbow. Turner's syndrome should be suspected in an individual who presents with primary amenorrhea, prepubescent secondary sexual characteristics, and sexually infantile external genitalia. The definitive diagnosis can be made with an **elevated FSH level and a karyotypic evaluation.** Other causes of hypergonadotropic hypogonadism are ovarian damage due to exposure to ionizing radiation, chemotherapy, inflammation, or torsion.

Hypogonadotropic hypogonadism (low FSH, low estrogen) is usually secondary to a **central defect. Hypothalamic dysfunction** may occur due to poor nutrition or eating disorders (anorexia nervosa, bulimia), extremes in exercise, and chronic illness or stress. Other causes are primary hypothyroidism, Cushing's syndrome, pituitary adenomas, and craniopharyngiomas (the most commonly associated neoplasm).

The diagnostic approach to delayed puberty begins with a meticulous history and physical examination. The history should query chronic illnesses, exercise and eating habits, and age at menarche of the patient's sisters and mother. The physical examination should search for signs of chronic illness, such as a goiter, or neurologic deficits, such as visual field defects indicative of cranial neoplasms. Skull imaging should be obtained to look for intracranial lesions. The laboratory evaluation should include serum measurements of FSH, prolactin, TSH, free T_4, and appropriate adrenal and gonadal steroids. A karyotype evaluation should be performed when the FSH level is elevated.

The management goals for those with delayed puberty are to initiate and sustain sexual maturation, prevent osteoporosis from hypoestrogenemia, and promote the full height potential. Hormonal therapy can be used to achieve these objectives. Combination **oral contraceptives provide the small amounts of estrogen needed to promote growth** and development and the **progestin** protects against endometrial cancer.

Comprehension Questions

[48.1] With gonadal dysgenesis, each of the following is generally present except:

    A. Primary amenorrhea
    B. Short stature
    C. Tanner stage IV breast development
    D. Osteoporosis
    E. Streaked ovaries

[48.2] Delayed puberty is defined as no secondary sexual characteristics by age:

    A. 10 years
    B. 12 years
    C. 14 years
    D. 16 years
    E. 18 years

[48.3] With gonadal dysgenesis, which of the following is usually elevated?

A. Follicle stimulating hormone levels
B. Estrogen levels
C. Progesterone levels
D. Prolactin levels
E. Thyroxine levels

[48.4] A 20-year-old individual with a 46,XY karyotype is noted to be sexually infantile phenotypic female and diagnosed as having gonadal dysgenesis. Which of the following is the most important treatment for this patient?

A. Progestin therapy to reduce osteoporosis
B. Estrogen and androgen therapy to enhance height
C. Progesterone therapy to prevent endometrial cancer
D. Gonadectomy
E. Estrogen therapy to initiate breast development

Answers

[48.1] **C.** Breast tissue is usually infantile with gonadal dysgenesis, since there is no estrogen produced. Breast tissue is a reflection of endogenous estrogen.

[48.2] **C.** Delayed puberty is defined as no secondary sexual characteristics by age 14 years.

[48.3] **A.** With gonadal dysgenesis, the FSH is elevated.

[48.4] **D.** The Y chromosome predisposes intraabdominal gonads to malignancy. Even a mosaic karyotype, such as 46,XX/46,XY, would predispose to gonadal malignancy.

CLINICAL PEARLS

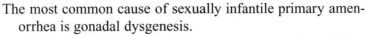 The most common cause of sexually infantile primary amenorrhea is gonadal dysgenesis.

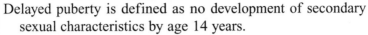 Delayed puberty is defined as no development of secondary sexual characteristics by age 14 years.

◈ The FSH level distinguishes ovarian failure from central nervous system dysfunction.

◈ The FSH level determines the gonadotropic state, and the ovarian estradiol level dictates the gonadal state.

◈ The most important initial test for primary amenorrhea with normal breast development is a pregnancy test.

REFERENCES

Mishell DR. Primary and secondary amenorrhea. In: Stenchever MA, Droegemueller W, Herbst AL, Mishell DR, eds. Comprehensive gynecology, 4th ed. St. Louis: Mosby-Year Book. 2001:1099–1124.

Buyalos RP. Puberty and disorders of pubertal development. In: Hacker NF and Moore JG, eds. Essentials of obstetrics and gynecology, 3rd ed. Philadelphia: Saunders. 1998:567–79.

A 20-year-old parous woman complains of right breast pain and fever. She states that 3 weeks previously, she underwent a normal spontaneous vaginal delivery. She had been breast-feeding without difficulty until 2 days ago, when she noted progressive pain, induration, and redness to the right breast. On examination, her temperature is 102°F, BP 100/70, and HR 110 bpm. Her neck is supple. Her right breast has induration on the upper outer region with redness and tenderness. There is also significant fluctuance noted in the breast tissue. The abdomen is nontender and there is no costovertebral angle tenderness. The pelvic examination is unremarkable.

◆ **What is the most likely diagnosis?**

◆ **What is your next step in therapy?**

◆ **What is the etiology of the condition?**

ANSWERS TO CASE 49: Breast Abscess and Mastitis

Summary: A 20-year-old breast-feeding woman who is 3 weeks' postpartum complains of right breast pain and fever of 2 days duration. She notes progressive pain, induration, and redness in the right breast. Her temperature is 102°F. There is also significant fluctuance noted in the right breast.

◆ **Most likely diagnosis:** Abscess of the right breast.

◆ **Next step in therapy:** Incision and drainage of the abscess and antibiotic therapy.

◆ **Etiology of the condition:** *Staphylococcus aureus.*

Analysis

Objectives

1. Know the clinical presentation of postpartum mastitis.
2. Know that *Staphylococcus aureus* is the most common etiology in postpartum mastitis.
3. Understand that the presence of fluctuance in the breast probably represents an abscess that needs incision and drainage.

Considerations

This woman is 3 weeks' postpartum with breast pain and fever. This is a typical presentation of a breast infection, since mastitis usually presents in the third or fourth postpartum week. Induration and redness of the breast accompanied by fever and chills are also consistent. The treatment for this condition is an antistaphylococcal agent, such as dicloxicillin. Provided that the offending agent is not methicillin resistant, improvement should be rapid. Affected women are instructed to continue to breast-feed or drain the breast by pump. This patient has fluctuance of the breast that speaks for an abscess, which usually requires surgical drainage and will not generally improve with antibiotics alone. If there is uncertainty about the diagnosis, ultrasound examination may be helpful in identifying a fluid collection.

APPROACH TO BREAST INFECTIONS

Definitions

Mastitis: Infection of the breast parenchyma typically caused by *Staphyloccocus aureus.*

Breast abscess: The presence of a collection of purulent material in the breast, which requires drainage.

Galactocele: A noninfected collection of milk due to a blocked mammary duct leading to a palpable mass and symptoms of breast pressure and pain.

Clinical Approach

Postpartum breast disorders and infections are common. They include cracked nipples, breast engorgement, mastitis, breast abscesses, and galactoceles. **Cracked nipples** usually arise from **dryness,** and may be exacerbated by harsh soap or water-soluble lotions. Treatment includes air-drying the nipples, the use of a nipple shield, or the application of an oil-based lotion.

Breast engorgement is usually noted during the **first week postpartum and is due to vascular congestion and milk accumulation.** The patient will generally complain of **breast pain** and induration, and may have a **low-grade fever. Infant feedings around-the-clock usually help to alleviate this condition.** Fever seldom persists for more than 12 to 24 hr. Treatment consists of a **breast binder, ice packs, and analgesics.**

Postpartum mastitis is an infection of the breast parenchyma, affecting about 2% of lactating women. These infections usually occur between the **second and fourth week after delivery.** Other signs and symptoms include **malaise, fever, chills, tachycardia, and a red,**

tender, swollen breast. Importantly, there should be **no fluctuance** of the breast, which would indicate abscess formation. The most commonly isolated organism is ***Staphylococcus aureus,*** **usually arising from the infant's nose and throat.** The treatment for mastitis should be prompt to prevent abscess formation, consisting of an antistaphylococcal agent, such as **dicloxicillin. Breast-feeding should be continued** to prevent the development of abscess.

About one in ten cases of mastitis is complicated by **abscess,** which should be suspected with **persistent fever after 48 hr of antibiotic therapy or the presence of a fluctuant mass.** Ultrasound examination may be performed to confirm the diagnosis. The purulent collection is best treated by **surgical drainage,** or alternatively by ultrasound-guided aspiration; antistaphylococcal antibiotics should also be used.

The **galactocele or milk-retention cyst** is caused by blockage of a milk duct. The milk accumulates in one or more breast lobes, leading to a nonerythematous fluctuant mass. They usually resolve spontaneously, but **may need aspiration.**

Comprehension Questions

[49.1] A 25-year-old woman who is breast-feeding notes fever, induration, and redness of the left breast. No fluctuance is noted. Each of the following statements is correct except:

A. The patient needs an incision and drainage procedure.
B. The etiology is most likely *Staphylococcus aureus.*
C. Oral dicloxicillin is an acceptable therapy.
D. The woman should continue to breast-feed.
E. The bacteria most likely came from the baby.

[49.2] A 22-year-old nulliparous woman is noted to have a tender, red, right breast and enlarged, tender axillary lymph nodes that have persisted despite antibiotics for 3 weeks. She denies manipulation of her breasts and is not lactating. Which of the following is the most appropriate next step?

A. Course of oral antibiotic therapy
B. Sonographic examination of the breasts

C. Mammographic examination of the breasts
D. Check the serum prolactin level
E. Biopsy of the breast

[49.3] Which of the following is the best treatment for a galactocele of the breast?

A. Oral antibiotic therapy
B. Oral antifungal therapy
C. Bromocriptine therapy
D. Aspiration
E. Mastectomy

[49.4]. Which of the following is the most common time period for the development of postpartum mastitis?

A. 2–3 days postpartum
B. 3–7 days postpartum
C. 1–2 weeks postpartum
D. 3–4 weeks postpartum
E. 4–6 weeks postpartum

Answers

[49.1] **A.** Because there is no fluctuance, the patient does not need incision and drainage.

[49.2] **E.** This woman has had persistent tenderness and redness of the breast despite not lactating and not having trauma to the breast; these symptoms have worsened despite antibiotic therapy. There is a concern about inflammatory breast carcinoma, and she should undergo biopsy.

[49.3] **D.** Often, a galactocele will require aspiration to prevent abscess formation.

[49.4] **D.** The most common time for postpartum mastitis to occur is 3 to 4 weeks after delivery.

CLINICAL PEARLS

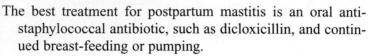
The best treatment for postpartum mastitis is an oral anti-staphylococcal antibiotic, such as dicloxicillin, and continued breast-feeding or pumping.

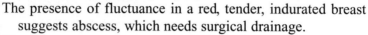
The presence of fluctuance in a red, tender, indurated breast suggests abscess, which needs surgical drainage.

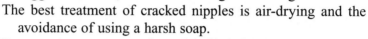
The best treatment of cracked nipples is air-drying and the avoidance of using a harsh soap.

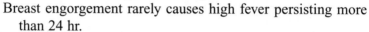
Breast engorgement rarely causes high fever persisting more than 24 hr.

REFERENCES

Cunningham FG, Gant NF, Leveno KJ, Gilstrap LC III, Hauth JC, Wenstrom KD. The puerperium. In: Williams obstetrics, 21st ed. New York: McGraw-Hill. 2001:413–415.

Ross MG, Hobel CJ. Normal labor, delivery, and the puerperium. In: Hacker NF and Moore JG, eds. Essentials of obstetrics and gynecology, 3rd ed. Philadelphia: Saunders. 1998:166.

A 19-year-old G2 Ab1 woman at 9 weeks' gestation by LMP underwent an induced abortion 2 days previously. Prior to the procedure, she did not have bleeding, pain, or passage of tissue. She had slight vaginal spotting for 1 day following the procedure, and otherwise has felt well. Histologic examination of the uterine curetting revealed no chorionic villi. On examination, her temperature is 98°F, BP 100/50, and HR 70 bpm. Her heart examination is normal, and lungs are clear bilaterally. Her abdomen shows no abdominal tenderness and no masses. The pelvic examination demonstrates a closed cervical os, a 4-weeks' sized nontender uterus, and no adnexal tenderness. Her pregnancy test is positive.

◆ **What is the most likely diagnosis?**

◆ **What is your probable therapy for this patient?**

ANSWERS TO CASE 50: Ectopic Pregnancy

Summary: A 19-year-old G2 Ab1 woman at 9 weeks' gestation underwent an induced abortion 2 days previously by uterine dilation and curettage. Histologic examination revealed no chorionic villi. Her physical examination is unremarkable. The pelvic examination demonstrates a small uterus, a closed cervix, and no adnexal tenderness.

◆ **Most likely diagnosis:** Ectopic pregnancy.

◆ **Probable therapy for this patient:** Methotrexate intramuscularly.

Analysis

Objectives

1. Understand that a pregnant woman with no chorionic villi on uterine curettage most likely has an ectopic pregnancy.
2. Understand the role of methotrexate in treating ectopic pregnancy.

Considerations

This 19-year-old woman had an elective abortion 2 days previously for what was suspected to be a 9-week pregnancy. When the tissue was analyzed on microscopy, there were no chorionic villi noted. Her examination is currently unremarkable. Several possibilities come to mind with this situation.

1. The patient has an intrauterine pregnancy (IUP), but the attempted curettage did not reach the pregnancy tissue.
2. The patient had an intrauterine pregnancy, which had spontaneously aborted, with complete passage of tissue prior to having the induced abortion.

3.   The patient has an ectopic pregnancy. The abortion (uterine curettage) did not reveal any chorionic villi because she does not have an intrauterine pregnancy.

Scenario 1 (current IUP) is not likely because her uterus is small and normal in shape. With an unsuccessful pregnancy termination, the operator usually encounters an incomplete evacuation of the pregnancy rather than completely missing the pregnancy altogether. A patient who has an incomplete evacuation of the uterus will usually present with crampy lower abdominal pain and vaginal spotting.

Scenario 2 (completed spontaneous abortion) is unlikely since the patient did not report passage of tissue or vaginal bleeding before the procedure. If the patient had complained of passage of blood clots or possibly tissue, this would be a viable alternative.

Hence, scenario 3 is the most likely diagnosis. Indeed, in situations where elective terminations are performed for presumed intrauterine pregnancies and no chorionic villi are identified, an extrauterine pregnancy is the most likely diagnosis. Because each of these scenarios is possible, the next steps would entail checking a quantitative hCG level and performing a transvaginal ultrasound examination to help to differentiate among the possibilities. If the transvaginal ultrasound reveals an intrauterine pregnancy, an unsuccessful abortion is the diagnosis. If the hCG level has fallen significantly since the initial hCG examination, a completed abortion is possible.

If an ectopic pregnancy is confirmed, based on elevated hCG levels and no evidence of an intrauterine pregnancy, the best therapy would likely be methotrexate.

APPROACH TO POSSIBLE ECTOPIC PREGNANCY

Definitions

Methotrexate: An antimetabolite chemotherapeutic agent that inhibits DNA synthesis, used also to treat ectopic pregnancies.

Chorionic villi: Development of the placental syncytiotrophoblasts and cytotrophoblasts to form a "brush border" for fetal–maternal diffusion.

Clinical Approach

See Explanations in Cases 7 and 30.

Comprehension Questions

[50.1] A 28-year-old woman has been given ovulation induction agents of human menopausal gonadotropin (FSH and LH) and becomes pregnant. On sonography, she is noted to have a viable intrauterine pregnancy as well as a pregnancy with fetal cardiac activity in the adnexa. Which of the following is the best therapy?

    A. Intramuscular methotrexate
    B. Oral methotrexate
    C. Surgical therapy
    D. Mifepristone (RU 486)
    E. Oral progestin therapy

[50.2] A 22-year-old woman is diagnosed with an ectopic pregnancy based on hCG levels, which have plateaued at 2900 mIU/mL and an endometrial biopsy showing no chorionic villi. In reviewing the options of therapy with the patient, the physician explains the mechanisms of action of methotrexate. Which one of the following is a correct statement about methotrexate?

    A. It interferes with mitosis phase of the cell cycle.
    B. It is obtained from the bark of the Pacific yew tree.
    C. It severs DNA strands between particular base pairs.
    D. It interferes with folate synthesis and DNA synthesis.
    E. It causes pulmonary fibrosis in about 5% of patients.

[50.3] A 22-year-old woman is given intramuscular methotrexate for a proven ectopic pregnancy. On the fourth day after therapy, she experiences crampy lower abdominal pain. Her blood pressure and heart rate are normal. The abdominal examination is unre-

markable. A transvaginal ultrasound examination shows no free
fluid. Which of the following is the best next step?

A. Immediate laparoscopy
B. Immediate exploratory laparotomy
C. Observation
D. Institution of folic acid
E. Follow serial progesterone levels

[50.4] A 25-year-old G1 P0 woman at 5 weeks' gestation receives oral
mifepristone (RU 486) and 2 days later receives oral misopros-
tol (cytotec). The next day, she has vaginal bleeding and passage
of tissue. She comes into the emergency room because of persistent cramping and vaginal bleeding. The tissue has a frond-
like, floating appearance in saline. Her cervical os is open.
Which of the following is the most likely diagnosis?

A. Incomplete abortion
B. Ectopic pregnancy
C. Molar pregnancy
D. Ruptured corpus luteum
E. Completed abortion

Answers

[50.1] **C.** The presence of fetal cardiac activity in ectopic pregnancy is
a relative contraindication to methotrexate use due to increased
risk of failure. Also, methotrexate would affect the IUP as well
as the ectopic pregnancy.

[50.2] **D.** Methotrexate interferes with S phase (DNA synthesis) by an-
tagonizing folate metabolism. Its main side effect is myelosup-
pression. Bleomycin is known for causing pulmonary fibrosis.

[50.3] **C.** Mild abdominal pain is very common after methotrexate, and
should be differentiated from intra-abdominal hemorrhage and
hypotension.

[50.4] **A.** The frond-like appearance is very suggestive of products of conception; the open cervical os is consistent with an incomplete abortion.

CLINICAL PEARLS

❖ When no chorionic villi are found on uterine curettage of a pregnant woman, the most likely etiology is ectopic pregnancy.

❖ Methotrexate inhibits DNA synthesis due to its interfering with folate metabolism.

❖ A relative contraindication to methotrexate use is an ectopic pregnancy larger than 3.5 cm or the presence of fetal cardiac activity in the tube.

REFERENCES

Mishell DR. Ectopic pregnancy. In: Stenchever MA, Droegemueller W, Herbst AL, Mishell DR, eds. Comprehensive gynecology, 4th ed. St. Louis: Mosby-Year Book. 2001:443–478.

Palmieri A, Moore GJ, DeCherney AH. Ectopic pregnancy. In: Hacker NF and Moore JG, eds. Essentials of obstetrics and gynecology, 3rd ed. Philadelphia: Saunders. 1998:487–498.

An 18-year-old G2 P1 at 35 weeks' gestation has a history of Graves' disease and is under treatment with oral propylthiouracil. She states that over the last day, she has been feeling as though her "heart is pounding." She also complains of nervousness, sweating, and diarrhea. On examination, her BP is 150/110, HR 140 bpm, RR 25/min, and temperature 100.8°F. The patient appears anxious, disoriented, and somewhat confused. The thyroid gland is mildly tender and enlarged. The cardiac examination reveals tachycardia with a III/VI systolic murmur. The fetal heart rate tracing shows a baseline in the 160 bpm range without decelerations. Deep tendon reflexes are 4+ with clonus. Her leukocyte count is 20,000/mm^3.

◆ **What is the most likely diagnosis?**

◆ **What is the best management for this condition?**

ANSWERS TO CASE 51: Thyroid Storm in Pregnancy

Summary: An 18-year-old G2 P1 at 35 weeks' gestation is taking PTU for Graves' disease. She has a 1-day history of palpitations, nervousness, sweating, and diarrhea. On examination, her BP is 150/110, HR 140 bpm, RR 25/min, and temperature 100.8°F. The patient appears anxious, disoriented, and somewhat confused. The thyroid is mildly tender and enlarged. Deep tendon reflexes are 4+ with clonus. She has a leukocytosis.

◆ **Most likely diagnosis:** Thyroid storm.

◆ **Best management for this condition:** A beta blocker (such as propranolol), corticosteroids, and PTU.

Analysis

Objectives

1. Know that the most common cause of hyperthyroidism in the United States is Graves' disease.
2. Recognize the clinical presentation and danger of thyroid storm.

Considerations

This 18-year-old woman at 35 weeks' gestation has a history of hyperthyroidism due to Graves' disease. In the United States, the **majority of hyperthyroidism is due to Graves' disease;** the clinical presentation is typically that of a **painless, uniformly enlarged thyroid gland with occasional proptosis.** She is being treated with propylthiouracil (PTU), which is the most commonly used medication for hyperthyroidism in pregnancy. For whatever reason, which is not stated, the patient has symptoms of increased thyrotoxicosis of 1-day duration. Some possible reasons include noncompliance with the medication, or a stressor, such as surgery or an illness. This woman not only has the nervousness and palpitations of hyperthyroidism, but also **autonomic instability, which**

is the hallmark of thyroid storm. Her blood pressure is 150/110 and her temperature is elevated. She is disoriented and markedly confused. Thyroid storm must be recognized because it carries a **significant risk of mortality.** The **therapy consists of a beta-blocking agent, such as propranolol, corticosteroids, and additional propylthiouracil.** In the nonpregnant patient, a saturated solution of potassium iodide (SSKI) oral drops may also be used; however, this agent may affect the fetal thyroid gland. Notably, the patient has a high white blood cell count. This fact is important since rarely, PTU can induce a bone marrow aplasia, leading to leukopenia, and sepsis.

APPROACH TO THYROTOXICOSIS IN PREGNANCY

Definitions

Hyperthyroidism: A syndrome caused by excess thyroid hormone, leading to nervousness, tachycardia, palpitations, weight loss, diarrhea, and heat intolerance.

Thyroid storm: Extreme thyrotoxicosis leading to central nervous system dysfunction (coma or delirium) and autonomic instability (hyperthermia, hypertension, or hypotension).

Graves' disease: The most common cause of thyrotoxicosis in the United States, leading to a diffusely enlarged goiter.

Free thyroxine (T$_4$): Unbound or biologically active thyroxine hormone.

Clinical Approach

Hyperthyroidism is rare in pregnancy, occurring in about 1 in 2000 pregnancies. Symptoms of thyrotoxicosis include tachycardia, heat intolerance, nausea, weight loss or failure to gain weight despite adequate food intake, thyromegaly, thyroid bruit, tremor, exophthalmos, and systolic hypertension. The most common cause of hyperthyroidism in pregnancy is **Graves' disease, an autoimmune disorder in which antibodies are produced which mimic the function of TSH.** These antibodies stimulate the thyroid gland to produce more thyroid hormone, leading to the symptoms responsible for thyrotoxicosis. The diagnosis of hyperthyroidism is confirmed in the presence of an **elevated free thyroxine and low serum TSH levels.** Treatment during pregnancy may be medical or surgical; however, generally, hyperthyroidism in pregnancy is managed medically. **Propylthiouracil (PTU) is generally accepted as the drug of choice** in pregnancy. PTU inhibits the peripheral conversion of T_4 to T_3 and does not cross the placenta readily. Methimazole is another option. Thyroidectomy is reserved for those patients who are noncompliant with or cannot tolerate medical therapy. Risks from surgery include vocal cord paralysis and hypoparathyroidism.

Thyroid storm is a rare but life-threatening complication of hyperthyroidism. Symptoms suggestive of storm include **altered mental status, hyperthermia, hypertension, and diarrhea.** Congestive heart failure can result from the effects of thyroxine on the myocardium. Because the mortality rate associated with thyroid storm is high, accurate early identification is crucial. These patients are best monitored in an **intensive care unit. Propylthiouracil** is administered by mouth or nasogastric tube. **Beta blockers** are used to control the symptoms of tachycardia; however, they should be used with caution in those patients with congestive heart failure. **Acetaminophen or cooling blankets** are used for hyperthermia. **Corticosteroids** may also be used to prevent the peripheral conversion of T_4 to T_3.

Comprehension Questions

[51.1] Which of the following best describes the effect of pregnancy on the thyroid hormones as compared with the nonpregnant state?

    A. Elevation of TSH levels
    B. Elevation of total thyroxine levels
    C. Decrease in thyroid-binding globulin levels
    D. Decrease in free T_4 levels
    E. No effect on TSH or total thyroxine levels

[51.2] A 15-year-old woman G1 P0 at 16 weeks' gestation complains of some intermittent palpitations, and feeling warm more often. Which of the following is the best screening test for hyperthyroidism?

A. Serum thyroid stimulating hormone (TSH) levels
B. Serum thyroid-binding globulin levels
C. Serum antithyroid antibody levels
D. Serum total thyroxine levels
E. Serum transferrin levels

[51.3] A 24-year-old woman delivered vaginally at term about 2 months previously. She was in good health until 1 week ago, when she began to complain of nervousness, tremulousness, and feeling warm. The TSH is 0.01 mIU/L. Which of the following is the most likely diagnosis?

A. Graves' disease
B. Destructive lymphocytic thyrotoxicosis
C. Multinodular thyrotoxicosis
D. Autonomous thyroid adenoma
E. Pheochromocytoma

[51.4] Which of the following is most consistent with hypothyroidism in pregnancy?

	TSH	Free Thyroxine	Thyroid-Binding Globulin	Total Thyroxine
A.	Unchanged	Elevated	Decreased	Unchanged
B.	Decreased	Elevated	Unchanged	Decreased
C.	Increased	Decreased	Elevated	Unchanged
D.	Unchanged	Decreased	Decreased	Elevated
E.	Unchanged	Unchanged	Unchanged	Decreased

Answers

[51.1] **B.** Total T_4 is increased in pregnancy, but free T_4 (which is biologically active) and TSH are unchanged.

[51.2] **A.** The TSH is considered the best screening test for hyperthyroidism. A low level suggests hyperthyroidism; an elevated level
suggests hypothyroidism.

[51.3] **B.** After delivery, the most likely diagnosis is destructive lymphocytic thyroiditis because the steroid levels are lower in this
period. Often, antimicrosomal antibodies are present.

[51.4] **C.** With hypothyroidism, the TSH is elevated, and the free T_4 is
decreased.

CLINICAL PEARLS

Graves' disease is the most common cause of hyperthyroidism
in pregnancy. Thyroid storm should be considered when
central nervous system dysfunction and autonomic instability are present. The treatments for thyroid storm in pregnancy include PTU, steroids, and beta blockers.

Pregnancy (or use of estrogens) causes total thyroxine to be
increased, free T_4 to be unchanged, TSH to be unchanged,
and thyroid-binding globulin to be increased.

Postpartum thyroiditis often occurs 1 to 4 months postpartum,
is associated with antimicrosomal antibodies, and can lead
to hypothyroidism.

REFERENCES

Cunningham FG, Gant NF, Leveno KJ, Gilstrap LC III, Hauth JC, Wenstrom KD.
Endocrine disorders. In: Williams obstetrics, 21st ed. New York: McGraw-Hill.
2001:1340–1344.

Nuwayhid B, Nguyen T, Khalife S. Medical complications of pregnancy. In: Hacker
NF and Moore JG, eds. Essentials of obstetrics and gynecology, 3rd ed. Philadelphia: Saunders Co. 1998:248–251.

An 18-year-old G1 P0 at 22 weeks' gestation has a positive *Chlamydia* DNA assay of the endocervix. She denies vaginal discharge, lower abdominal pain, or fever. On examination, her BP is 110/70, HR 70 bpm, and she is afebrile. Her heart and lung examinations are normal. Her abdomen is nontender and gravid. The fundal height is 20 cm. Fetal heart tones are in the 140 bpm range. The gonorrhea culture is negative and the Pap smear result is normal.

⬥ **What is your next step in therapy?**

ANSWERS TO CASE 52: Chlamydial Cervicitis in Pregnancy

Summary: An 18-year-old G1 P0 at 22 weeks' gestation has a positive *Chlamydia* DNA assay of the endocervix. She denies lower abdominal pain and is afebrile. Her abdomen is nontender and gravid. The gonorrhea culture is negative.

◆ **Next step in therapy:** Oral erythromycin, azithromycin, or amoxicillin.

Analysis

Objectives

1. Understand that *Chlamydia trachomatis* is a common cause of cervicitis.
2. Know that tetracyclines (doxycycline also) are contraindicated in pregnancy.
3. Know that chlamydial infections may lead to neonatal pneumonia or conjunctivitis if untreated.

Considerations

This 18-year-old nulliparous woman at 22 weeks' gestation has a positive DNA test for *Chlamydia.* These types of tests are often utilized because of their high sensitivity and specificity yet lower cost as compared with chlamydial cultures. This patient has a chlamydial infection, which is more common than gonorrheal involvement; accordingly, her gonorrheal culture was negative. Chlamydial endocervical infection has not been proven to cause adverse problems with pregnancy, such as preterm labor or preterm premature rupture of membranes. It has been implicated in neonatal conjunctivitis and pneumonia. Interestingly, the erythromycin eye ointment given at birth does not prevent chlamydial conjunctivitis, although it does protect against gonococcal eye infection. Babies with documented chlamydial ophthalmic infections are given oral erythromycin for 14 days. Because it is mainly neonatal disease that is the issue, an important time to screen for the organism would be the third trimester, close to the time of delivery. Treatment includes erythromycin or amoxicillin for 7 days or azithromycin as a one-time dose.

APPROACH TO CERVICITIS IN PREGNANCY

Definitions

Chlamydial neonate infection: Conjunctivitis or pneumonia acquired by inoculation during the birth process.

Tetracycline effect: Tetracycline compounds, such as doxycycline, taken by pregnant women can lead to staining of the fetal teeth.

Clinical Approach

Chlamydia trachomatis **is an obligate intracellular organism** with several serotypes. It is one of the **most common sexually transmitted organisms in the United States,** causing **urethritis, mucopurulent cervicitis, and late postpartum endometritis.** Vertical transmission may occur during the labor and delivery process, leading to neonatal **conjunctivitis or pneumonia.** It is unclear whether chlamydial infection of the cervix is associated with preterm labor or preterm rupture of membranes; thus, the main concern is for the neonate. Eye prophylaxis is effective for preventing gonococcal conjunctivitis but **not** chlamydial involvement. **Late postpartum endometritis,** occurring 2 to 3 weeks after delivery, is associated with chlamydial disease.

Usually, chlamydial infections are asymptomatic, although they **may cause mucopurulent cervicitis or urethritis.** The discharge is often difficult to detect because of the increased cervical mucus in pregnancy. Direct fluorescent antibody tests and DNA detection tests using polymerase chain reaction (PCR) are highly sensitive and specific, and less costly than culture. Treatment includes **oral erythromycin, amoxicillin, or azithromycin. Tetracycline is contraindicated in pregnancy** because of the possibility of staining of the neonatal teeth. Because reinfection is common, repeat testing is prudent in the third trimester.

Gonococcal infection may complicate pregnancy, especially in teens or those with a history of sexually transmitted disease. Gonococcal cervicitis is associated with **abortion, preterm labor, preterm premature rupture of membranes, and postpartum infection. Disseminated gonococcal** disease is more common in the pregnant woman, presenting as **pustular skin lesions, arthralgias, and septic arthritis.** *Chlamydia* commonly is present in a patient who is infected with gonorrhea. Thus, the usual treatment for gonococcal cervicitis is **ceftriaxone intramuscularly and an additional antibiotic for *Chlamydia trachomatis,* such as erythromycin.**

Comprehension Questions

[52.1] Each of the following is a characteristic of chlamydial infection except:

    A. Has a characteristic appearance on Gram's stain
    B. Has a propensity for transitional and columnar epithelium
    C. Causes neonatal pneumonia; may be subclinical, presenting as failure to gain weight or chronic cough
    D. Is one of the leading causes of blindness worldwide

[52.2] Which of the following statements is true regarding *Chlamydia trachomatis* infections?

    A. The organism has a fairly rapid replication cycle, about 6 hr
    B. Is an obligate intracellular organism
    C. Erythromycin eye drops are an effective means of preventing chlamydial conjunctivitis
    D. Is associated with acute early endometritis
    E. Is a cause of infectious arthritis

[52.3] Each of the following is an acceptable treatment for chlamydial cervicitis in pregnancy except:

A. Azithromycin
B. Erythromycin estolate
C. Amoxicillin
D. Erythromycin ethylsuccinate

[52.4] Which of the following is *Chlamydia trachomatis* least likely to cause?

A. Urethritis
B. Cervicitis
C. Perihepatitis
D. Bartholinitis
E. Vaginitis

Answers

[52.1] **A.** *Chlamydia* is not typically seen on Gram's stain, since it is an intracellular organism. It does have a propensity for columnar and transitional epithelium.

[52.2] **B.** *Chlamydia* is an obligate intracellular organism, is associated with late postpartum endometritis, and has a long replication cycle.

[52.3] **B.** Erythromycin estolate can lead to liver dysfunction in pregnancy; thus the estolate salt is contraindicated in pregnant women.

[52.4] **E.** *Chlamydia* is associated with cervicitis and urethritis, and not vaginitis.

CLINICAL PEARLS

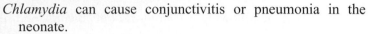 The best treatments for chlamydial cervicitis in pregnancy are erythromycin, azithromycin, and amoxicillin.

Chlamydia can cause conjunctivitis or pneumonia in the neonate.

Ophthalmic antibiotics administered to the neonate help to prevent gonococcal disease but not chlamydial conjunctivitis.

REFERENCES

Cunningham FG, Gant NF, Leveno KJ, Gilstrap LC III, Hauth JC, Wenstrom KD. Sexually transmitted diseases. In: Williams obstetrics, 21st ed. New York: McGraw-Hill. 2001:1492–1494.

Goodman JR. AIDS and infectious diseases in pregnancy. In: Hacker NF and Moore JG, eds. Essentials of obstetrics and gynecology, 3rd ed. Philadelphia: Saunders. 1998:219.

A 24-year-old G2 P1 woman at 22 weeks' gestation complains of an episode of myalgias and low-grade fever 1 month ago. Her 2-year-old son had high fever and "red cheeks." On examination, her BP is 110/60, HR 82 bpm, and she is afebrile. The heart and lung examinations are normal. The fundal height is 28 cm and fetal parts are difficult to palpate.

◆ **What is the most likely diagnosis?**

◆ **What is the most likely mechanism?**

ANSWERS TO CASE 53: Parvovirus Infection in Pregnancy

Summary: A 24-year-old G2 P1 woman at 22 weeks' gestation complains of an episode of myalgias and low-grade fever 1 month ago. Her 2-year-old son had high fever and "red cheeks." The fundal height is 28 cm and fetal parts are difficult to palpate.

◆ **Most likely diagnosis:** Hydramnios, with probable fetal hydrops due to parvovirus B19 infection.

◆ **Most likely mechanism:** Fetal anemia due to neonatal parvovirus infection, which inhibits bone marrow erythrocyte production.

Analysis

Objectives

1. Know the clinical presentation of parvovirus infection in children and adults.
2. Understand the possible effects of parvovirus B19 infection on the pregnancy.
3. Know the clinical presentation of hydramnios.

Considerations

This 22-year-old woman presents with a history of myalgias and low-grade fever. Her 2-year-old son had "red cheeks" and a high fever. This illustrates the difference in the clinical presentation of parvovirus B19 infection in an adult versus that of a child. **Adults rarely have high fever, but more often have malaise, arthralgias and myalgias, and a reticular (lacy) faint rash** that comes and goes. In contrast, **children often develop the classic "slapped cheek"** appearance and high fever, which is the manifestation of "fifth disease." Parvovirus infections in pregnancy may cause a fetal infection, which may lead to suppression of the erythrocyte precursors of the bone marrow. Severe fetal anemia may result, leading to fetal hydrops. One of the earliest signs of fetal

Table 53–1
CAUSES OF HYDRAMNIOS

Fetal central nervous system anomalies
Fetal gastrointestinal tract malformations
Fetal chromosomal abnormalities
Fetal nonimmune hydrops
Maternal diabetes
Isoimmunization
Multiple gestation
Syphilis

hydrops is hydramnios, or excess amniotic fluid (see Table 53–1 for causes of hydramnios). This patient's uterine size is greater than that predicted by her dates, and fetal parts are difficult to palpate, which are classic findings of hydramnios. An ultrasound examination would confirm the fetal and amniotic fluid effects.

APPROACH TO SUSPECTED FIFTH DISEASE IN PREGNANCY

Definitions

Fifth disease: Illness caused by a single-stranded DNA virus, parvovirus B19, also known as erythema infectiosum.
Fetal hydrops: A serious condition of excess fluid in body cavities, such as ascites, skin edema, pericardial effusion, and/or pleural effusion.
Hydramnios (or polyhydramnios):   Excess amniotic fluid.

Clinical Approach

Parvovirus B19 infection usually causes minimal or no symptoms in the adult, but may lead to devastating consequences for the fetus. A small, single-stranded DNA virus, parvovirus B19 causes a red "slapped cheek" appearance and fever in children; adults usually are

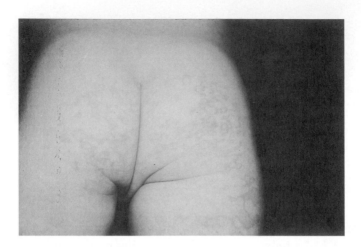

Figure 53–1.   **Fifth disease.** Lacy reticular rash of erythema infectiosum (fifth disease).

(Reproduced, with permission, from Braunwald E, et al, eds. Harrison's principles of internal medicine, 15th ed. New York: McGraw-Hill; 2001: 2416.)

less symptomatic and often have myalgias, and a **characteristic lacy reticular rash, which comes and goes** (Figure 53–1). **School-aged children** are commonly affected, and frequently transmit the virus to adults. Specific IgM antibody confirms the diagnosis. The virus may cause **an aplastic anemia by destroying erythroid precursors.**

Parvovirus infection may lead to fetal abortion, stillbirth, and hydrops. Hydrops fetalis is defined as excess fluid located in two or more fetal body cavities, and many times is associated with hydramnios; pregnancies less than 20 weeks' gestation are at particular risk. Theories about the mechanism of the hydrops include the observation that **the severe anemia may cause heart failure,** or induction of the hematopoietic centers in the liver to replace normal liver tissue, leading to low serum protein. The anemia is usually transient. For severely affected fetuses, **intrauterine transfusion** is one option, while mild cases may sometimes be observed. Other causes of fetal anemia are isoimmunization, such as an Rh-negative woman who is sensitized to develop anti-D antibodies, a large fetal-to-maternal hemorrhage, or thalassemia.

Comprehension Questions

[53.1] Which of the following is least likely to cause fetal anemia?

A. Abruptio placentae
B. Fifth disease
C. Rh isoimmunization
D. Intrauterine growth restriction

[53.2] In each of the following clinical situations, which of the following etiologies of fetal anemia is due to a bone marrow process?

A. Rh disease
B. Fifth disease
C. Anti-Duffy antibodies
D. HELLP (hemolysis elevated liver enzymes, low platelets) syndrome
E. Immune thrombocytopenia purpura

[53.3] A 22-year-old schoolteacher at 28 weeks' gestation has a history of a faint rash and low-grade fever. She states that fifth disease is spreading in her school. Which of the following is the best method of diagnosing an infection of fifth disease in the patient?

A. Fetal sonography
B. Fetal bone marrow sampling
C. IgG and IgM serology
D. Viral culture
E. Peripheral leukocyte count

[53.4] A 23-year-old woman at 26 weeks' gestation is noted to have hydramnios with an amniotic fluid index (AFI) of 35 cm. Which of the following examinations is/are indicated to evaluate the underlying etiology (more than more answer may be correct)?

A. Ultrasound to assess for anencephaly
B. 3-hr glucose tolerance test
C. Fetal sonography to assess for fetal tachyarrythmias
D. Ultrasound examination to assess for a "double bubble" sign
E. Indirect Coombs' test
F. Ultrasound examination to assess for fetal renal abnormalities

Answers

[53.1] **D.** IUGR usually leads to polycythemia; the other processes may cause fetal anemia.

[53.2] **B.** With fifth disease, it is bone marrow effects that lead to anemia.

[53.3] **C.** IgM and IgG serology is one method to diagnose acute fifth disease.

[53.4] **A, B, C, D,** and **E.** Duodenal atresia (double-bubble sign) and anencephaly are associated with hydramnios due to inhibition of fetal swallowing. Fetal cardiac arrhythmias often cause fetal hydrops, including hydramnios. Gestational diabetes and isoimmunization may also lead to hydramnios. Fetal renal anomalies usually lead to oligohydramnios.

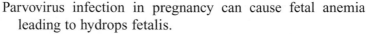

CLINICAL PEARLS

❖ Parvovirus infection in pregnancy can cause fetal anemia leading to hydrops fetalis.

❖ Hydramnios is one of the earliest manifestations of fetal hydrops.

❖ A parvovirus infection in the adult commonly leads to subtle findings of myalgias, malaise, and the reticular rash, whereas an infected child often has high fever and a "slapped cheek" appearance.

❖ Some causes of hydramnios include gestational diabetes, isoimmunization, syphilis, fetal cardiac arrhythmias, and fetal intestinal atresias.

REFERENCES

Cunningham FG, Gant NF, Leveno KJ, Gilstrap LC III, Hauth JC, Wenstrom KD. Abnormalities of the fetal membranes and amniotic fluid. In: Williams obstetrics, 21st ed. New York: McGraw-Hill. 2001:817–821.

Surrey ES, Lu JKH, Toot PJ. The menstrual cycle, ovulation, fertilization, implantation, and the placenta. In: Hacker NF and Moore JG, eds. Essentials of obstetrics and gynecology, 3rd ed. Philadelphia: Saunders. 1998:74.

A 22-year-old nulliparous woman presents to the physician's office with a 4- to 5-day history of fever, malaise, and sores on her vulva. She experiences discomfort, especially when she is sitting. She denies a history of prior episodes of vulvar sores or ulcers. She recalls that her last episode of sexual intercourse was 2 weeks ago. On examination, her BP is 120/78, HR 80/min, and temperature is afebrile. Her heart and lung examinations are normal. Inspection of the vulva region reveals multiple, shallow vulvar ulcers 5 to 10 mm in diameter on the labia majora and minora. The inguinal lymph nodes are enlarged bilaterally and nontender.

◆ **What is your next diagnostic step?**

◆ **What is the most likely diagnosis?**

ANSWERS TO CASE 54: Herpes Simplex Virus Infection

Summary: A 22-year-old nulliparous woman, who last had intercourse 2 weeks previously, complains of a 4- to 5-day history of fever, malaise, and painful vulvar sores. She has multiple shallow, vulvar ulcers 5 to 10 mm in diameter on the labia majora and minora, as well as inguinal adenopathy.

◆ **Next diagnostic step:** Viral culture.

◆ **Most likely diagnosis:** Herpes simplex virus (HSV).

Analysis

Objectives

1. Know the classic presentation of primary herpes simplex virus, which includes systemic symptoms.
2. Understand that viral culture is the gold standard in the diagnosis of HSV.
3. Understand the natural history of herpes simplex virus infections, and the tendency for recurrence.

Considerations

This 22-year-old woman complains of significant pain in the vulvar region. Her last episode of intercourse was 2 weeks ago, which is the typical incubation period for herpes simplex virus (7 to 10 days). This patient has systemic symptoms, malaise, and fever, which is consistent with a primary infection. Notably, the viral load is much higher with the primary episode. The description of the lesions are classic for HSV, that is, groups of vesicles that subsequently ulcerate on an erythematous base. The virus remains dormant in the dorsal ganglia of the nerve roots and can cause intermittent outbreaks. Because of its predilection for nerves, patients many times will complain of paresthesias, burning, or tingling prior to the outbreak of the vesicles. Viral culture is the most sensitive method of diagnosis. Upon clinical diagnosis, acyclovir may be helpful in reducing the duration of symptoms.

APPROACH TO SUSPECTED HERPES SIMPLEX VIRUS

Definitions

Genital herpes: An incurable sexually transmitted disease caused by herpes simplex virus.

Primary genital herpes infection: Initial herpes simplex infection, which usually causes systemic symptoms, such as fever, adenopathy, and malaise, as well as local symptoms of vulvar pain, vesicles that ulcerate, and inguinal adenopathy.

Recurrent genital herpes infection: Reactivation of the herpes simplex virus, which lays dormant in the sacral dorsal root ganglia, leading to local symptoms, such as vulvar burning, pain, and vesicles and ulcers.

Clinical Approach

Genital herpes is a **recurrent sexually transmitted disease** that currently has no cure. There are two types, HSV-1 and HSV-2. HSV-1 usually affects the epithelium in the oral or facial region (above the waist); whereas HSV-2 usually affects the genital region, (below the waist). However, up to one-third of the time, the "above-the-waist versus below-the-waist" rule does not hold true. HSV is the most common cause of infectious vulvar ulcers in the United States.

Primary genital infection has both local and systemic effects. It usually affects people between the ages of 15 and 35 years. After an **incubation period of 3 to 7 days,** the herpes infection will usually induce **paresthesias** of vulvar skin, then cause vesicles to form, which become shallow ulcers. Often, the vagina, cervix, and perineal area may be involved. The ulcers of the primary infection may persist for 2 to 6 weeks, and viral shedding will generally continue for 2 to 3 weeks after lesions appear. Local symptoms include pruritus, inguinal adenopathy, vulvar pain, and discharge. About three-quarters of affected patients will have systemic symptoms, which include malaise, myalgias, and fever. Rarely, the virus may cause CNS infection (herpes encephalitis) with a mortality rate of 50%.

After the primary infection, the herpes virus lies dormant in the dorsal root ganglia, typically in the sacral (S2 to S4) region. Triggers for reactivation include sunlight, fever, menses, emotional stress, and local trauma. **Recurrent disease is mostly local and unilateral, and symptoms are much less severe, lasting approximately 1 week.** Often, a prodromal phase, with symptoms of vulvar burning, tenderness, and pruritus, occurs a few hr to 5 days before an outbreak. Viral shedding typically lasts for only 5 days.

The diagnosis of HSV infection is first suspected by clinical clues. The history may include **vulvar burning, tingling, or pain.** The lesions, which are shallow and eroded on an erythematous base, are painful to the touch. The **"gold standard"** diagnostic test is isolation of the **virus by a cell culture.** A specimen should be obtained by swabbing at the base of an open vesicle. Overt lesions that are not ulcerative should be unroofed and the fluid sampled. The cultures generally become positive 2 to 4 days after inoculation. Newer methods include polymerase chain reaction (PCR) and DNA hybridization, which have equivalent accuracy. Cultures for other sexually transmitted diseases should be obtained on examination. Women should be advised to abstain from sexual intercourse from the time of the prodromal symptoms or when lesions appear until they have re-epithelialized.

In the **pregnant woman,** practitioners usually **allow a vaginal delivery** if at the time of labor, there are no lesions (ulcers or vesicles) noted in the cervix, vagina, or vulva, and the patient **denies prodromal symptoms.** Cesarean delivery should be performed if primary or recurrent lesions are present near the time of labor, when the membranes are ruptured, or if there are prodromal symptoms.

The **nucleoside analogues, acyclovir, valacyclovir, and famcyclovir,** inhibit viral DNA replication. The two latter have increased bioavailability, allowing for less frequent dosing to achieve the same therapeutic benefits. Although each is available in oral, topical, and intravenous preparations, the topical preparation generally is not recommended since it is less effective and may lead to inoculation of other sites. Oral agents are most commonly used to decrease the duration of primary infection, or suppression of recurrent episodes. Severe infection requiring hospitalization or affecting immunocompromised women, such as with HIV infection, may require intravenous acyclovir.

Comprehension Questions

[54.1] Each of the following statements about HSV is true except:

    A. HSV is a DNA virus.
    B. Genital herpes infections are usually caused by HSV type 2.
    C. The ulcers of HSV usually do not leave scars upon healing.
    D. The most sensitive test for HSV is the Tzanck smear.

[54.2] Which best describes valacyclovir as compared to acyclovir?

    A. Greater bioavailability
    B. Requires more frequent dosing per day
    C. Achieves a cure versus suppression
    D. Has less side effects

[54.3] A 20-year-old woman is at 38 weeks' gestation and presents with rupture of membranes. She has a history of herpes simplex virus infections. There are no lesions noted of the cervix, vagina, vulva, or perineal areas. She complains of a slight tingling sensation of the vulvar area but no burning. Which of the following is the best management?

    A. Counsel patient and offer cesarean delivery
    B. Expectant management
    C. Oxytocin induction of labor
    D. Intravenous acyclovir and allowing vaginal delivery
    E. Vulvar scraping for Zanck smear

[54.4] As compared to recurrent herpes infections, each of the following statements about the typical primary episode of herpes simplex virus infection is true except:

A. Higher viral load
B. Longer duration of viral shedding
C. Less infectious potential
D. More often systemic symptoms

Answers

[54.1] **D.** Viral culture and PCR testing are the best diagnostic examinations.

[54.2] **A.** Valacyclovir has more bioavailability than acyclovir.

[54.3] **A.** Perineal burning suggests HSV viral shedding, and the patient should be counseled and offered cesarean delivery.

[54.4] **C.** Primary, first-episode HSV has more infectious potential, more systemic symptoms, and lasts longer.

CLINICAL PEARLS

 The most common cause of infectious vulvar ulcer disease in the United States is herpes simplex virus.

 Acyclovir is indicated to suppress frequent recurrences during the year.

 Primary HSV is a systemic disease; recurrent HSV is generally a local process.

 Often, infected women complain of neurologic symptoms, such as tingling, burning, or itching at the skin site, before vesicles break out.

REFERENCES

Droegemuller W. Infections of the lower genital tract. In: Stenchever MA, Droegemueller W, Herbst AL, Mishell DR, eds. Comprehensive gynecology, 4th ed.
St. Louis: Mosby-Year Book. 2001:641–706.

Lebherz TB. Infectious and benign diseases of the vagina, cervix, and vulva. In:
Hacker NF and Moore JG, eds. Essentials of obstetrics and gynecology, 3rd ed.
Philadelphia: Saunders. 1998:393–411.

A 24-year-old G1 P1 woman underwent a low transverse cesarean section 2 days ago for arrest of active phase of labor. She required oxytocin and an internal uterine pressure catheter. Her baby weighed 8 lb 9 oz. The past medical and surgical histories were unremarkable. She denies a cough or dysuria. On examination, the temperature is 102°F, HR 80/min, BP 120/70, and RR 12/min. The breasts are nontender. The lungs are clear to auscultation. There is no costovertebral angle tenderness. The abdomen reveals that the skin incision is without erythema. The uterine fundus is firm, at the level of the umbilicus, and somewhat tender. No lower extremity cords are palpated.

◆ **What is the most likely diagnosis?**

◆ **What is the most likely etiology of the condition?**

◆ **What is the best therapy for the condition?**

ANSWERS TO CASE 55: Postpartum Endomyometritis

Summary: A 24-year-old G1 P1 woman, who underwent a cesarean delivery 2 days previously for arrest of labor, has a fever of 102°F. She denies cough or dysuria. There are no abnormalities of the breasts, lungs, costovertebral region, or skin incision. The uterine fundus is somewhat tender.

◆ **Most likely diagnosis:** Endomyometritis.

◆ **Most likely etiology of the condition:** Ascending infection of vaginal organisms (anaerobic predominance but also gram-negative rods).

◆ **Best therapy for the condition:** Intravenous antibiotics with anaerobic coverage (for example, gentamicin and clindamycin).

Analysis

Objectives

1. Know that the most common cause of fever for a woman who has undergone cesarean delivery is endomyometritis.
2. Know the mechanism of the endomyometritis, that is, ascending infection of "polymicrobial" vaginal organisms.
3. Know the differential diagnosis of fever in the woman who has undergone cesarean delivery include mastitis, wound infection, and pyelonephritis.

Considerations

This 24-year-old woman underwent cesarean delivery for arrest of labor. She presumably had a long labor, an intrauterine pressure catheter, and numerous vaginal examinations. These are all risk factors for the development of **postpartum endomyometritis.** On examination, she has a fever to 102°F. The scenario reveals that there are no abnormalities of the breasts, which rules out mastitis. The lungs are normal to auscultation, which speaks against atelectasis; in the obstetric patient, **atelectasis is an uncommon** cause of postoperative fever since the majority of cesarean deliveries are performed under regional anesthesia. This patient's wound appears normal. There is no costovertebral angle tenderness, so the likelihood of pyelonephritis is low. Urinary tract infections involving only the bladder do not usually cause fever. The uterus is only somewhat tender, which does not overtly point to endomyometritis. However, when the remainder of the examination does not reveal a focus, the majority of women who have fever after cesarean delivery have endomyometritis.

APPROACH TO FEVER AFTER CESAREAN DELIVERY

Definitions

Febrile morbidity: Temperature after cesarean delivery equal to or greater than 38°C (100.4°F) taken on two occasions at least 6 hr apart, exclusive of the first 24 hr.
Endomyometritis: Infection of the decidua, myometrium, and, sometimes, the parametrial tissues.
Septic pelvic thrombophlebitis: Bacterial infection of pelvic venous thrombi, usually involving the ovarian vein.

Clinical Approach

A woman who has **febrile morbidity after cesarean delivery most likely has endomyometritis.** The mechanism of infection is ascension of bacteria, a mixture of organisms from the normal vaginal flora. In other words, postcesarean delivery infection is almost always "polymicrobial," with a mix of both aerobic and anaerobic bacteria. The uterine incision site, being devitalized and containing foreign material (i.e., suture), is commonly the site for infection. Typically, the fever occurs on postoperative day 2. When intra-amniotic infection occurs during labor, the fever usually continues postpartum. The patient may complain of

abdominal tenderness or a foul-smelling lochia. Uterine tenderness is common. Broad-spectrum antimicrobial therapy especially with **anaerobic coverage** is important. **Intravenous gentamicin and clindamycin** is a well-studied regimen and effective in 90% of cases. Other choices include extended penicillins or cephalosporins. The fever usually improves significantly after 48 hr of antimicrobial therapy. **Enterococcal** infection may be one reason for nonresponse; **ampicillin** is the treatment for this organism and often is added if fever persists after 48 hr of therapy.

Another cause of fever after cesarean delivery is **wound infection.** Prophylactic antibiotics given during surgery decrease the incidence. When a patient fails to respond to antibiotic therapy, wound infection is the most likely etiology. The fever usually occurs on postoperative day 4. **Erythema or drainage may be present in the wound site.** The organisms are often the same as those involved with endomyometritis. The treatment includes surgical opening of the wound (and dressing changes) and antimicrobial agents. The fascia must be inspected for integrity.

Septic pelvic thrombophlebitis (SPT) is a rare, bacterial infection affecting thrombosed pelvic veins, usually the ovarian vessels. The bacterial infection at the placental implantation site spreads to the ovarian venous plexuses or to the common iliac veins, sometimes extending to

Table 55–1
APPROACH TO POSTPARTUM FEVER

Evaluate for pulmonary etiology: Cough? Atelectesis?

Evaluate for pyelonephritis: Costovertebral angle tenderness? Dysuria? Pyuria?

Evaluate for breast engorgement: Are breasts engorged, tender, red?

Evaluate for wound infection: Is the wound indurated, erythematous? Is there drainage?

Evaluate for endometritis: Is the uterus tender? Foul-smelling lochia?

If endometritis, begin intravenous gentamicin and clindamycin.

If no response in 48 hr, re-evaluate and if endometritis is still considered, add ampicillin for enterococcus coverage.

If no response after 48 hr of triple antibiotics, re-evaluate (especially look for wound infection). Consider CT imaging to assess for abscess, hematoma, or septic pelvic thrombophlebitis.

---

the inferior vena cava. Women with SPT may have a **hectic fever and look well, or sometimes have a palpable pelvic mass.** The diagnosis may be confirmed by a CT scan or MRI. Treatment includes both antimicrobial and heparin therapy.

Other considerations in a febrile postpartum woman should include pyelonephritis (fever, flank tenderness, leukocytes in the urine), pelvic abscess or infected pelvic hematoma, and breast engorgement (Table 55–1).

Comprehension Questions

[55.1] A 30-year-old G1 P1 who underwent a cesarean section 3 days previously has a fever of 101°F. The wound is indurated and erythematous. Which of the following is the best management?

A. Initiation of intravenous ampicillin
B. Initiation of intravenous heparin
C. Placement of a warm compress on the wound
D. Opening of the wound

[55.2] Each of the following is a risk factor for postpartum endomyometritis except:

A. Numerous vaginal examinations
B. Bacterial vaginosis
C. Internal uterine pressure monitors
D. Prolonged rupture of membranes
E. Precipitous labor

[55.3] Which of the following bacteria is most commonly isolated in endomyometritis complicating patients who have undergone cesarean delivery?

A. *Bacteroides* species
B. *Staphylococcus aureus*
C. Group B streptococcus
D. *E. coli*

[55.4] A 22-year-old woman who underwent cesarean delivery has persistent fever of 102°F, despite the use of triple antibiotic therapy (ampicillin, gentamicin, and clindamycin). The urinalysis, wound, breasts, and uterine fundus are normal on examination. A CT scan of the pelvis is suggestive of septic pelvic thrombophlebitis. Which of the following is the best therapy for this condition?

A. Continued triple antibiotic therapy
B. Discontinue antibiotic therapy and initiate intravenous heparin
C. Continue antibiotic therapy and begin intravenous heparin
D. Surgical embolectomy
E. Streptokinase therapy

Answers

[55.1] **D.** The best treatment for a wound infection is opening of the wound.

[55.2] **E.** Long labor and not precipitous labor is a risk factor for postpartum endometritis.

[55.3] **A.** Anaerobic bacteria are the most commonly isolated, especially *Bacteroides* species.

[55.4] **C.** The best treatment for septic pelvic thrombophlebitis is antibiotics and heparin.

CLINICAL PEARLS

◈ The most common cause of fever after cesarean delivery is endomyometritis.

◈ The major organisms responsible for postcesarean endomyometritis are anaerobic bacteria.

◈ Atelectesis is rare in obstetric patients due to the large number of women who have regional anesthesia.

REFERENCES

Cunningham FG, Gant NF, Leveno KJ, Gilstrap LC III, Hauth JC, Wenstrom KD. Puerperal infection. In: Williams obstetrics, 21st ed. New York: McGraw-Hill. 2001:673–677.

Hayashi RII. Postpartum hemorrhage and puerperal sepsis. In: Hacker NF and Moore JG, eds. Essentials of obstetrics and gynecology, 3rd ed. Philadelphia: Saunders. 1998:339–342.

A 31-year-old woman comes in for a well-woman examination. Her last menstrual period was 2 weeks ago. She has no significant past medical or surgical history. She denies having been treated for sexually transmitted diseases. On examination, her BP is 130/70, IIR 70/min, and temperature is afebrile. Her thyroid is normal on palpation. Her heart and lung examinations are within normal limits. The abdomen is nontender and without masses. Examination of the external genitalia reveals a nontender, firm, ulcerated lesion approximately 1 cm in diameter, with raised borders and an indurated base. Bilateral inguinal lymph nodes are also noted that are nontender. Her pregnancy test is negative.

◆ **What is the most likely diagnosis?**

◆ **What is your next step in diagnosis?**

◆ **What is the best therapy for this condition?**

ANSWERS TO CASE 56: Syphilitic Chancre

Summary: A 31-year-old woman who comes in for a well-woman examination is noted to have a nontender, firm, 1-cm ulcerated lesion of the vulva; it has raised borders and an indurated base. She also has bilateral nontender inguinal lymphadenopathy.

◆ **Most likely diagnosis:** Syphilis (primary chancre).

◆ **Next step in diagnosis:** Syphilis serology (RPR or VDRL) and, if negative, darkfield microscopy.

◆ **Best therapy for this condition:** Intramuscular penicillin.

Analysis

Objectives

1. Know the classic appearance and presentation of the chancre lesion of primary syphilis.
2. Know that penicillin is the treatment of choice for syphilis.
3. Understand that the antibody tests (VDRL or RPR) may not yet turn positive with early syphilitic disease and that darkfield microscopy would then be the diagnostic test of choice.

Considerations

This 31-year-old woman came in for a well-woman examination. It was unexpected to find the lesion in the vulva area. The patient denies any history of sexually transmitted diseases. Nevertheless, she has the classic lesion of primary syphilis, the painless chancre. It is typically a **nontender ulcer with clean appearing edges,** often accompanied by painless inguinal adenopathy. In practice, the next step would be serology to assess for a non-treponemal antibody test, such as the RPR or VDRL test. Occasionally, the patient will have a negative non-treponemal test, in which case the next step is a scraping of the lesion for **darkfield microscopy.** Primary syphilis usually manifests itself within 2 to 6 weeks after inoculation. The treatment for syphilis that is less than 1-yr duration is one set of injections of a long-acting penicillin. If this patient were older, for instance, in her postmenopausal years, squamous cell carcinoma of the vulva would be considered. If the lesion were painful, herpes simplex virus would be the most common diagnosis.

APPROACH TO INFECTIOUS VULVAR ULCERS

Definitions

Non-treponemal tests: Nonspecific antitreponemal antibody test, such as the Venereal Disease Research Laboratory (VDRL) or rapid plasma reagin (RPR) tests. These titers will fall with effective treatment.

Specific serologic tests: Antibody tests that are directed against the treponemal organism such as the MHA-TP (microhemagglutinin antibody against *Treponema pallidum*) and FTA-ABS (fluorescent-labeled treponemal antibody absorption) tests. These tests will remain positive for life after infection.

Clinical Approach (Figure 56–1)

The three most common infectious causes of vulvar ulcers in the United States are herpes simplex virus, syphilis, and chancroid.

Herpes simplex virus is a recurrent sexually transmitted disease, for which there is no cure. This organism is highly contagious, and it is thought that 20% of women in their childbearing years are infected. There are two types of herpes viruses, HSV type I and type II. Type I usually causes infections in the oral region, and type II in the genital region, however, cross-infection may occur. Recurrence is greater with HSV type II. The **primary episode is usually a systemic** as well as local disease, with the woman often complaining of fever or general malaise. Local infection typically induces paresthesias before vesicles

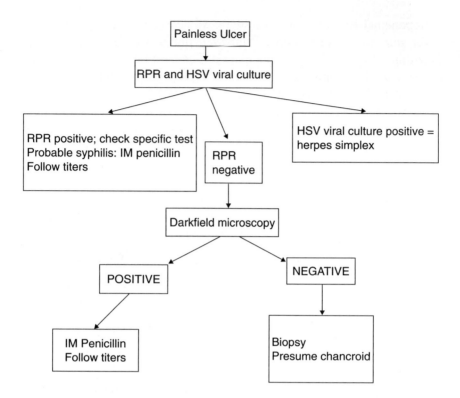

Figure 56–1.   Algorithm for the assessment of vulvar ulcers.

erupt on a red base. After the primary episode, the recurrent disease is local, with less severe symptoms. The recurrent herpes ulcers are small and superficial, and do not usually scar. The **best diagnostic test is viral culture.** Rarely, the infections may be severe enough to warrant hospitalization, such as with encephalopathy or urinary retention. Treatment for immunosuppressed individuals often requires intravenous acyclovir therapy; **oral acyclovir is effective in suppressing frequent recurrences.**

   Syphilis, caused by the bacteria *Treponema pallidum,* may induce a chronic infection. The organism is extremely tightly wound, and too thin to be seen on light microscopy. The typical incubation period is 10 to 90 days. The disease can be divided up into primary, secondary, latent, and tertiary stages. Primary syphilis classically presents as the indurated, nontender chancre. The ulcer usually arises 3 weeks after ex-

posure and disappears spontaneously after 2 to 6 weeks without therapy. Non-treponemal tests (such as the RPR or VDRL) sometimes do
not become positive with the appearance of the chancre; if the serology
is negative in the face of a painless ulcer, then darkfield microscopy is
the best diagnostic step.

Secondary syphilis usually is systemic, occurring about 9 weeks
after the primary chancre. The classic **macular papular rash over the
body including the palms and soles** of the feet, or the flat lesion of
condylomata lata on the vulva may be seen (Figure 56–2). These lesions have a high concentration of spirochetes.

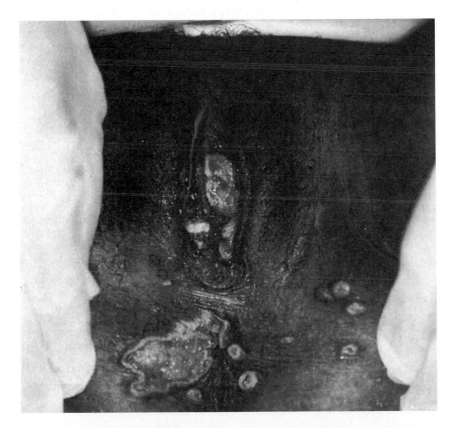

Figure 56–2.   Genital condyloma lata of secondary syphilis.

(Reproduced, with permission, from Cunningham FG et al. Williams obstetrics, 21st ed. New
York: McGraw-Hill; 2001: 1487.)

Latency of varying duration occurs after secondary disease. If untreated, about one-third of women may proceed into tertiary syphilis, which may affect the cardiovascular system or central nervous system. Optic atrophy, tabes dorsalis, and aortic aneurysms are some of the manifestations. Penicillin is the treatment of choice for syphilis. Because of the long replication time, prolonged therapy is required. For example, a long-acting penicillin, benzathine penicillin G, is often used. One injection of 2.4 million units intramuscularly is standard treatment for early disease (primary, secondary, and latent up to 1 year of duration). Patients with late latent syphilis (greater than 1 year) should be treated with a total of 7.2 million units intramuscularly divided as 2.4 million units every week for a total of three courses. For women allergic to penicillin, oral erythromycin or doxycycline may be used (Table 56–1). **In pregnancy, penicillin is the only known effective treatment to prevent congenital syphilis.**

Neurosyphilis requires more intensive therapy, usually **intravenous penicillin.**

After therapy, the non-treponemal test is followed quantitatively every 3 months for at least 1 year. An appropriate response is a fourfold fall in titers in 3 months, and a negative titer in 1 year. When the titer does not fall appropriately, one possible etiology is neurosyphilis, which may be diagnosed by lumbar puncture.

Chancroid is a sexually transmitted disease, usually manifesting a **soft, tender ulcer** of the vulva. It is more common in males than fe-

Table 56–1
TREATMENT FOR SYPHILIS

DURATION	TREATMENT
Primary, secondary, early latent (less than 1 year)	Penicillin 2.4 M units IM
Late latent (> 1 year), or unknown duration	Penicillin 2.4 M units IM every week × 3 doses
Neurosyphilis	IV Penicillin × 4–6 doses

From the CDC 2002 Guidelines for treatment of sexually transmitted diseases.

males. The typical ulcer is **tender, with ragged edges on a necrotic base.** Tender lymphadenopathy may also coexist with these infections. The etiologic organism is ***Haemophilus ducreyi,*** a small gram-negative rod. Gram's stain usually reveals the **classic "school of fish."** After ruling out syphilis and herpes, chancroid should be suspected. Biopsy and/or culture helps to establish the diagnosis. Treatment includes **oral azithromycin or intramuscular ceftriaxone.**

Comprehension Questions

[56.1] A 19-year-old woman is noted to have a RPR titer of 1:16, and the confirmatory (MHA-TP) test is positive. She had no history of syphilis. She is treated with benzathine penicillin 2.4 million units intramuscularly. Three months after therapy, she is noted to have an RPR titer of 1:2. The next month (4 months after treatment), the titer is 1:1. Two months later, 6 months after treatment, the repeat RPR is noted be 1:32. Which of the following is the most likely diagnosis?

A. Resistant organism
B. Inadequately treated syphilis
C. Laboratory error
D. Reinfection
E. Systemic lupus erythematosus

[56.2] Each of the following statement about *Treponema pallidum* is correct except:

A. It is a spirochete.
B. Gram's stain is not a very sensitive method of diagnosis.
C. It causes neonatal disease mainly by direct inoculation of the baby by the genital lesion.
D. Alternative treatments include doxycycline and erythromycin.

[56.3] An 18-year-old G1 P0 at 14 weeks' gestation is noted to have a positive RPR with a positive confirmatory MHA-TP test. The patient states that she is allergic to penicillin, with hives and swelling of the tongue and throat in the past. Which of the following is the most appropriate next step?

A. Desensitize and treat with penicillin
B. Oral erythromycin
C. Oral doxycycline
D. Pretreat with prednisone, then administer penicillin
E. Intramuscular ceftriaxone

[56.4] A 29-year-old woman is noted to have a persistently elevated RPR titer of 1:32, despite treatment with benzathine penicillin 2.4 million units each week for a total of 3 weeks. She complains of slight dizziness and a clumsy gait of 6 months duration. Which of the following is the best test to diagnose neurosyphilis?

A. Plain x-ray films of the skull
B. Electroencephalograph (EEG)
C. CT scan of the head
D. Lumbar puncture
E. Psychiatric evaluation

Answers

[56.1] **D.** When the RPR titers respond abruptly to therapy and then suddenly rise, the most likely scenario is reinfection.

[56.2] **C.** Transplacental infection is the most common method of vertical transmission.

[56.3] **A.** Penicillin is the best treatment for syphilis in pregnancy. When a pregnant woman with syphilis is allergic to penicillin, she should undergo desensitization and receive penicillin.

[56.4] **D.** Cerebrospinal fluid for RPR may point toward neurosyphilis although there is no definitive test.

CLINICAL PEARLS

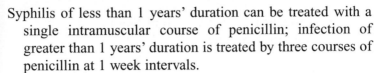 Syphilis of less than 1 years' duration can be treated with a single intramuscular course of penicillin; infection of greater than 1 years' duration is treated by three courses of penicillin at 1 week intervals.

The nontender ulcer with indurated edges is typical for the chancre lesion of primary syphilis. If serology is negative, then darkfield examination warranted.

The best treatment for syphilis in pregnancy is penicillin.

Pregnant women with syphilis and an allergy to penicillin should undergo penicillin desensitization and then receive penicillin.

The three most common infectious vulvar ulcers in the United States are herpes simplex virus, syphilis, and chancroid.

REFERENCES

Droegemuller W. Infections of the lower genital tract. In: Stenchever MA, Droege-mueller W, Herbst AL, Mishell DR, eds. Comprehensive gynecology, 4th ed. St. Louis: Mosby Year Book. 2001;641–706.

Lebherz TB. Infectious and benign diseases of the vagina, cervix, and vulva. In: Hacker NF and Moore JG, eds. Essentials of obstetrics and gynecology, 3rd ed. Philadelphia: Saunders. 1998:393–411.

Centers for Disease Control and Prevention. 2002 Guidelines for treatment of sexually transmitted diseases. 2002;51(RR06):13–32.

A 24-year-old woman G2 P1 at 30 weeks' gestation was admitted 2 days ago for premature rupture of membranes. Her antenatal history has been unremarkable. She states that her baby is moving normally and she denies any fever or chills. Her past medical and surgical histories are unremarkable. On examination, her temperature is 100.8°F, BP 100/60, and HR 90/min. Her lungs are clear to auscultation. No costovertebral angle tenderness is found. The uterine fundus is 30 cm and is slightly tender. No lower extremity cords are palpated. The fetal heart tones are persistently in the 170 to 175 bpm range without decelerations.

◆ **What is the most likely diagnosis?**

◆ **What is the best management for this patient?**

◆ **What is the most likely etiology of this condition?**

ANSWERS TO CASE 57: Intra-amniotic Infection

Summary: A 24-year-old G2 P1 woman at 30 weeks' gestation was admitted 2 days ago for premature rupture of membranes. Her temperature is 100.8°F. The uterine fundus is slightly tender. There is persistent fetal tachycardia in the 170 to 175 bpm range.

◆ **Most likely diagnosis:** Intra-amniotic infection (chorioamnionitis).

◆ **Best management for this patient:** Intravenous antibiotics (ampicillin and gentamicin) and induction of labor.

◆ **Etiology of this condition:** Ascending infection from vaginal organisms.

Analysis

Objectives

1. Know that infection and labor are the two most common acute complications of preterm premature rupture of membranes.
2. Know the clinical presentation of intra-amniotic infection, and that fetal tachycardia is an early sign of this infection.
3. Understand that broad-spectrum antibiotic therapy and delivery are the appropriate treatment of intra-amniotic infection.

Considerations

This 24-year-old woman at 30 weeks' gestation has preterm premature rupture of membranes. Upon presentation to the hospital, the practitioner should assess for infection; in the absence of signs of infection, corticosteroid therapy should be administered to reduce the risk of respiratory distress syndrome (RDS). Additionally, broad-spectrum antibiotic therapy is given to help reduce the incidence of intra-amniotic infection. Because the risk of prematurity outweighed the risk of infection, expectant management was chosen for this patient. After 2 days in the hospital, the patient developed a fever, mild uterine tenderness, and fetal tachycardia. These symptoms are consistent with intra-amniotic infection. Upon recognition of this diagnosis, the patient should be given intravenous antibiotic therapy, such as ampicillin and gentamicin. Neonates are most commonly affected by group B streptococci and gram-negative enteric organisms such as *E. coli*. **Delivery is also an important aspect of therapy for both neonatal and maternal well-being.** A vaginal delivery is acceptable, so that induction of labor was chosen in this case.

APPROACH TO PRETERM PROM

Preterm premature rupture of membranes (PPROM) is defined as rupture of membranes prior to the onset of labor and at less than 37 weeks' of pregnancy. This complication occurs in about 1% of all pregnancies. **Approximately one-third of preterm births are associated with PPROM.** Risk factors are noted in Table 57–1.

The history consistent with PPROM is that of a **loss or "gush" of fluid per vagina,** which is very accurate and should be taken seriously. The diagnosis is confirmed with a speculum examination showing the **pooling of amniotic fluid in the posterior vaginal vault, alkaline changes of the vaginal fluid, and a ferning pattern** of the fluid when seen on microscopy. Occasionally, the speculum examination may be

Table 57–1
RISK FACTORS FOR PPROM

Lower socioeconomic status
Sexually transmitted diseases
Cigarette smoking
Cervical conization
Emergency cerclage
Multiple gestation
Hydramnios
Placental abruption

negative, but clinical suspicion is high; in these cases, an ultrasound examination revealing **oligohydramnios** is consistent with PPROM.

The outcome is dependent on the gestational age. Approximately half of patients with PPROM will go into labor within 48 hr, and 90% within 1 week. Complications of preterm delivery, such as **respiratory distress syndrome,** are common. Other complications include chorioamnionitis, placental abruption, and necrotizing enterocolitis.

Chorioamnionitis affects about 1% of all pregnancies, and 7 to 10% of those with PPROM with prolonged rupture of membranes. **Maternal fever, maternal tachycardia, uterine tenderness, and malodorous vaginal discharge** are some clinical indicators. An **early sign is fetal tachycardia,** a baseline heart rate of greater than 160 bpm.

The treatment of PPROM is controversial. **Prior to 32 weeks' gestation, antenatal steroids** may be given to enhance fetal lung maturity in the absence of overt infection. Broad-spectrum antibiotic therapy has been shown to delay delivery and decrease the incidence of chorioamnionitis. Expectant management is undertaken when the risk of infection is thought to be less than the risk of prematurity. After a gestational age of 34 to 35 weeks, the treatment is usually delivery. Some of the risks of expectant management include stillbirth, cord accident, infection, and abruption. When infection is apparent, broad-spectrum antibiotics, such as intravenous **ampicillin and gentamicin,** should be initiated and labor should be induced. Also, the infant should be delivered when there is evidence of fetal lung maturity, such as by the presence of phosphatidyl glycerol (PG) on the vaginal pool amniotic fluid.

Comprehension Questions

[57.1] A 33-year-old G1 P0 at 30 weeks' gestation is admitted for preterm premature rupture of membranes. Each of the following statements is correct except:

   A. Intramuscular corticosteroid therapy should be given to enhance fetal lung maturity if there is no evidence of infection.

   B. Broad-spectrum antibiotic therapy is indicated only with maternal fever.

   C. Labor is the most common acute complication to be expected.

D. Bacterial vaginosis is a risk factor for preterm premature rupture of membranes.

[57.2] A 30-year-old G2 P1 woman at 28 weeks' gestation with preterm premature rupture of membranes is suspected of having intra-amniotic infection based on fetal tachycardia. The maternal temperature is normal. Which of the following is the most accurate method to confirm the intra-amniotic infection?

A. Serum maternal leukocyte count
B. Speculum examination of the vaginal discharge
C. Amniotic fluid Gram's stain by amniocentesis
D. Palpation of the maternal uterus
E. Height of oral temperature

[57.3] An 18-year-old Hispanic G1 P0 woman has a clinical presentation of intra-amniotic infection. She denies any leakage of fluid per vagina, and repeated speculum examinations fail to identify rupture of membranes. Which of the following organisms is most likely to be the underlying etiology?

A. Group B streptococci
B. *Listeria monocytogenes*
C. *Clostridia difficile*
D. *Chlamydia trachomatis*
E. *E. coli*

[57.4] A 36-year-old woman at 16 weeks' gestation undergoes a genetic amniocentesis for being of advanced maternal age. Shortly after the procedure, she feels leakage of fluid per vagina. Rupture of membranes is confirmed. Each of the following statements is true regarding her condition except:

A. The chances of the membranes resealing is much higher after amniocentesis versus with spontaneous rupture of membranes.
B. If there is continued severe oligohydramnios, the baby has is a high likelihood of developing pulmonary hypoplasia.
C. Severe oligohydramnios that is prolonged can lead to fetal renal abnormalities.
D. The risk of rupture of membranes with genetic amniocentesis is about 0.3 to 0.5%.

Answers

[57.1] **B.** Antibiotics should be given to prolong the pregnancy and decrease the risk of infection.

[57.2] **C.** An amniocentesis revealing organisms on Gram's stain is diagnostic of infection.

[57.3] **B.** *Listeria* may induce a chorioamnionitis without rupture of membranes; the mechanism is transplacental spread. A history of ingesting unpastuerized milk products (such as some varieties of goat cheese) should raise clinical suspicion of *Listeria* as a possibility.

[57.4] **C.** It is fetal renal anomalies that lead to oligohydramnios, and not vice versa. Severe oligohydramnios at an early gestational age can cause pulmonary hypoplasia.

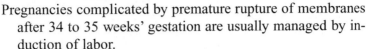

CLINICAL PEARLS

 Pregnancies complicated by premature rupture of membranes after 34 to 35 weeks' gestation are usually managed by induction of labor.

 Pregnancies with PPROM less than 32 weeks' gestation are usually managed expectantly.

 The earliest sign of chorioamnionitis (intra-amniotic infection) is usually fetal tachycardia.

 Pregnancies complicated by PPROM and chorioamnionitis should be treated with broad-spectrum antibiotics (like ampicillin and gentamicin) and delivery.

REFERENCES

Cunningham FG, Gant NF, Leveno KJ, Gilstrap LC III, Hauth JC, Wenstrom KD. Preterm birth. In: Williams obstetrics, 21st ed. New York: McGraw-Hill. 2001:704–708.

Hobel CJ. Preterm labor and premature rupture of membranes. In: Hacker NF and Moore JG, eds. Essentials of obstetrics and gynecology, 3rd ed. Philadelphia: Saunders. 1998:319–323.

American College of Obstetricians and Gynecologists. Premature rupture of membranes. Practice Bulletin 1, June 1998.

An 18-year-old nulliparous woman complains of a vaginal discharge with a fishy odor over the past 2 weeks. She states that the odor is especially prominent after intercourse. Her last menstrual period was 3 weeks ago. She denies being treated for vaginitis or sexually transmitted diseases. She is in good health. She takes no medications other than an oral contraceptive agent. On examination, her BP is 110/70, HR 80/min, and temperature is afebrile. The thyroid is normal to palpation. The heart and lung examinations are normal. Her breasts are Tanner stage V as is the pubic and axillary hair. The external genitalia are normal; the speculum examination reveals a homogeneous, white vaginal discharge and a fishy odor. No erythema or lesions of the vagina are noted.

◆ **What is the most likely diagnosis?**

◆ **What is the best treatment for this condition?**

ANSWERS TO CASE 58: Bacterial Vaginosis

Summary: An 18-year-old nulliparous woman complains of a fishy vaginal discharge, which is worse after intercourse. The speculum examination reveals a homogeneous, white vaginal discharge and a fishy odor. No erythema or lesions of the vagina are noted.

◆ **Most likely diagnosis:** Bacterial vaginosis.

◆ **Best treatment for this condition:** Metronidazole orally or vaginally; clindamycin is an alternative.

Analysis

Objectives

1. Know the three common infectious causes of vaginitis or vaginosis.
2. Know the diagnostic criteria for bacterial vaginosis (BV).
3. Know the treatments for the corresponding causes of vaginitis and vaginosis.

Considerations

This 18-year-old woman complains of a **vaginal discharge that has a fishy odor, which is the most common symptom of bacterial vaginosis.** The discharge associated with BV has a typical white, **homogenous** vaginal coating, described like "spilled milk over the tissue." The pH is not given in this scenario. Also, although a whiff test is not performed with KOH, the **worsening** of the discharge **after intercourse** is presumably due to the alkaline semen. The vaginal epithelium is not erythematous or inflamed, which also fits with bacterial vaginosis. Of the three most common causes of infectious vaginal discharge (*Candida, Trichomonas,* and BV), bacterial vaginosis is the one etiology that is not inflammatory; there is a predominance of anaerobic bacteria rather than a true infection. Hence, antibiotic therapy aimed at anaerobes, such as metronidazole or clindamycin is appropriate.

APPROACH TO VAGINAL INFECTIONS

The three most common types of vaginal infections are bacterial vaginosis, trichomonal vaginitis, and candidal vulvovaginitis (Table 58–1).

Bacterial vaginosis is not a true infection, but rather an overgrowth of anaerobic bacteria, which replaces the normal lactobacilli of the vagina. Although it may be sexually transmitted, this is not always the case. The most common symptom is a **fishy odor,** often exacerbated by menses or intercourse, since both of these situations introduce an alkaline substance. The vaginal pH is elevated above normal. The addition of potassium hydroxide (KOH) leads to the release of amines, causing a fishy odor (whiff test). There is no inflammatory reaction; hence, the patient will not complain of swelling or irritation, and typically, the microscopic examination does not usually reveal leukocytes. Microscopy of the discharge in normal saline (wet mount) typically shows **clue cells** (Figure 58–1), which are bacteria adherent to the ex-

Table 58–1
CHARACTERISTICS OF VARIOUS VAGINAL INFECTIONS

	BACTERIAL VAGINOSIS	TRICHOMONAL VAGINITIS	CANDIDAL VULVOVAGINITIS
Appearance	Homogenous, white discharge	Frothy, yellow to green	Curdy, lumpy
Vaginal pH	> 4.5	> 4.5	< 4.5
Whiff test (fishy odor with KOH)	++++	++	None
Microscopy	Clue cells	Trichomonads	Pseudohyphae
Treatment	Metronidazole	Metronidazole	Oral diflucan or imidazole cream

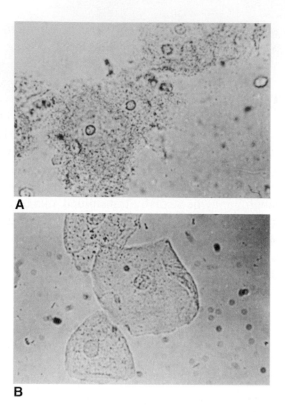

Figure 58–1.   Vaginal epithelial "clue cells." Clue cells (A) with the granular appearance are contrasted to normal cells (B).

(Reproduced, with permission, from Braunwald E, et al, eds. Harrison's principles of internal medicine, 15th ed. New York: McGraw-Hill. 2001: 844.)

ternal surfaces of epithelial cells. Bacterial vaginosis is associated with genital tract infection, such as endometritis, pelvic inflammatory disease, and pregnancy complications, such as preterm delivery and preterm premature rupture of membranes. Treatment includes oral or vaginal metronidazole.

Trichomonas vaginalis is a single-cell anaerobic flagellated protozoa that induces an intense **inflammatory** reaction. It is a common sexually transmitted disease. *T. vaginalis* can survive for up to 6 hours on a wet surface. Aside from causing infection of the vagina, this organism can also inhabit the urethra or Skene's glands. The most common symptom associated with trichomoniasis is a profuse vaginal discharge or vaginal irritation. Intense inflammation of the vagina or cervix may be noted, with the classic punctate lesions of the cervix **(strawberry cervix)**. A fishy odor is common with this disorder, which is somewhat exacerbated with KOH. Microscopy in saline will often display **mobile, flagellated organisms.** If the wet mount is cold or there are excess leukocytes present, the movement of the trichomonads may be inhibited. Optimal treatment consists of a fairly high dose of **metronidazole** (2 g orally) as a one-time dose, with the partner treated as well. Resistant cases may require the same dose every day for 7 days.

Candidal vaginitis is usually caused by the fungus, *Candida albicans,* although other species may be causative. The lactobacilli in the vagina inhibit fungal growth; thus, **antibiotic therapy** may decrease the lactobacilli concentration, leading to *Candida* overgrowth. Diabetes mellitus, which suppresses immune function, may also predispose patients to these infections. Candidiasis is usually not a sexually transmitted disease. The patient usually presents with **intense vulvar or vaginal burning, irritation, and swelling.** Dyspareunia may also be a prominent complaint. The discharge usually appears **curdy or like cottage cheese,** in contrast to the homogenous discharge of bacterial vaginosis. The pH of the vagina is typically normal (less than 4.5). The microscopic diagnosis is confirmed by identification of the hyphae or pseudohyphae after the discharge is mixed with potassium hydroxide. The KOH solution lyses the leukocytes and erythrocytes, making identification of the candidal organisms easier. Treatment includes oral diflucan or topical imidazoles, such as terconazole (Terazol), or miconazole (Monistat).

Comprehension Questions

[58.1] Each of the following is consistent with bacterial vaginosis except:

    A. pH less than 4.5
    B. Homogenous vaginal discharge
    C. Predominance of anaerobes
    D. Positive whiff test

[58.2] A 26-year-old woman taking antibiotics for cystitis complains of itching, burning, and a yellowish vaginal discharge. Which of the following is the best therapy?

    A. Metronidazole
    B. Erythromycin
    C. Fluconazole
    D. Hydrocortisone
    E. Clindamycin

[58.3] Which of the following organisms may be isolated from a wet surface 6 hours after inoculation?

    A. *Candida albicans*
    B. *Trichomonas vaginalis*
    C. *Gardenerella* species
    D. *Peptostreptococci*

[58.4] A 27-year-old woman complains of a fishy odor and a vaginal discharge. The speculum examination reveals an erythematous vagina and punctations of the cervix. Which is the most likely diagnosis?

    A. Candidal vaginitis
    B. Trichomonal vaginitis
    C. Bacterial vaginosis
    D. Human papilloma virus
    E. Herpes simplex virus

Answers

[58.1] **A.** The vaginal pH in BV is usually > 4.5.

[58.2] **C.** After antibiotic therapy, candidal organisms often proliferate and may induce an overt infection.

[58.3] **B.** *Trichomonas vaginalis* is a hardy organism and may be isolated from a wet surface up to 6 hr after inoculation.

[58.4] **B.** The strawberry cervix is a classic finding of the inflammatory punctations induced by trichomoniasis.

CLINICAL PEARLS

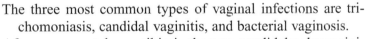 The three most common types of vaginal infections are trichomoniasis, candidal vaginitis, and bacterial vaginosis.

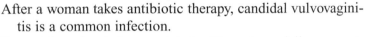 After a woman takes antibiotic therapy, candidal vulvovaginitis is a common infection.

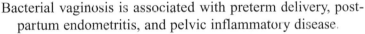 Bacterial vaginosis is associated with preterm delivery, postpartum endometritis, and pelvic inflammatory disease.

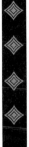 Trichomonal vaginitis is associated with an intense inflammatory process and may induce punctations of the cervix known as "strawberry cervix."

REFERENCES

Droegemuller W. Infections of the lower genital tract. In: Stenchever MA, Droegemueller W, Herbst AL, Mishell DR, eds. Comprehensive gynecology, 4th ed. St. Louis: Mosby-Year Book. 2001:641–706.

Lebherz TB. Infectious and benign diseases of vagina, cervix, and vulva. In: Hacker NF and Moore JG, eds. Essentials of obstetrics and gynecology, 3rd ed. Philadelphia: Saunders. 1998:393–399.

A 42-year-old parous woman has noticed increasing hair growth on her face and abdomen over the past 8 months. She denies the use of steroid medications, weight changes, or a family history of hirsutism. Her menses previously had been monthly, and now occur every 35 to 70 days. Her past medical and surgical histories are unremarkable. On examination, her thyroid is normal to palpation. She has excess facial hair and male pattern hair on her abdomen. Acne is also noted on the face. The cardiac and pulmonary examinations are normal. The abdominal examination reveals no masses or tenderness. Examination of the external genitalia reveals possible clitoromegaly. Pelvic examination shows a normal uterus and cervix and an 8-cm, right adnexal mass.

◆ **What is the most likely diagnosis?**

◆ **What is the probable management?**

ANSWERS TO CASE 59: Hirsutism, Sertoli–Leydig Cell Tumor

Summary: A 42-year-old woman with an 8-month history of increasing hirsutism and irregular menses. She denies the use of steroid medications, weight changes, or a family history of hirsutism. Pelvic examination shows an 8-cm, right adnexal mass.

◆ **Most likely diagnosis:** An ovarian tumor, probable Sertoli–Leydig cell tumor.

◆ **Probable management:** Ovarian cancer (surgical) staging.

Analysis

Objectives

1. Understand the differential diagnosis of hirsutism.
2. Know the work-up and approach to a woman with virilism and hirsutism.
3. Know the typical history and physical examination for the various causes of hirsutism.

Considerations

This 42-year-old woman has the onset of excess male-pattern hair over the past 6 months, as well as features of virilism (clitoromegaly). This is evidence of excess androgens. The **rapid onset speaks of a tumor.** Adrenal or ovarian tumors are possibilities. This woman has a large adnexal mass, and so the diagnosis is straightforward. She has irregular menses because of the androgen effect of inhibiting ovulation. The patient does not have the stigmata of Cushing's disease, such as hypertension, buffalo hump, abdominal striae, and central obesity. Likewise, she does not take any medications containing anabolic steroids. **Polycystic ovarian syndrome (PCOS) is probably the most common cause of hyperandrogenism,** but it does not fit this patient's clinical presentation. PCOS usually presents with a gradual onset of hirsutism and irregular menses **since menarche.** A Sertoli–Leydig cell tumor of the ovary is a solid stromal type of tumor, the androgen counterpart of granulosa-theca cell tumor. These tumors are usually of low malignant potential and slow growing, but nevertheless may metastasize and often recur. Hence, surgical staging is the treatment of choice.

APPROACH TO HIRSUTISM

Hirsutism should be viewed as both an endocrine and cosmetic problem. It is most commonly associated with **anovulation;** however, other causes of increased androgen levels need to be ruled out, such as **adrenal and ovarian diseases.** The most sensitive marker of excess androgen production is hirsutism, followed by acne, oily skin, increased libido, and virilization. Virilization consists of clitoromegaly, deepening of the voice, balding, increased muscle mass, and male body habitus. Adrenal hyperplasia or androgen-secreting tumors of the adrenal gland or ovary are causes of virilization. The treatment depends on the underlying etiology.

The pattern of hair growth is genetically predetermined. Differences in hair growth between ethnic groups are secondary to variations in hair follicle concentration and 5-alpha-reductase activity. Hair growth can be divided into three phases: anagen (growing phase), catagen (involution phase), and telogen (quiescent phase). Hair length is determined by the length of the anagen phase, and the stability of hair is determined by the length of the telogen phase. Hair found on the face, axilla, chest, breast, pubic area, and anterior thighs are termed "sex hair" because they respond to sex hormones. Androgens (especially testosterone) initiate growth of and increase the diameter and pigmentation of "sex hair." Androgens may be produced by the ovary, adrenal gland, or by peripheral conversion. Dehydroepiandrosterone sulfate **(DHEA-S)** is derived almost exclusively from the **adrenal gland.** Dihydrotestosterone (DHT) is metabolized from testosterone by 5-alpha-reductase; an increased activity of 5-alpha-reductase leads to an increase in DHT and stimulation of hair growth. The majority of testosterone is bound to sex hormone-binding globulin (SHBG) and it is the unbound portion that is primarily responsible for androgenicity. Hyperandrogenism decreases SHBG, and thus, exacerbates hirsutism.

The appearance and cosmetic changes associated with hirsutism depend on the number of follicles present, ratio of growth to resting phases, asynchrony of growth cycles, and thickness and degree of pigmentation of individual hairs. The history should focus on the **onset and duration of symptoms** (faster growth is associated with tumors of adrenal and ovary, whereas slow onset since menarche is more likely polycystic ovarian syndrome). The severity of symptoms should be characterized (for example, virilization is rare and is usually associated with androgen-secreting tumors). The regularity of the menses and symptoms of thyroid disease should also be sought. The physical examination should focus on the location of hair growth and its severity, thyromegaly, body shape and habitus, the presence of breast discharge, skin changes (acanthosis or abdominal striae), adnexal or abdominal masses, and the external genitalia. Helpful laboratory tests include assays for serum **testosterone, dihydroepiandrostenedione sulfate (DHEA-S), 17-hydroxyprogesterone (which is elevated with congenital adrenal hyperplasia), prolactin, and TSH.** A markedly elevated **testosterone** level suggests an androgen-secreting ovarian tumor, such as a **Sertoli–Leydig cell tumor.** With a high **DHEA-S level,** the examiner should be suspicious of an **adrenal process,** such as adrenal hyperplasia or a tumor.

The differential diagnosis for hirsutism (Table 59–1) includes anovulation, late onset adrenal hyperplasia, androgen-secreting tumors (adrenal or ovarian in origin), Cushing's disease, medications, thyroid disease, and hyperprolactinemia. Treatment depends on the etiology; however, in general, the goal is to decrease the amount of DHT available. This can be accomplished by inhibiting adrenal or ovarian androgen secretion, changing SHBG binding, impairing peripheral conversion of androgen to active androgen, and inhibiting activity at target tissues. Treatment options include weight loss, combined oral contraception pills, spironolactone (a diuretic that is an androgen antagonist), progesterone-containing medications, electrolysis, waxing, and shaving. The patient must warned that there is a slow response to treatment with medications (an average of 6 months). To help with more immediate results, nonmedical therapies (waxing and shaving) may be used initially until the new medication begins to work effectively.

Table 59–1
DIFFERENTIAL DIAGNOSIS OF HIRSUTISM

DISEASE	HISTORY	PHYSICAL EXAMINATION	LABORATORY TEST	TREATMENT
Cushing's syndrome	Glucose intolerance	Hypertension, buffalo hump, central obesity	Dexamethasone suppression test	Surgical
Adrenal tumor	Rapid onset virilism	Abdominal mass	DHEA-S	Surgical
Congenital adrenal hyperplasia	Ambiguous genitalia; family history	Hypotension	Elevated 17-hydroxy-progesterone	Replace cortisol and mineral-corticoid
Polycystic ovarian syndrome	Onset since menarche	Hirsutism; rarely virilization	Elevated LH versus FSH ratio	Oral contraceptive pills
Sertoli–Leydig cell tumor	Rapid onset	Hirsutism, virilism, adnexal mass	Elevated testosterone level	Surgical

Comprehension Questions

[59.1] A 6-year-old girl is noted to have breast development and vaginal spotting. No abnormal hair growth is noted. A 10-cm ovarian mass is palpated on rectal examination. Which of the following is the most likely diagnosis?

A. Benign cystic tumor (dermoid)
B. Idiopathic precocious puberty
C. Sertoli–Leydig cell tumor
D. Congenital adrenal hyperplasia
E. Granulosa-theca cell tumor

[59.2] A 15-year-old G0 P0 complains of increasing hair over her face and chest. She also has a deepening voice and clitoromegaly.

There have been two neonatal deaths in the family. Which of the following is the best diagnostic test for the likely diagnosis?

A. Testosterone level
B. Dexamethasone suppression test
C. 17-hydroxyprogesterone level
D. LH and FSH levels
E. Karyotype

[59.3] A 22-year-old nulliparous woman with irregular menses of 7 years' duration complains of primary infertility. She has a family history of diabetes. She has mild hirsutism on examination. Which of the following is the most likely therapy?

A. Cortisol and mineralcorticoid replacement
B. Excision of an adrenal tumor
C. Surgical excision of an ovarian tumor
D. Oral clomiphene citrate
E. Intrauterine insemination

[59.4] A 24-year-old woman complains of bothersome hirsutism and skipping periods. She does not have evidence of voice changes, hair loss, or clitoromegaly. The pelvic examination does not reveal adnexal masses. The serum DHEA-S, testosterone, and 17-hydroxyprogesterone levels are normal. The LH to FSH ratio is 2:1. Which of the following is the most likely diagnosis?

A. Polycystic ovarian syndrome
B. Familial hirsutism
C. Ovarian tumor
D. Adrenal tumor
E. Cushing's syndrome

Answers

[59.1] **E.** Isosexual (no virilization) precocious puberty with an adnexal mass is usually a granulosa cell tumor of the ovary.

[59.2] **C.** The most common neonatal endocrine cause of death (salt wasting) is congenital adrenal hyperplasia (21-hydroxylase deficiency).

[59.3] **D.** Probable PCO syndrome; the initial treatment for infertility is clomiphene citrate.

[59.4] **A.** Polycystic ovarian syndrome is the most common cause of hirsutism and irregular menses. Treatment may be spironolactone (androgen antagonist) and oral contraceptives. Familial hirsutism usually is not associated with oligomenorrhea or an abnormal LH to FSH ratio.

CLINICAL PEARLS

The rapid onset of hirsutism or virilization usually indicates the presence of an androgen-secreting tumor.

The most common cause of hirsutism and irregular menses is polycystic ovarian syndrome.

The most common cause of ambiguous genitalia in the newborn is congenital adrenal hyperplasia.

Hyperandrogenism in the face of an adnexal mass usually indicates a Sertoli–Leydig cell tumor of the ovary, and is treated surgically.

REFERENCES

Chang JR. Virilism and hirsutism. In: Hacker NF and Moore JG, eds. Essentials of obstetrics and gynecology, 3rd ed. Philadelphia: Saunders. 1998:594–601.

Herbst AL. Neoplastic diseases of the ovary. In: Stenchever MA, Droegemueller W, Herbst AL, Mishell DR, eds. Comprehensive gynecology, 4th ed. St. Louis: Mosby-Year Book. 2001:955–998.

A 20-year-old G1 P0 woman at 16 weeks' gestation by last menstrual period has received a serum maternal alpha-fetoprotein test that returned as 2.8 multiples of the median. She is fairly sure of her last menstrual period and has regular menses. She denies a family history of congenital anomalies or chromosomal abnormalities. On examination, her BP is 100/70, HR 70/min, and temp afebrile. The heart and lung examinations are normal. The fundal height is midway between the symphysis pubis and the umbilicus. Fetal heart tones are in the range of 140 bpm.

❖ **What is your next diagnostic step?**

ANSWERS TO CASE 60: Serum Screening in Pregnancy

Summary: A 20-year-old G1 P0 woman at 16 weeks' gestation by a fairly certain last menstrual period has received a serum maternal alpha-fetoprotein test that returned as 2.8 multiples of the median.

◆ **Next diagnostic step:** Basic obstetric ultrasound examination to assess for dates and multiple gestation.

Analysis

Objectives

1. Understand that the most common causes of abnormal serum screening are wrong dates and multiple gestation.
2. Know that an elevated maternal serum alpha-fetoprotein (msAFP) level may be associated with an open neural tube defect.
3. Know that a low msAFP level may be associated with fetal Down syndrome.

Considerations

This patient is at 16 weeks by a fairly certain last menstrual period, which is consistent with the clinical examination. The gestational age window of 16 to 20 weeks is the appropriate time to screen with serum testing. The msAFP returned as 2.8 multiples of the median (MOM), which exceeds the usual cut-off of 2.0 or 2.5 MOM. The interpretation of the msAFP depends on gestational age and number of fetuses. The components of a certain last menstrual period are: 1) patient sure of date of last menstrual period (LMP), 2) regular menses, 3) LMP was normal, 4) patient has had no spotting or bleeding after LMP. The uterine size correlates with the dates. At 16 weeks' gestation, the fundus is between the symphysis pubis and the umbilicus. At 20 weeks' gestation, the fundal height is generally at the level of the umbilicus. Although this patient has a sure LMP and size and date consistency, there is still a significant risk of a dating abnormality or a multifetal gestation. Hence, the next appropriate step is the basic ultrasound examination. If there is a dating error, the msAFP result would be recalculated based on the corrected gestational age. If the msAFP is still abnormally elevated, then at an early gestational age such as 16 weeks, repeating the serum test is an option. For women with abnormally elevated msAFP at a later gestational age, such as 20 weeks, genetic counseling and referral for amniocentesis may be considered.

APPROACH TO ABNORMAL SERUM SCREENING IN PREGNANCY

Definitions

Alpha-fetoprotein: A glycoprotein made by the fetal liver, analogous to the adult albumin.

Neural tube defect: Failure of closure of the embryonic neural folds leading to an absent cranium and cerebral hemispheres (anencephaly) or nonclosure of the vertebral arches (spina bifida).

Open neural tube defect: A neural tube defect that is not covered by skin.

Maternal serum alpha-fetoprotein: Alpha-fetoprotein level drawn from maternal blood; this may be elevated due to increased amniotic fluid alpha-fetoprotein.

Trisomy screen: Two or three serum markers that may indicate an increased risk of chromosomal abnormalities. A common combination includes maternal serum alpha-fetoprotein, human chorionic gonadotropin, and unconjugated estriol.

Clinical Approach

The triple (or trisomy) screen is used in pregnant women between 15 and 21 weeks' gestation to identify those pregnancies that may be complicated by **neural tube defects, Down syndrome, or trisomy 18.** It is a multiple marker test, and the term "triple" is often used to denote that it analyzes three chemicals in the maternal serum to determine the risk for neural tube defects or fetal aneuploidy: alpha-fetoprotein (AFP), human chorionic gonadotropin (hCG), and unconjugated estriol. The trisomy screen is typically not performed on women at high risk for aneuploidy, such as those women over the age of 35 years, referred to as advanced maternal age. They are usually offered genetic amniocentesis.

Alpha-fetoprotein is a glycoprotein synthesized initially by the fetal yolk sac and then later by the fetal gastrointestinal tract and liver. It passes into the maternal circulation by diffusion through the chorioamniotic membranes. When there is an opening in the fetus not covered by skin, levels of AFP increase in the amniotic fluid and maternal serum. Maternal serum AFP is measured in multiples of the median (MOM). Different laboratories have different cut-off levels for abnormal; in general, **levels greater than 2.0 to 2.5 MOM are suspicious for neural tube defects and warrant further evaluation.** However, an abnormally elevated serum AFP level does not necessarily coincide with fetal neural tube defects. Other causes of elevated maternal serum AFP are listed in Table 60–1.

In contrast to neural tube defects, which have an abnormally elevated maternal serum AFP, those pregnancies complicated **by Down syndrome have a low maternal serum AFP.** Again, other causes of abnormally decreased levels of AFP have been identified and are listed in Table 60–2. Unconjugated estriol is also decreased in fetuses with Down syndrome. **Human chorionic gonadotropin, however, is elevated** in these fetuses. By combining these serum chemicals into a mul-

Table 60–1
CAUSES OF ELEVATED MSAFP

Underestimation of gestational age
Multiple gestation
Neural tube defects
Abdominal wall defects
Cystic hygroma
Fetal skin defects
Sacrococcygeal teratoma
Decreased maternal weight
Oligohydramnios

Table 60–2
CAUSES OF LOW MSAFP

Overestimation of gestational age
Chromosomal trisomies
Molar pregnancy
Fetal death
Increased maternal weight

tiple marker screening test, approximately 60% of all Down syndrome pregnancies can be identified. **With trisomy 18, all of the serum markers are abnormally low.**

The **first step** in the management of an abnormal triple screen is a **basic ultrasound** to determine the correct gestational age, to identify the possibility of multiple gestation, and to exclude fetal demise. The most common cause of abnormal serum screening is wrong dating. If the risk of trisomy or neural tube defects is still increased after a basic sonogram, amniocentesis or targeted ultrasound is offered. A targeted examination can correctly identify fetuses with neural tube defects by direct visualization of the fetal head and spine. Furthermore, ultrasound may also detect those fetuses suspicious for having Down syndrome by identification of a thickened nuchal fold, shortened femur length, or echogenic bowel. Other conditions associated with an abnormally high or low maternal serum AFP, such as abdominal wall defects, oligohydramnios, and fetal skin defects, can be identified with ultrasound.

Because high-resolution sonography can detect up to 95% of neural tube defects, some practitioners will not proceed with invasive testing for an elevated msAFP. However, when **amniocentesis is chosen** for an elevated msAFP, the amniotic fluid is tested for AFP levels. Fetal karyotype is also obtained through amniocentesis, which will identify fetal aneuploidy, such as the trisomies. Fetal loss rate from an amniocentesis is about 0.5%. Other complications include rupture of membranes and chorioamnionitis.

The identification of a fetus affected by a neural tube defect or a chromosomal abnormality can be an ethical and moral dilemma for the parents, whose previous hopes and dreams for having a "normal" child are now extinguished. The parents should not be forced into any decision but should be provided information in an unbiased fashion.

Comprehension Questions

[60.1] An elevated msAFP is usually seen in each of the following circumstances except:

A. Twin pregnancy
B. Fetal anencephaly
C. Fetal macrosomia
D. Fetal omphalocele
E. Fetomaternal hemorrhage

[60.2] Which of the following is *least* likely to cause low msAFP levels?

A. Dating error
B. Fetal demise
C. Molar pregnancy
D. Congenital nephrosis

[60.3] A 22-year-old woman G2 P1 at 25 weeks' gestation with a sure last menstrual period asks for serum screening. The patient's sister has one child with Down syndrome and, otherwise, there is no family history of anomalies or genetic disorders. Which of the following is the most appropriate response?

A. Amniocentesis is the appropriate test.
B. Serum screening should be performed.
C. Explain to the patient that it is too late for serum screening, but that her risk for Down syndrome is not much higher than her age-related risk.
D. The patient being only 22 years of age does not need serum screening.
E. The patient has a 25% chance of her baby having Down syndrome.

[60.4] Which of the following is associated with an unexplained elevated msAFP?

A. Increased incidence of stillbirth
B. Gestational diabetes
C. Placenta previa
D. Molar pregnancy
E. Down syndrome

Answers

[60.1] **C.** Fetal macrosomia does not elevate the msAFP.

[60.2] **D.** Congenital nephrosis means protein being excreted by the fetal kidneys, primarily alpha-fetoprotein.

[60.3] **C.** The window for serum screening is usually between 15 and 21 weeks, so that her gestational age of 25 weeks is too late. The history of her sister having a baby with Down syndrome confers only a very small if any increased risk for her own pregnancy. If the patient herself had a prior baby with Down syndrome, the risk would be substantially increased, and genetic counseling with possible amniocentesis for karyotype would be appropriate.

[60.4] **A.** Pregnancies with elevated msAFP, which after evaluation are unexplained, are at increased risk for stillbirth, growth restriction, preeclampsia, and placental abruption.

CLINICAL PEARLS

◈ The most common cause of abnormal triple screening is wrong dates.

◈ The next step in the evaluation of abnormal triple screening is the basic ultrasound.

◈ Up to 95% of neural tube defects are detectable by targeted sonography.

◈ About 60% of Down syndrome cases are detected with the triple screen with an elevated human chorionic gonadotropin level, low msAFP, and low unconjugated estriol.

◈ An elevated msAFP suggests a neural tube defect, but there are many other etiologies.

REFERENCES

Cunningham FG, Gant NF, Leveno KJ, Gilstrap LC III, Hauth JC, Wenstrom KD. Prenatal diagnosis and fetal therapy. In: Williams obstetrics, 21st ed. New York: McGraw-Hill. 2001:979–987.

Fox M, Garber A. Genetic evaluation and teratology. In: Hacker NF and Moore JG, eds. Essentials of obstetrics and gynecology, 3rd ed. Philadelphia: Saunders. 1998:123–130.

Listing
of
Cases

LISTING BY CASE NUMBER

LISTING BY DISORDER (ALPHABETICAL)

INDEX

Page numbers followed by f or t refer to figures and tables respectively.